Back pain, incapacity for work and social security benefits: an international literature review and analysis

by

Gordon Waddell DSc, MD, FRCS
Consultant

Mansel Aylward BSc, MD, FFPM
Chief Medical Adviser and Medical Director

Philip Sawney BSc, MRCGP, DDAM
Principal Medical Adviser

Department for Work and Pensions
Adelphi
1–11 John Adam Street
London WC2N 6HT

The ROYAL
SOCIETY of
MEDICINE
PRESS Limited

Sponsored by an educational grant from
Corporate Medical Group, UK Department for Work and Pensions

The authors are responsible for the scientific content and for the views expressed, which are not necessarily those of the sponsor, of the Royal Society of Medicine or of the Royal Society of Medicine Press Ltd.

Declaration of interest: Professor Gordon Waddell is retained at times by the Department for Work and Pensions (DWP) as an independent consultant. Professor Mansel Aylward and Dr Philip Sawney are full-time employees of the DWP and established Senior Civil Servants. This review and analysis was not commissioned by the DWP or its predecessor the Department of Social Security (DSS). No remuneration has been received by Professor Waddell from the DWP (DSS) specifically in respect of the work undertaken in preparing this review and analysis. The views expressed are entirely those of the authors and do not necessarily represent the official view of the UK DWP or HM Government policy.

British Library Cataloguing in Publication Data
A catalogue record for this book is available from the British Library

ISBN 1-85315-542-X

Typeset by Phoenix Photosetting, Chatham, Kent
Printed in Great Britain by Ebenezer Baylis, The Trinity Press, Worcester

Contents

Preface

The aims of this book are:

- To review the literature and available data on social security arrangements, developments and trends in different EU and OECD countries, using back pain as an example
- To integrate this with a modern, biopsychosocial model of pain and disability
- To provide a factual and theoretical background to the social security debate on disability and incapacity benefits.

Non-specific low back pain and disability is used as a prime example of a subjective health complaint which is largely dependent on self-report, is often influenced by psychological and social factors, and typifies current social security problems. Back pain is now one of the most common reasons for chronic disability and incapacity for work in adults of working age and may serve as a good example for other common musculoskeletal disorders, pains and psychosomatic complaints. None of these concepts is unique to back pain: it is just that in many areas they have been studied and quantified most in patients with back pain. This is probably because back pain and disability is so common, it has been a problem area for so long, it was recognised early on that the medical model and treatment did not fully explain or resolve the problem, and it provides a readily available and relatively homogeneous group to study. However, many of the ideas were developed from and are equally applicable to other musculoskeletal disorders, other pains, stress-related and mental health disorders. The biopsychosocial model was developed from mental health and has since been applied to virtually every type of health condition.

This is an expert rather than a systematic review. As can be seen from the reference list, much of the material is from the 'grey literature' of government, agency and private foundation publications, which is not indexed in the standard, electronic databases. The review was therefore heavily dependent on hand searching, citation tracking and personal databases. There are administrative data and material from unpublished, internal reports, largely obtained through personal contacts. It is impossible to check the completeness of retrieval: suffice to say that this review took about 4 years to complete and no previous review has managed to collect more than a small proportion of the present material. The inclusion criteria for 'social security material relevant to back pain' were deliberately elastic and nothing found was excluded except on grounds of relevance. (Although inevitably there was selection of how much general background material on social security to include.) The major limitation is that only material available in English was included, although several colleagues kindly translated key items of information. As far as possible, the accuracy of the material was confirmed through more than one source or through personal contact(s), but the scientific quality is extremely variable. However, social policy is not a scientific matter. There was a particular problem with the closing date for a review of this magnitude, requiring access to policy and administrative material, and dependent on personal contact. For different countries, this generally varied from 1998 to 2000. Where we understand there may be significant, recent developments, attention is drawn in a footnote. From the nature of the material, systematic methods of data extraction were also inappropriate. This is therefore a narrative review, although it includes as much as possible of the raw data and sources, so that readers may access them directly. We have also tried to make it clear when we are making personal comment or interpretation. Waddell & Waddell (2000) and Waddell & Norlund (2000) provide further information on the preliminary literature-search strategies.

Gordon Waddell,
Mansel Aylward
and Philip Sawney
July 2002

Acknowledgements

We are grateful to the Department for Work and Pensions (DWP), Analytical Services Division for assistance throughout with DWP administrative statistics. Staff of the DWP Library, The Adelphi, London and of Glasgow University Library helped trace sources and material.

Many colleagues and friends in the DWP and around the world also helped with data and comments, but bear no responsibility for how we have presented and interpreted the material: Patrick Attard, Tom Bendix, Dag Bruusgaard, Kim Burton, Roy Carey, Alan Clayton, Phil Cox, Peter Croft, Peter Dewis, Peter Donceel, Lynn Elder, Nortin Hadler, Tommy Hansson, Bruce Harris, Moira Henderson, Peter James, Nick Kendall, Egon Jonsson, Even Laerum, James Latham, Annette Leclerc, Clem Leech, Len Matheson, Eliz McDowell, Catherine McGeoghan, George Mendelson, Alf Nachemson, Tony Newman-Taylor, Nick Niven-Jenkins, Anders Norlund, Lars Oderbeck, Rienk Prins, Heiner Raspe, Inger Scheel, Ben Stayte, Paul Stidolph, Roger Thomas, Holger Ursin, Ernie Volinn, Barbara Webster, Peter Wright and Mary Wyatt.

Abbreviations

AA	Attendance Allowance
ADL	Activities of daily living
CRS	Commonwealth Rehabilitation Service
DfEE	Department for Education and Employment
DLA	Disability Living Allowance
DoH	Department of Health
DSP	Disability Support Pension
DSS	Department of Social Security
DWA	Disability Working Allowance
DWP	Department for Work and Pensions
ERC	Earnings-related compensation
EU	European Union
IB	Incapacity Benefit
IIDB	Industrial Injury Disablement Benefit
IS	Income Support
ISdp	Income Support with disability premium
IVB	Invalidity Benefit
LBP	Low back pain
NI	National Insurance
RMS	Regional Medical Service
SB	Sickness Benefit
SDA	Severe Disablement Allowance
SSA	Social Security Administration (US)
SSDI	Social Security Disability Insurance (US)
SSI	Supplemental Security Income (US)
SSP	Statutory Sick Pay
TUC	Trade Union Congress
VR	Vocational rehabilitation

1   Low back pain, disability and social support

Medical background: low back pain and disability

In current western society, low back pain (LBP) is generally regarded as a health problem, although this review will show that this is only one, and not necessarily the most valid or important, perspective.

Epidemiology

The most recent Omnibus Survey conducted in the UK in March–June 1998 (ONS 1998) found that 40% of adults said they had suffered from back pain in the preceding 12 months. A third of those with back pain said that it had restricted their activities in the previous 4 weeks. Of those aged 16–64 who were employed, 5% said they had taken time off work in the previous 4 weeks because of back pain, although only 2% had received a medical sick certificate. Of those aged 16–64 who were not employed, 13% gave back pain as one of the reasons. These statistics are broadly consistent with various previous surveys (Waddell 1998).

There are no *a priori* reasons to expect any variation in the physical basis or pathology of back pain in different European countries or over time, although there is no direct evidence for this.

Raspe (1993) has suggested that there may be some national variation in the reporting of LBP. Table 1.1 shows the reported prevalence in different surveys from various European (EU) countries (Raspe 1993), although these figures must be interpreted with caution because there was considerable variation in survey designs and the exact questions used. Table 1.2 shows a more careful prospective comparison of the UK and Germany in which the surveys and questions were made as similar as possible [P Croft, personal

TABLE 1.1   National variation in self-reported prevalence of low back pain

	Point prevalence (%)	Life-time prevalence (%)
UK	15	51
Denmark	14	62
Switzerland	—	54
The Netherlands	26	55
Sweden	31	61–66
Finland	32	75
West Germany	31–42	81

Based on national surveys reviewed by Raspe (1993).

TABLE 1.2   Comparison of the prevalence of self-reported back pain and disability in the UK and Germany by gender

	Prevalence (%)			Mean pain intensity	Mean Disability (ADL)
	Point	1-year	Life-time	0–100	0–100
Men					
UK	12–19	27–40	57–66	41–57	6–15
East Germany	21–36	63–67	63–67	40–61	11–15
West Germany	29–45	60–82	60–82	50–55	14–21
Women					
UK	19–31	28–54	53–74	50–58	13–20
East Germany	34–49	77–83	88–89	47–59	20–28
West Germany	40–52	77–84	85–91	54–57	26–32

ADL = activities of daily living.

Based on data from Raspe et al [P Croft, personal communication, 2002 (Raspe H, Matthis C, Croft P, O'Neill. Back pain in the United Kingdom and Germany—are the British tougher? Unpublished report)].

communication, 2002 (Raspe H, Matthis C, Croft P, O'Neill. Back pain in the United Kingdom and Germany—are the British tougher? Unpublished report)]. These surveys were carried out in four to six centres in each country, with considerable variation between centres as shown by the ranges in Table 1.2. Nevertheless, there was a systematic variation between the UK and Germany and to a lesser extent between West and East Germany. The UK consistently showed the lowest and West Germany the highest point, period and life-time prevalence of reported back pain. The differences were not accounted for by national demographic or risk factors. Paradoxically, there was no difference in reported intensity of pain, but the UK also had lower and West Germany higher levels of self-reported low back disability. This was not unique to back pain, as there were similar patterns of self perceptions of general health status, consistent with a cited telephone survey in Germany, Belgium, the Netherlands, France and Spain, in which Germans reported the highest prevalence of health concerns, serious illness, chronic disease and handicap. [However, there are also similar regional variations within countries, e.g. Walsh et al (1992).] Although Raspe et al [P Croft, personal communication, 2002 (Raspe H, Matthis C, Croft P, O'Neill. Pain in the United Kingdom and Germany—are the British tougher? Unpublished report)] made every effort to standardise the surveys and questions, some of the differences could still be explained by subtle linguistic nuances and usage. For example, despite the use of a drawing to define the lower back in both questionnaires, one of the authors still questioned whether the area included in 'back pain' is comparable in normal usage in the two countries. Nevertheless, Raspe et al [P Croft, personal communication, 2002 (Raspe H, Matthis C, Croft P, O'Neill. Pain in the United Kingdom and Germany—are the British tougher? Unpublished report)] suggested that the most likely explanation for the findings was national differences in the perception and reporting of pain and comparable sensory and emotional experiences. Perhaps surprisingly, the UK and West Germany seemed to be the two extremes of a European range between low back 'toughness' and 'catastrophising' (Waddell 1998).

Walsh *et al* (1992) and Lau *et al* (1995) used identical clinical questionnaires about LBP and disability in population surveys in the UK and Hong Kong (Table 1.3). They found that the prevalence of reported symptoms in Hong Kong was only about 70% that in the UK, while that of self-reported low back disability was only about a quarter or a third. They suggested that the lower prevalence of back complaints in Hong Kong might be due to differences in people's threshold for reporting symptoms and that 'perhaps the Hong Kong Chinese are less conscious of their back pain than their British counterparts'.

King & Coles (1992) found even more marked variation in self-reported pain in adolescents in different European countries, ranging from 3% for girls aged 15 in Finland to 22% in Belgium (Table 1.4).

Table 1.5 shows that the prevalence of 'work-related' back pain varies from 13 to 37% in selected EU countries. However, this is based entirely on self-report and is very much a matter of perception (Waddell 1998). There is no evidence of any biological variation in different countries that can be attributed to occupation.

TABLE 1.3 Comparison of the prevalence of self-reported back pain and disability in the UK and Hong Kong

	Prevalence (%)		Low back pain making it impossible to put on socks or tights		Disability score > 9/16	
	1-year	Life-time	1-year	Life-time	1-year	Life-time
UK	34.2	55.1	3.3	9.4	4.3	12.1
Hong Kong	22.1	39.7	1.1	4.5	0.9	3.0

From Lau *et al* (1995).

TABLE 1.4 Percentage of adolescents reporting back pain 'often' in the past 6 months in different countries

	Age 11		Age 13		Age 15	
	Boys	Girls	Boys	Girls	Boys	Girls
Finland	1	2	1	1	2	3
Poland	2	3	2	4	2	5
Austria	3	3	5	8	8	8
Scotland	4	5	6	8	9	10
Spain	4	8	5	9	7	12
Wales	5	8	6	9	8	13
Norway	3	3	5	10	10	13
Hungary	4	5	4	8	6	14
Canada	8	8	12	14	12	16
Belgium	7	7	8	13	9	22

Based on data from King & Coles (1992).

TABLE 1.5   Prevalence of self-reported work-related low back pain (LBP)

	'Work-related LBP' (%)
Belgium	21
Denmark	30
East and West Germany	30 and 37
France	29
Ireland	13
The Netherlands	32
UK	23
Finland	33

Based on data from Paoli (1997).

A recent report in the *British Medical Journal* (Palmer *et al* 2000) suggested that there has been a dramatic increase in the prevalence of back pain in Britain between the late 1980s and late 1990s. Walsh *et al* (1992) and Palmer *et al* (2000) carried out two different population surveys in the UK in 1987–88 and 1997–98. These were each based on large samples selected in a similar manner, with wide geographical coverage and similar responses rates. However, the primary purpose of the two surveys was different, the first being directly primarily to the epidemiology of back pain and the second to occupational vibration and associated health effects. The sampling was based on different family doctor practices and the authors did not state whether they allowed for possible clustering effects. Both surveys incorporated two identical questions about back pain lasting 24 hours or longer in the previous 12 months and whether it had made it impossible to put on socks, stockings or tights. Palmer *et al* (2000) found that the 1-year prevalence of back pain increased from 35.4 to 49.1% (95% CI for the increase: 10.6–15.1%, although this statistical estimate of confidence is spurious because it relates solely to the random error due to the sample size and does not consider systematic error due to the experimental design). The trend was consistent across all ages in both men and women and also within social class and regions of the country. In contrast, however, the prevalence of back pain making it impossible to put on socks, stockings or tights showed no change. Palmer *et al* (2000) suggested this demonstrated a true increase in the prevalence of less disabling back pain, even if there was no greater incidence of severe back disease. They hypothesised how these findings might relate to trends of sickness absence and social security benefits, without considering how this could account for the discrepancies in the findings between pain and disability. Some risk factors for back pain, such as monotonous sedentary work or dissatisfaction with work place, could have increased even if others such as manual handling have declined, although changed risk factors could not explain such a sharp rise over such a short period affecting different population groups so evenly (Croft 2000). Rather, Palmer *et al* (2000) suggested that the most likely explanation of their findings was cultural change which had led to a greater awareness of more minor back symptoms and greater willingness to report them, although that was apparently a *post hoc* explanation without any other evidence to support it.

An accompanying editorial by Croft (2000) further explored possible cultural changes, and suggested that any explanation must strike a balance between the reality of pain for the sufferer, the evidence that mechanical factors including work can precipitate or aggravate symptoms, the equally strong evidence that distress and dissatisfaction with work or life may aggravate and perpetuate back pain and disability, and the possibility that part of the problem was that public attention was increasingly drawn to the back during the 1990s. He further suggested that the challenge now is how to change the culture and the beliefs and at the same time keep faith with the person with the pain.

However, this report by Palmer et al (2000) is an isolated finding which is contrary to all the other epidemiological evidence.

An historical review by Allan & Waddell (1989) concluded that human beings have had back pain throughout recorded history, and that it is no more common or severe than it has always been.

International epidemiological studies show conflicting evidence of any change in the prevalence of back pain. Raspe (1993) found that the point prevalence of LBP in 23 sub-national surveys published between 1969 and 1991 varied from 15 to 42% and suggested that it was higher in the more recent studies. However, at this time he failed to allow for the fact that the earlier studies were mainly in countries with lower prevalence while the most recent studies were dominated by West Germany which, as noted above, has the highest prevalence in Europe. Leboeuf-Yde & Lauritsen (1995) reviewed 26 Nordic studies from 1954 through 1992 and found no definite trend but considered that apparent differences were probably due mainly to the wording of the questions. Because of the problems of comparing different surveys in different countries, however, it is more useful to look at identical surveys repeated over time in the same country.

Three detailed and identical Omnibus Surveys of the prevalence of back pain in Britain between 1993 and 1998 showed no significant change in the prevalence of back pain or disability over this period (Table 1.6). A more recent survey in 2000 (Working Backs Scotland, unpublished data) found a broadly comparable 12-month prevalence of 35%, although this was data from Scotland only which tended to show a slightly lower prevalence in the Omnibus Surveys and the wording of the question was not identical.

Leino et al (1994) analysed identical questions in annual surveys in Finland from 1978 to 1992 and found that the prevalence of back pain remained unchanged. Leino (personal

TABLE 1.6   Prevalence of back pain in Britain 1993–1998

	March–June (1993) (%)	March–June 1996 (%)	March–June 1998 (%)
12-month prevalence	37	40	40
Restricted activities in previous 4 weeks[1]	30	30	33
Time off work in previous 4 weeks[2]	6	5	5
Medical sick certification in previous 4 weeks[2]	—	4	2

[1] Of those with back pain.
[2] Of those with back pain and employed.
From Mason (1994), Department of Health (1999).

communication 2000) has made a preliminary analysis of the same data for 1985–1995 which showed a slight decrease in the prevalence of back pain, taking into account age, occupation-based social class (or educational level), some life-style factors (smoking, body mass index), the occurrence of 'stress' symptoms, and unemployment in a crude manner. However, as Finland experienced a dramatic economic recession and unemployment during the first half of the 1990s, these findings will not be published until a more detailed analysis of the data from 1985 to 1999 is completed. In another time series from Finland, the Work Environment Survey in 1977, 1984, 1990 and 1997 also showed a slight decline in low back symptoms but an increase in neck–shoulder symptoms [with crude results published in Finnish by Lehto et al (1998)]. Swedish national surveys from 1975 to 1995 do not provide separate data on neck or back pain, but show a decrease in subjective reports of problems of the locomotor system, of which back and neck pain form a large part (SCB 1997).

The prevalence of limiting long-term illness and disability reported in the UK General Household Surveys increased very slightly from about 15 to 17% between 1975 and 1995, although this fluctuated and there was no clear trend. This must be interpreted against a more dramatic rise from 21 to 35% for all self-reported illness over the same period, despite gradually improving objective health parameters. Disability data from the Labour Force Surveys suggested that the number of people of working age reporting a long-term health problem or disability which affected their working life increased gradually from about 10 to 14% of the population of working age between 1984 and 1997–1998, partly due to an increase in the number of older workers, although also due to changes in the definition and wording of the questions. However, a Labour Force Survey Technical Report (June 1998) suggested this rise was probably due mainly to changing attitudes towards and increased awareness of disability rather than any 'real' change in the level of disability.

Similarly, there is no clear evidence of any increase in the number of work-related back injuries. UK data from the Health and Safety Executive, which is entirely about reported accidents and nothing to do with compensation claims or benefits, shows no definite trend (Hodgson et al 1993). Most other data from the US, Australia, New Zealand and Japan is about claims or awards for compensation, which may be quite different from the actual injury rate. (This is discussed in the appropriate country sections in Chapter 4.)

Hansson & Hansson (2001) reported results from the ISSA study of employed men and women aged 18–60 who were sick-listed for a minimum of 90 days due to back pain in Sweden, Denmark, the Netherlands, Germany, Israel and the US. The majority of medical interventions took place in the first year. Apart from a few 'local' treatments, e.g. medical baths in Germany, there were only marginal differences in the types and frequencies of treatments in the different countries. Surgery within the first 90 days ranged from 6% in Sweden, 9–11% in Denmark, Germany and Israel, 18% in the Netherlands and 32% in the US (these apparently high incidences being in the selected groups of patients who were sick-listed for at least 3 months). There was little evidence that any medical treatment had any significant effect on return to work within the first year, apart from surgery, and even then only in Sweden and Denmark.

To summarise the epidemiology:

- There are no *a priori* reasons to expect any variation in the biological basis or pathology of LBP in the countries being compared or over the time period under consideration. Heavy occupational demands on the back have generally decreased over the last generation or two (during which there has been a major increase in the number of people on long-term sickness absence and social security benefits for back pain), although there is no evidence of any positive or negative change in psychosocial aspects of work
- There is moderate evidence that there is significant variation in the prevalence of self-reported back pain in different countries:
  - There is strong evidence that there has been no significant change, although there is limited conflicting evidence of an increase, in the self-reported prevalence of back pain over the last decade or two (during which there has been a major increase in the number of people on long-term sickness absence and social security benefits for back pain)
  - There is limited and conflicting evidence which suggests there may be some increase in self-reported low back disability
  - There is considerable agreement, although little direct evidence, that these variations are most likely due to cultural variation in the self-reporting of low back symptoms
- As will be seen later (see p000), there is strong evidence that the amount of long-term sickness absence and social security benefits for back problems increased considerably in all the countries reviewed between about the 1970s and the early–mid 90s. There is preliminary evidence that this trend may have stopped in the last few years, at least in some settings. These trends appear to be associated with social and social security changes rather than any biological change in the back or any variation in medical treatment.

Medical conditions and impairment

In the UK, the social security system uses the term *loss of faculty* in place of impairment, but the definition and usage is identical.

The first modern (Prussian) approaches to social security were based on a very biomedical, disease model, which works well for clear-cut physical pathology such as an amputation or blindness. The International Classification of Impairments, Disabilities and Handicaps (ICIDH) (WHO 1980) definitions of impairment and disability reflected this approach (Figure 1.1).

This assumes a linear relationship between disease and disability and works well for clear-cut physical pathology such as amputation or blindness. It still forms the framework for how most health professionals, patients, members of the public and policy makers think about disability.

ICIDH (WHO 1980) defined impairment as 'any loss or abnormality of anatomical, physiological or psychological structure or function'. The most recent edition of the American Medical

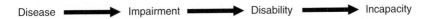

Disease ➡ Impairment ➡ Disability ➡ Incapacity

Figure 1.1 Medical model of disability

Association *Guides to the Evaluation of Permanent Impairment* (Cocchiarella & Andersson 2000) defines impairment very similarly as 'a loss, loss of use, or derangement of any body part, organ system or organ function'. The US Social Security Administration (SSA) operationalises this as 'an anatomical, physiological or psychological abnormality that can be shown by medically acceptable, clinical and laboratory diagnostic techniques' (SSA 2001). However, these definitions imply there may be two fundamentally different kinds of physical impairment:

- Pathological or anatomical loss or abnormality of structure
- Physiological loss or limitation of function.

The main demand of most North American jurisdictions, like SSA, is that physical impairment should be a matter of objective evidence. This whole approach is based on a medical model and a traditional orthopaedic approach to back pain and medical evaluation, which have always focused on tissue damage and structural impairment.

The AMA *Guides* assess lumbar impairment by the Diagnosis-Related Estimates or the Range-of-Motion methods, both of which reflect a traditional orthopaedic approach that works best for patients with fractures, radiculopathy or neurological findings and is of limited relevance to patients with chronic non-specific LBP.

Several studies of physical impairment in non-specific LBP (Waddell *et al* 1992, AMA 1993, Moffroid *et al* 1992, 1994) demonstrate that:

- There is frequently no clinical or radiological evidence of any permanent anatomical or structural impairment
- Clinical evaluation provides a measure of current physiological impairment or functional limitation associated with pain
- These findings are a measure of performance, and depend on effort
- This impairment has the potential to recover.

In the context of pain, physiological loss of function may be more relevant than any lasting physical damage and could still meet the definition of impairment. These studies demonstrate 'functional limitations' associated with pain or disuse or, more graphically, 'inability to do' because of pain. This is more consistent with the new International Classification of Functioning, Disability and Health (ICIDH-2) emphasis on 'body functions' rather than impairments (WHO 2000). It is also a matter of perspective—whether these findings are regarded as physiological impairment or as clinical observations of performance. In any event, performance in these tests will depend on how the individual reacts to pain, on motivation and on effort, just as much as on the underlying physical or physiological disorder. It is not possible to interpret 'inability to do' in purely physical terms. The main proviso remains that it should be possible to demonstrate any such loss of function objectively.

Matheson *et al* (2000) attempted to reconcile the medical model of work disability and the demands of the US SSA for sequential causal links from medical condition to incapacity for work, but admitted this does not always work in practice. In reality, different patients follow different assessment 'tracks' from pathology and diagnosis, to structural or functional impairment to occupational disability (Figure 1.2). In some conditions, e.g. cardiovascular

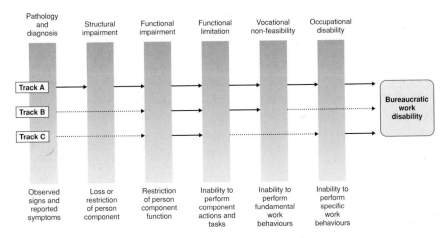

Figure 1.2 Assessment 'tracks' between pathology and occupational disability

Reproduced with permission from Matheson et al (2000)

disease, every stage can be assessed. In others, e.g. pain, and mental and behavioural disorders, it is only possible to assess physiological impairment and disability and then to imply incapacity for work. Perhaps in recognition of these conceptual problems, most North American jurisdictions make a clear distinction between the assessment of impairment and incapacity for work. Impairment is medically-determined loss of structure or function of part of the body, but the final decision on disability rating and sickness benefits is a legal or administrative responsibility (Drewry 1896, Cocchiarella & Andersson 2000). For more than a century, all parties in the US have considered this to be 'a useful division of responsibility'. Medical evidence on impairment is only one factor that the social security, Workers' Compensation or legal systems take into account in determining disability. Determination of disability considers the claimant's own evidence, their circumstances and needs, the physical demands of their jobs, their own report of pain and suffering, and their credibility, and reflects the interaction between impairment and socio-economic factors.

Greenwood (2000), in the context of North American Workers' Compensation, pointed out that in theory compensation is directed to need, i.e. incapacity for work based on clear medical evidence. However, 'the reality is that any disability programme is highly dynamic and malleable because the popular concept of disability is broader than official statements or definitions of disability. Thus, the basic legal construct of disability becomes socially manipulated, becoming a *de facto* economic construct with an inherent tendency to expand. Proof of disability is therefore not so clear'.

Pain and disability

The fundamental limitation to this approach to impairment, well illustrated by LBP, is that pain and disability are subjective.

Pain is defined by the International Association for the Study of Pain as 'an unpleasant sensory and emotional experience associated with actual or potential tissue damage, or described in terms of such damage' (Merskey 1979). Ultimately, pain is a symptom. There are no clinical signs of chronic pain. Pain may be a clinical diagnosis, but it rarely by itself establishes a pathological diagnosis. Pain is not the same as disability. Despite some attempts, there is no good argument that pain is an impairment. It is not possible to assess pain directly, but only the person with the pain. Assessment always depends on the individual's report of their subjective experience, so the report of pain always depends on how the individual thinks and feels about their pain and communicates it.

The WHO (1980) defined disability as 'any restriction or lack (resulting from an impairment) of ability to perform an activity in the manner or within the range considered normal for a human being'. The 5th edition of the *Guides to the Evaluation of Permanent Impairment* (Cocchiarella & Andersson 2000) defines disability as 'an alteration of an individual's capacity to meet personal, social or occupational demands because of an impairment'. The new International Classification of Functioning, Disability and Health (ICF) changes the emphasis to *activity* and *activity limitation*, which is 'a difficulty in the performance, accomplishment, or completion of an activity at the level of the person. Difficulty encompasses all the ways in which the doing of the activity may be affected' (WHO 2000). ICF also emphasises that activity limitation must be seen in the individual and social context, and that body function and structure, activities and participation are interactive rather than linearly related (Table 1.7). Activity is further defined as 'Something a person does, ranging from very basic elementary or simple to complex. Difficulties in performing activities occur when there is a qualitative or quantitative alteration in the way in which activities are carried out'. Chapter 18 on pain in the 5th edition of the AMA *Guides* (Cocchiarella & Andersson 2000) uses the concept of 'pain-related activity restrictions'.

ICF emphasises that disability encompasses all of these inter-related and interacting biopsychosocial dimensions. An individual's functioning or disability in a particular situation depends on complex interactions between their health condition and their context, including environmental and personal factors.

TABLE 1.7 ICF classification of functional states across three dimensions

---

Body functions: physiological and psychological functions of body systems
Impairments: problems in body function or structure such as a significant deviation or loss

Activity: execution of a task or action by an individual
Participation: involvement in a life situation
Activity limitations: difficulties an individual may have in executing activities. [This is equivalent to the WHO (1980) definition of disability, i.e. 'restricted activity' but removes the assumption that it is 'resulting from an impairment']
Participation restrictions: problems an individual may experience in involvement in life situations. [This is equivalent to the WHO (1980) definition of handicap]

Environmental factors: external features of the physical, social and attitudinal world which can have an impact on the individual's performance in a given domain

---

From WHO (2000).

However, pain-related activity limitations and low back disability depend as much on psychosocial factors as on the physical condition of the back, and can only be understood and managed by a biopsychosocial model (Waddell 2002a, Figure 1.3).

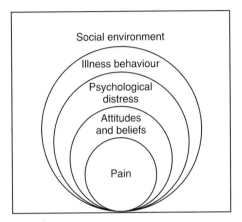

Figure 1.3 A biopsychosocial model of low back pain and disability

Reproduced with permission from Waddell (1998)

There are close links between physiological and psychological events:

- Non-specific LBP seems to be mainly a matter of disturbed function or painful musculoskeletal dysfunction
- Disability is limited activity. It is a matter of which activities the individual does (or does not do) and of altered performance
- Pain behaviour or illness behaviour is also a matter of what the individual does (or does not do)
- Disability may involve both physical dysfunction and illness behaviour, which in a sense are simply two sides of the same coin. Behaviour always involves motor and physiological activity; and physiological processes always have behavioural expressions. Function changes at both physiological and social levels
- Clinical assessment of disability usually relies on the patient's own report, so again is subjective and open to the same influences as the report of pain.

LBP and disability are clearly related, but they are not the same and the link between them is much weaker than often assumed. Severity of LBP only accounts for about 10% of the variance of the associated disability (Figure 1.4) (Waddell & Main 1984, Gallacher et al 1995, Turk & Okifuji 1996). It is therefore important to make a very clear distinction between pain and disability conceptually, in clinical practice, and as the basis for sick certification and social security benefits. Pain is a symptom; disability is restricted activity; incapacity for work is another issue.

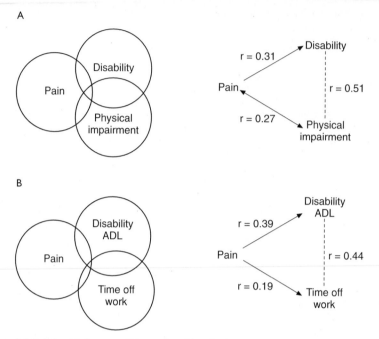

Figure 1.4 Relationship between (A) severity of low back pain, disability and physical impairment and (B) severity of low back pain, disability [activities of daily living (ADL)] and time off work. r = correlation coefficient, where r = 0 means that there is no relationship and r = 1 means that there is 100% correlation. Approximately, r = 0.30 means 10% in common, and r = 0.50 means 25% in common

Fordyce (1995) considered further the nature of impairment and disability associated with LBP from a biopsychosocial perspective. The problem is that it is not possible to assess back pain, but only the person with the pain. Pain, suffering and pain behaviour all confound questions of impairment and disability. Disability may mean either restricted activity or simply reduced activity, but observation of performance cannot distinguish between these. Reduced performance may reflect actual loss of capacity, or the individual may stop before they reach their physical limits, or their performance may be inhibited by pain, or they may not even attempt the activity because of expectations of pain. Fordyce (1995) defined a 'state of disability—is when a person prematurely terminates an activity, under-performs or declines to undertake it'. The concept and measure of disability cannot be independent of performance. It is not possible to separate body and mind. Physical defects affect the person's beliefs and expectations about their situation. On the other hand, beliefs and expectations help to shape the impact of physical defects on activity. The extent to which psychological and social processes can influence physical activity should not be under-estimated, and vice versa. Concepts of impairment and disability must allow for this dynamic interaction. Disability is not only a question of physical impairment, but of behaviour and performance, too. Performance depends on anatomical and physiological capacities, but also on psychological and social resources. Performance depends on effort. Testing itself may cause pain and inhibit performance. As an over-simplification, ability may be set by physiological limits but performance is set by psychological limits.

Distinction may also be made between:

- Functional limitations—what one cannot do
- Functional restrictions—what one should not do (because it may be harmful or dangerous)
- Residual functional capacity—what one *can* still do.

The last distinction raises issues of potential for rehabilitation, retraining and re-integration; of disabled people in the work place and in the community; and of the need to integrate medical and social models of sickness and disability.

There is a major difference in applying these concepts in European and US social security systems. In the US, both the SSA and Workers' Compensation systems are still based on the biomedical model, seek medical evidence on impairment and place considerable emphasis on objective clinical and laboratory evidence to support disability evaluation. In contrast, social security systems in most European countries, including Germany, now take a more holistic approach and place more emphasis on the claimant's symptoms and disability and on overall medical judgements, rather than on objective medical assessment of impairment.

Social support or compensation for disability is directed primarily to wage replacement for *incapacity for work*. For example, the US SSA (1995) operationalises disability as 'the inability to engage in any substantially gainful activity by reason of any medically determinable physical or mental impairment'. In practice, this means total incapacity for any form of work, and assessment of that incapacity must be based on medical evidence of impairment, although administrative definitions and the degree of required incapacity varies in different countries and jurisdictions. However, incapacity for work is only one aspect of disability, even if it is quite reasonably the focus of financial support and particularly wage replacement.

In the UK, the social security system has a unique term *disablement*, used for a number of social security benefits such as Severe Disablement Allowance (SDA) and Industrial Injury Disablement Benefit (IIDB). It is not quite the same as disability. Disablement is defined as 'the limiting, loss or absence of capacity of an individual to meet personal, social or occupational demands, or to meet statutory or regulatory requirements'. It is the overall effect of the disabilities on the power to enjoy a normal life. Recognition and assessment of disablement rests upon quantification of the effects of loss(es) of faculty. In practice, this requires demonstration of loss of faculty, and then quantification of the effects of this loss of faculty, and these effects include elements of both disability and handicap. However, disablement does not fully address the social factors inherent in the WHO definition of handicap. Levels of disablement are prescribed for certain conditions, e.g. loss of a hand or foot is 100% disablement, while registered blind or partially sighted is 80% disablement (which is the threshold for certain benefits).

It remains to be seen when or to what extent these modern concepts as now embodied in the new International Classification of Functioning (WHO 2000) will influence the understanding and evaluation of disability on both sides of the Atlantic.

Modern understanding and management of low back pain and disability

Traditional management of LBP was based on orthopaedic principles. LBP was regarded as an injury or related to degenerative changes in the spine, both of which were often assumed to be occupationally based. It was assumed that LBP equalled disability, that the role of health care was simply to treat the pain, and (assuming treatment produced a 'cure') this would automatically get people back to work. The fundamental strategy of management was by rest and it was often advised that activity should be limited until the pain completely settled. Because it was often assumed that work was the cause of the pain, an implicit part of treatment was to avoid work because it might aggravate the condition or cause re-injury, and so continued pain automatically meant incapacity. All of these assumptions supported routine sick certification for LBP.

However, there were a number of major flaws in the logic of this approach (Waddell 1998):

- 60–80% of adults get LBP at some time in their lives, and often have some persistent or recurrent symptoms. Most low back symptoms are subjective and non-specific, with very little evidence of any significant musculoskeletal injury or damage. Most X-ray and scan findings of 'degeneration' are normal age-related changes which bear little relationship to clinical symptoms
- LBP can be occupational in the sense that it is common in adults of working age, frequently affects capacity for work, and presents to occupational health care, but there is increasing scientific question about the extent to which it is actually *caused* by work. The scientific evidence shows that physical demands of work (bending and twisting, lifting, manual materials handling, and exposure to whole body vibration) can be associated with the onset or aggravation of back symptoms and reported 'injuries' but they do not generally produce lasting damage. Overall, they are less important than other individual, non-occupational and unidentified factors (Waddell & Burton 2000)
- Pain and disability are linked, but the relationship between any objective evidence of impairment, LBP, disability and incapacity for work is weak (Figure 1.3)
- There is no evidence of any permanent physical impairment associated with chronic, non-specific LBP. There is always at least the potential to recover and rehabilitate. It may be questioned whether non-specific LBP in itself is a sufficient basis for permanent total incapacity
- The exponential increase in sickness absence, sick certification and sickness benefit associated with LBP has occurred without any evidence of any change in spinal pathology or the physical basis of LBP
- There is no evidence that rest is an effective treatment for LBP, and increasing evidence that it may actually increase and prolong disability.

Modern, evidence-based, clinical guidelines (Bigos et al 1994, CSAG 1994a, RCGP 1999) stress the need for clear differential diagnosis between the few patients with possible serious spinal pathology such as tumour or infection (1–2%), those with specific clinical symptoms and objective clinical and radiological evidence of a nerve root lesion (5–10%), and the large majority with non-specific LBP. For simple back pain, they recommend that the most effective clinical management is:

- Reassurance that there is no serious disease and that most back pain settles quite quickly
- Simple symptomatic measures to relieve or control pain
- Avoiding over-investigation, 'labelling' and medicalisation
- Advice to continue ordinary activities as normally as possible.

Recent, evidence-based, occupational health guidelines (Carter & Birrell 2000) stress that, whatever its cause, back pain is a common occupational problem and that workers, employers and health professionals must all work together to deal with it and prevent unnecessary disability. They advise that workers with back pain should remain at work if possible or return to work at an early stage and do not need to wait until they are completely pain free. Employers and occupational health professionals should provide help and support for the individual to recover and return to their normal activities as quickly and safely as possible. The scientific evidence confirms that this general approach leads to shorter periods of work loss, fewer recurrences and less work loss over the following year. The danger is that the longer anyone is off work with back pain, the greater the risk of chronic pain and disability and the lower their chance of ever returning to work. By 6 weeks off work, there is a 10–40% risk (depending on circumstances) of still being off work at 1 year. By 6–12 months off work, there is a 90% chance of never returning to any form of work in the foreseeable future.

This modern understanding of back pain carries a number of implications for the present analysis of social security:

- There is increasing evidence and acceptance that LBP, and particularly chronic LBP and disability, can only be understood and managed according to a biopsychosocial model which allows for psychological and social influences as well as the physical condition of the back
- 60–80% of adults get LBP at some time and often have some persistent or recurrent symptoms, but most of them deal with it themselves most of the time without any health care, sickness absence or social security benefits. There is little demonstrable difference in the nature or severity of the pain in those who deal with it themselves and in those who seek health care and receive sick certification
- 20–50% of acute attacks of LBP are reported to start with an 'injury', although this is usually an ordinary everyday activity such as bending or lifting. However, there is usually no other medical evidence of any lasting physical damage and on a balance of probabilities it is not possible to distinguish injury and non-injury, or work-related and non-work-related LBP
- Pain is a very subjective and personal experience. Clinical assessment and management of LBP are based largely on subjective reports of symptoms, which do not necessarily bear much relationship to physical impairment or incapacity for work
- LBP may start as a physical problem in the back, but 'if left untampered' the natural history is good and most symptoms should settle sufficiently to allow return to work quite rapidly, even if some persisting symptoms and recurrences are common. There is

no evidence of any permanent structural damage in most patients with chronic LBP. The clinical findings generally consist mainly of physiological impairment or disturbed function due to pain, which retains the potential to recover even after many years

● There is now considerable evidence that the best management strategy for acute LBP is to stay as active as possible and to continue ordinary activities as normally as possible. This leads to faster recovery and less chronic disability. It does not increase the risk of 're-injury', but actually leads to fewer recurrences. There is also growing evidence that the best management for sub-acute and chronic LBP is re-activation, rehabilitation and return to work.

Development of chronic low back pain and incapacity

There is now extensive evidence that although back pain arises from a physical problem in the back, the development of chronic pain and disability and incapacity for work depends more on psychosocial factors (Waddell 1998):

● The symptom of back pain arises from a physical problem in the back and nociception
● The key to chronic pain and disability may be failure of acute pain to recover as it would normally be expected to do, rather than the development of a different syndrome
● As pain becomes chronic (and this process may start within 3–8 weeks), attitudes and beliefs, psychological distress and illness behaviour may become increasingly important and may aggravate and perpetuate the severity of symptoms and disability
● This all occurs within a social context, involving social interactions with others, including in particular family, work, health care and the social security system.

There is now extensive evidence that by the sub-acute stage (4–12 weeks), non-medical and psychosocial factors are stronger predictors of chronic LBP and disability than any biomedical information (Waddell 1998). The Accident Rehabilitation & Compensation Insurance Corporation in New Zealand has developed a guide to assessing psychosocial risk factors or predictors for chronicity (Kendall et al 1997). These include clinical and psychological features such as:

● Beliefs that back pain is harmful or potentially severely disabling
● Fear-avoidance behaviour (avoiding a movement or activity due to misplaced anticipation of pain) and reduced activity levels
● Psychological distress, low mood and withdrawal from social interactions
● Expectations that relief depends on passive treatments rather than personal action.

The New Zealand guide also identifies a number of social issues around the family, occupation and compensation. Main & Spanswick (2000) suggest that these occupational and social issues may be divided into:

● Individual 'perceptions' of work and incapacity
● 'System' issues.

It is now recognised that these psychosocial issues are not confined to and are not just the consequence of chronic pain. Rather, they occur at a much earlier stage than previously realised and play an important role in the development and maintenance of chronic pain and disability (Waddell 1998). Main & Spanswick (2000) extend this logic to a clinical management perspective in which these psychosocial issues may also become 'obstacles to recovery'. The psychological and individual perception issues can be addressed in the clinical management of the individual worker and are potentially remediable. The system issues are more fixed and depend on changing employers, conditions of employment, labour market conditions, and compensation or social security systems.

Low back pain was a 20th century health-care disaster (Waddell 1998). Within a generation or so, in all western countries, there has been an epidemic of chronic disability attributed to non-specific LBP and an increase in associated sick certification and disability and incapacity benefits, for which there is no good medical explanation and which appears to be largely a social phenomenon. We need a better understanding and new clinical management of LBP and disability, but society also needs to reconsider the medical basis for disability, sick certification and incapacity benefits. LBP may be a good exemplar for other forms of non-specific and psychosomatic symptoms and incapacity.

Co-morbidity

Back pain is the third most common bodily symptom, after headache and tiredness, so it is not surprising that people with back pain often report other complaints. The Nuprin Pain Report in the US (Taylor & Curran 1985) found that 90% of those with frequent back pain had multiple pains, although 50% of them said back pain was the 'most troublesome'. Many clinical and epidemiological studies show that up to 60% of people with LBP also report some neck symptoms. Makela (1993) found that many chronic musculoskeletal pains go together. The association was particularly strong between back pain, neck pain and osteoarthritis of the hips and knees, although inflammatory joint disorders were quite separate.

Bergenudd (1989) and Bergenudd & Nilsson (1994) found that back pain was the most common locomotor complaint in 55-year-old men and women in Sweden, but was often associated with other pains (Table 1.8).

TABLE 1.8 Association of back pain and other pains

	Men (%)	Women (%)
Back pain	28	30
Shoulder pain	13	15
Knee pain	8	13
Hip pain	4	4
	Of those with back pain (%)	
Back pain alone	14	
Back pain and shoulder pain	7	
Back pain and knee pain	5	
Back pain and hip pain	3	

Based on data from Bergenudd (1989).

The South Manchester Study in the UK confirmed the close association between the presence of other pains and the likelihood of developing new back pain (Table 1.9).

TABLE 1.9 Back pain as part of general pain complaints

No back pain at baseline; number of other pains at baseline	% who develop new back pain in next 12 months
0	23.6
1 area	38.7
2 areas	37.8
3 areas	40.5

Based on data from the South Manchester Study (P Croft, personal communication).

Hurwitz & Morgenstern (1997) analysed the 1989 US National Health Interview Survey and also found that a disabling non-back co-morbidity produced an odds ratio of 2.21 (95% CI 2.09–2.34) for a disabling back condition. Yelin (1997) analysed the 1992 US Health and Retirement Survey of persons aged 51–61 years: 59% had one or more musculoskeletal morbidity and 38% of these had at least one co-morbid condition. Those with musculoskeletal conditions and co-morbidity had 15% lower family income and 35% fewer assets, while those with musculoskeletal conditions and no co-morbidity were not significantly different from average.

Men and women who attend their family doctor with back pain also attend more frequently with other problems. Porter & Hibbert (1986) found that 17% of men who consulted their family doctor with back pain also consulted about neck pain at some time. Patients who consulted with back pain and neck pain, but not sciatica, were also more likely to consult with stress and mental disorders—or, at least, they were more likely to get a diagnosis of stress and mental disorders. Psychological distress also led to an increased risk of reporting back pain.

Hill & Trist (1962) provided one of the earliest reports on 'consideration of industrial accidents as a means of withdrawal from the work situation' in 'a study of their relation to other absences in an iron and steel works'. They pointed out that industrial 'accidents' seemed frequently to be related to the personal characteristics of those sustaining them. Workers who had absences from work due to 'accidents' also had a significantly higher number of sick-certificated and other absences. They suggested that having accidents, going sick and other forms of absence from work may be different forms of negative reaction, implying a poor relationship between the worker and his or her employing institution which was not always fully acknowledged. They could not assess the frequency or importance of these influences from their data, but at that early date argued the need for a psychosocial approach to industrial accidents. Interestingly, at the time of their analysis (1947–1951) back injuries only accounted for 3% of all work-related accidents to heavy manual labourers in a UK iron and steel works.

In Britain, 53% of new recipients of Invalidity Benefit reported more than one long-term health problem (Erens & Ghate 1993). A review of social security disability pensions awarded for LBP in Sweden in 1996 found that 40% of recipients also had neck pain and 25% had an additional psychiatric or psychosomatic diagnosis (Waddell & Norlund 2000).

In summary, from an epidemiological and social security perspective, neck and back pain are not discrete clinical problems, but are often associated with other pains, co-morbidities, psychological and stress-related symptoms, and work-related or other social problems. From a social security perspective, LBP has many features in common with other musculoskeletal complaints, and with psychological and stress-related conditions. Aylward (2000), from an historical perspective, has noted the similarities between low back disability and the chronic fatigue syndrome.

Social background

Waddell & Waddell (2000) reviewed >6000 medical and scientific titles and abstracts and identified 470 studies about social influences on LBP and disability. These provide extensive evidence that the following social influences are important, although the strength of the evidence and the magnitude of the effect varies:

- *Culture:* neck and back pain are common to all societies but different cultural groups do not seem to perceive or respond to this pain in the same way. Attitudes and beliefs about the pain, expectations and the meanings attached to pain seem to vary in different societies and over time. Culture may be associated with how people express pain and emotions, pain behaviour, and whether and how they communicate their pain to others, including health professionals. It may be associated with how they seek and respond to treatment. Unfortunately, despite the probable importance of cultural influences on back pain, there is little evidence on which cultural issues are most important, how they operate or how they can be modified
- *Family:* much of the family research is weak methodologically, many of the results are inconclusive, and most of the available evidence is about chronic pain in general. Despite these limitations, available evidence suggests that family influences may be associated with treatment outcome and the development and maintenance of chronic pain and disability. For most routine patients with back pain, good family and social support may be associated with better recovery and less disability, but for a small minority of chronic pain patients, a history of physical or sexual abuse, or spouse re-inforcement may be associated with more chronic pain and disability. Unfortunately, despite the potential importance of family issues, there is little evidence on exactly which family influences are most important, how they operate or how they can be modified
- *Social class:* there is conflicting evidence for a relationship between the prevalence of back pain and lower social class, and any association is probably weak. There is strong and consistent evidence that back pain is associated with more work loss in people of lower social class. The relationship to social class is most consistent in men. The problem with interpreting these findings is understanding what 'social class' means. Social class is a very crude index, which deals with a host of social, educational, occupational,

economic, life-style and psychosocial influences, and corresponding social attitudes and behaviour, any or all of which may bear a relationship to work loss associated with back pain. It is probably partly a matter of manual work, particularly in men. It is probably also a matter of social disadvantage in both men and women, although it is not clear exactly which aspects of this disadvantage are important or how they affect back pain

- *Job satisfaction and psychosocial aspects of work:* in a separate, unpublished meta-analysis, Waddell & Waddell (2000) also reviewed 69 studies on job satisfaction and psychosocial aspects of work in relation to neck and back pain. There are some theories but limited evidence that psychosocial aspects of work affect the physical condition of the back or actually *cause* neck or back pain. About half the studies show that individual psychosocial aspects of work, particularly low job satisfaction, high demand/intensity and low social support at work, are associated with how people *report* neck and back pain on questionnaires, although the odd ratios are generally only 1.5–2.0 which, because of the statistical properties of odds ratios, is roughly equivalent to an increased prevalence from 40 to about 50%. Job satisfaction and high job demand/intensity also show odds ratios of about 1.5 for health care and sick listing. Monotonous work, low job control and low job clarity show generally non-significant or very weak associations. There is insufficient evidence to support any theoretical model of demand–control interaction for LBP. These psychosocial aspects of work may be better conceptualised as psychosocial influences rather than as causal 'risk factors'
- *Industrial relations:* there is limited but suggestive evidence that good and bad industrial relations can be associated with altered rates of reporting low back injuries and the amount of sickness absence
- *Litigation:* most of the commonly quoted literature is in fact about Workers' Compensation and there is limited and conflicting evidence on adversarial litigation. Most studies are on selected clinical series, often from highly selected referral situations, and it is difficult to generalise from the results. There is considerable legal evidence that litigation may influence reports of symptoms and disability and the clinical presentation in the medico-legal context, but in the clinical situation it does not appear to be associated with any significant increase in the severity of pain or distress. There is insufficient evidence to assess whether or to what extent litigation may be associated with any difference in clinical outcomes, disability or return to work.

Waddell & Waddell (2000) concluded that there is extensive, although scientifically often poor quality, evidence that social factors may influence the reporting of back pain, pain behaviour, disability, and sickness absence. There is suggestive evidence that some of these interactions may be potentially powerful and at least in some situations may be more important than any physical abnormality in the neck or back. On the evidence available, and remembering the limitations and weaknesses of much of this evidence, it may be hypothesised that the key social influences lie in the area of individual, group and society in general's attitudes and beliefs about work, about back pain and its relationship to work, about sickness absence and about social security benefits.

Biopsychosocial model of disability

Waddell (2002a) reviewed models of disability and concluded:

1. Incapacity benefits have risen in all developed countries in the past few decades, despite improvement in most objective measures of health. Most of this rise is accounted for by non-specific and subjective health complaints like back pain, musculoskeletal complaints, mental conditions and stress

2. It is important to make a clear distinction between symptoms and disability conceptually, in clinical practice, and as the basis for sick certification and social benefits. Pain is a subjective symptom; disability is restricted activity; incapacity for work is another matter—and the relationship between them is much weaker than generally assumed

3. The medical model of disability (Figure 1.1) was developed for serious medical conditions such as amputation, paralysis or blindness, where it still has considerable validity provided due allowance is made for the individual and their situation. However, this model does not work well for more subjective health complaints where it is difficult to define or measure any objective disease or impairment. Bodily symptoms generally arise from a physical source, but there is increasing evidence that the development and maintenance of chronic pain, chronic disability and particularly chronic incapacity for work depend even more on psychological, behavioural and social factors

4. The medical model underpins a false dichotomy between the 'deserving' disabled (who have a clear, objective medical condition causing obvious incapacity for work, who are the stereotype of 'the disabled' and who form the basis of political protest in any welfare debate) or if they do not have such a medical condition then they may be regarded as 'undeserving' (which implies conscious choice, lack of motivation, abuse and even fraud). In reality, somewhere in the region of 15–25% of Incapacity Benefit recipients have such a clear medical condition. At the other extreme, probably <5% involve frank abuse or fraud. For the 70% between, the situation is more complex and cannot be understood in purely medical terms. This does not mean they do not have any health problem, but rather that they do not have a serious medical condition and what health problem they do have is insufficient *in itself* to explain fully their incapacity

5. In reaction to the limitations of the medical model and as part of the fight for disabled rights, disability groups have proposed an alternative 'social model of disability'. This essentially argues that many of the restrictions suffered by disabled people lie not in the individual's impairment but are imposed by the way society is organised for able-bodied living. Society fails to make due allowance and arrangements which would enable disabled people to fulfil the ability and potential they do retain. This may best be described as a social disadvantage and exclusion model or, with more obvious political overtones, a 'social oppression model'

6. However, this is only one of a number of possible social models, e.g. the 'cultural model' (which may be defined as the collective attitudes, beliefs and behaviour that characterise a particular social group over time); the economic and social insurance model; and various social models of absence from work

7. Each of these medical and social models reflects a particular perspective on disability: each has some validity and they all need to be taken into account. There is now accumulating evidence that disability can only be understood and managed by a biopsychosocial model that includes *all* the physical, psychological and social issues that influence disability and incapacity for work (Figure 1.3)

8. Disability depends on the individual, their health condition and their social situation, and on the powerful and complex interactions between them. This is a 'complex system' which cannot be reduced to the sum of its parts, but the interactions produce new properties, characteristics and effects. So an apparently simple intervention on one element of the model does not necessarily have a direct and predictable effect. Rather, any intervention may influence the complex interactions in unforeseen ways with more indirect effects, as occurs with many health and social policy initiatives

9. The biopsychosocial model provides the basis for more appropriate and effective health care and social management of disability. In clinical management, it shifts the focus from treating disease to dealing with all the human aspects of illness, and from a primary focus on pain to equal emphasis on disability. In occupational health, it provides a framework to: guide evaluation and management; identify obstacles to return to work; develop targeted interventions to overcome these obstacles; and design effective rehabilitation services. Health and social policy solutions to the problem (as opposed to control mechanisms designed simply to restrain expenditure) must allow for the health and (in)capacity of the individual *and* the pressures and constraints of their occupational and socio-economic environment *and* the interactions between them. They must address the individual, psychosocial and system obstacles to return to work, and provide the resources and support required to overcome them. They must change the culture of the benefits system

10. This demands a new, more complex, but more balanced and more human understanding of disability.

Historical background to social support

Co-operation and mutual support in adversity are among the earliest and most fundamental hallmarks of human society and civilisation. In earlier times and in less developed countries today, social support for sickness and disability was from the family. Indeed, even in the most highly developed welfare states today, much basic support for sickness and disability still comes from the family. Family assessment of need and agreement about providing this support depend on many family issues and dynamics apart from the medical state of the invalid; and may be much more generous, or harsh, or idiosyncratic than any social security administration could ever be.

Through history, society has developed two distinct but linked forms of support for the injured, sick and disabled (Allan & Waddell 1989):

● Compensation
● Social security.

Compensation

Ancient compensation codes from the cradle of civilisation in the Middle East, e.g. the Code of Hammurabi (circa 1750 BC), the Code of Eshunna (circa 1700 BC) and the Law of Moses (circa 800 BC), pre-date written history. The original concept was simply retribution: 'an eye for an eye; tooth for tooth; hand for hand; foot for foot', but the Babylonian kingdom of Eshunna provided financial compensation for loss of life or limb while in the service of the state. Examples of Eshunna compensation included 60 shekels for the loss of an eye and 30 shekels for the loss of an ear. Most intriguing, they also included 10 shekels for a slap in the face, a fascinating reflection on the value of the dignity of state officials! By the 2nd and 3rd centuries AD, the oral laws of Israel were written down in the *Mishna* and the fourth book compiled the civil law—the *Nezikin* or *Damages*. More or less structured scales of financial compensation eventually became embodied in common law of all countries and still remain the basis of civil litigation for personal damages.

During the early stages of the industrial revolution a worker could claim compensation from an employer or fellow employee for accidental injury, but this depended on proving someone was to blame for the accident. These legal rights were limited, and in practice civil litigation was difficult and expensive. Employers had powerful legal defences to exonerate them. No claim was possible if the accident was due to 'ordinary risk' in the course of employment or to an Act of God. Nor could a worker claim if he had been even partly to blame for the accident, which was 'contributory negligence'. The 'fellow–servant' doctrine meant that the employer was not responsible for negligence by another worker. These legal defences became known as the 'unholy trinity'. Even more unjust, any legal case stopped with the death of the worker and his dependents then had no claim. The first case of a worker successfully suing his employer for a work injury in England was not until 1836, but it was not until after the passage of legislation limiting these defences in the latter part of the 19th century that successful litigation for employment-related injury became more frequent. Even then, the law on contributory negligence was not actually repealed until 1945 and that on the 'fellow–servant' doctrine in 1948, while risk in the normal course of employment was not finally disposed of until a House of Lords' decision in 1992.

One of the key elements of the industrial revolution was the building of the railroads. The world's first railway line opened in England in 1825 and the carriage bore the legend 'a public service free of danger', but rapid and uncontrolled growth of the railways led to casualties on a scale unprecedented except in war. In a single year, 1145 people died and 3038 were injured working or travelling on the railways in Britain and public anxiety led to legislation. When the Berlin–Potsdam railway opened in 1838 the Prussian government made the railway companies legally responsible for accidents. In England the Fatal Accidents Act of 1846 first gave the right of compensation to the family of a person killed in an accident. The Employers' Liability Act of 1880 went some way to abolish the 'fellow–servant' doctrine, and started compulsory insurance, but it was still necessary to prove fault which limited its value. By 1886, the Employers Liability Assurance Corporation recorded 10,217 accidents but only 24% of the individuals involved made any claim and only 12% actually received any compensation.

The new laws eventually led to a spate of legal and medical activity. Some of the injuries were severe and fully justified compensation, but there was soon a problem of many claims for more minor injuries. Some of these claimants had subjective symptoms without much objective evidence of injury and 'sprains and strains' of the back were soon a leading example. The limitations of medical examination made the problem worse. 'Lawyers and judges appear to have a pretty generally formed opinion that a doctor's statement concerning disability of the lower back is largely a matter of guesswork' (Wentworth 1916). As legislation extended the scope of compensation, so the scale of the problem grew. By 1915, 'pain in the back as a result of injury is the most frequent affection for which compensation is demanded from the casualty company'. King (1915) summed up the dilemma neatly: 'Lumbago is a condition of most frequent occurrence. The labourer however seldom suffers from the pain of lumbago but is a frequent victim of pain in the back due to injury'.

Wesely (2001) reviewed the medical reaction and pre-occupation with the detection of malingering (Collie 1913, Jones & Llewellyn 1917). Through history, malingering (the false or fraudulent simulation or exaggeration of physical or mental disease or defect) had been a matter of attempted evasion of military or social responsibilities. After the development of social insurance in the late 19th and early 20th centuries, the whole focus shifted to illness for which economic compensation was sought. Wentworth (1916) summed up what many doctors in civil litigation still feel today: 'Exaggeration is as common as malingering is rare'. Assessment became medicalised, doctors became the referees and gatekeepers for social insurance, and many approached the task with enthusiasm. The new arrangements were an affront to their conservative, middle-class values, potentially provided licence and support for idleness, and this offended Darwinian principles. Then, as now, it was argued that work was getting easier and serious or fatal accidents were becoming less frequent, so there was no physical reason why 'incapacity' and claims for compensation were increasing. Others took a more lenient view, recognising the 'weakness of the working man' and suggesting it was not his fault. 'It is easy to trace the mental process of a patient who, after a hard previous day's work, honestly concludes that the lumbago of today had its origin in the employment of yesterday. Such an individual is scarcely a malingerer, but rather the victim of a false conception, the more deep rooted often because of tactless disputes at previous examinations' (Conn 1922)—the forerunner of genetic and psychological theories. In any event, medical assessment became antagonistic with the patient/claimant versus the insurance doctor (usually a physician or surgeon) and some doctors became detectives in the game of diagnosing 'malingering', while others were 'on the side of the working man' but who 'let the side down'.

World War I crystallised the debate in the UK, France and Germany (Wesely 2001). Examining doctors were now acting on behalf of the nation in a time of national emergency and 'malingering' was a court martial offence which at least in theory carried the death penalty. However, psychologists and psychiatrists were now also involved and 'shell shock' provoked a debate on traumatic shock. In Germany, the neurologist Oppenheim supported the theory of 'traumatic neurosis', but lost to the large majority of psychiatrists who considered it was either hysteria or malingering. After the war, the debate in the UK followed the same course and Collie (the authority on malingering) was appointed head of the 'neurasthenia board'. The dilemma remained: psychological versus malingering and fraud; courage versus cowardice; and rights versus duty?

Another 20 years and World War II led to much more far-reaching social change and the development of a greatly expanded welfare state. Over the next few decades, in many countries there was a progressive increase in the number of claims of incapacity. LBP was one of the most common examples, now supported by medical concepts of ruptured discs. Yet in many cases the fundamental debate remained: psychological magnification versus exaggeration and fraud?

Social security

Present forms of social support for sickness and invalidity date from the social, industrial and medical revolutions of the 19th century. There had been war pensions for disabled soldiers since Greek times, but now society also began to care for 'the wounded soldiers of industry'. As national wealth and income rose, there was gradual acceptance that society had a responsibility to provide care for all the sick and disabled, and the goal of welfare then gradually evolved from dealing with absolute destitution to alleviating poverty.

Ploug & Kvist (1996) described four phases in the development of western-European welfare states. The first phase, up to about 1883, was prior to state intervention. The second was from about 1883 to 1914 when the state intervened. The third was between the two world wars when social policy changed from insurance systems for workers to national insurance systems for larger population groups. The fourth was from 1945 to 1975 when most systems expanded to include health care, support for families and social services. The first phase was concerned with stopping outright destitution, the second and third stages with alleviating poverty, and the fourth with preventing poverty. Arguably, social security should now increasingly be about promoting opportunity and developing potential (UK Government Green Paper 1998a).

In agrarian societies, prior to the industrial revolution, there was no unemployment or retirement in the modern sense. In the first phase, before the industrial revolution and state intervention, welfare was only concerned with tackling outright destitution. During the Middle Ages, social support for the destitute took the form of charity, initially led by the church and religious bodies under the codified church 'Canon Law'. Exactly 400 years ago— in 1598 and 1601—the 'Poor Laws' were passed in feudal Elizabethan England and remained in force until the 20th century. This was the first recognition that the state had any interest in preventing destitution, raising taxes to do so and ensuring that there was an administrative framework to deliver help. At the same time it provided a mechanism for the state to control the poor and outlaw begging. Early forms of social security in the towns consisted of mutual aid among members of the craft guilds, mainly in the event of sickness, and in rural areas in the form of landowners' obligations towards farm workers and tenant farmers. However, this was a very patchy social safety net. In the towns, for example, it normally only covered well-paid tradesmen. Poverty was regarded as self-induced and the local councils gave grudging relief to the poor. A UK *Royal Commission on the Poor Laws* in 1834 was set up to reform the Poor Laws, which re-asserted the basic Elizabethan principles, although it adapted them to the developing industrial society and was an early attempt to control processes of social change. It took the view that dependency on the state should be discouraged, that people supported by parishes should not be 'eligible' for the same standard of living as the poorest labourer, it opposed cash assistance and proposed that access to assistance should be deliberately harsh. Assistance was not a right for people of working age, but subject to conditions of behaviour. At various times poor relief was associated with forced labour, forfeiture of citizenship rights, the right to marry and the right to vote. At its strictest, anyone receiving relief had to leave their family and go to live and work in the 'workhouse'. These were deliberate social policy attempts to control the poor and maintain law and order. The rules of entitlement were designed to discourage all but the most needy and desperate, and to minimise sloth and malingering. Even worse, according to religious beliefs of the times, hopes of resurrection depended on 'proper burial', so if the poor were condemned to a pauper's funeral they might be damned through all eternity.

As early as 1722, the UK parliament introduced a motion for compulsory insurance which was approved by the House of Commons but defeated in the House of Lords. During the French Revolution in 1794 there was an attempt to develop legislation for a universal pension scheme but this was never implemented. It may be that there simply was not the economic base, public support or political will to provide a more general social security scheme until after the social, industrial and economic developments of the 19th and early 20th centuries. From one perspective, these social policy initiatives were a natural development to cope with the changes in working and living conditions following urbanisation and industrialisation. Alternatively, they may be seen as a reaction from 19th century politicians to the democratisation process and emergence of labour movements.

Ploug & Kvist (1996) summarised the major social changes in western Europe during the 19th century resulting from agrarian reforms and the industrial revolution. In almost all countries the population doubled. Ever increasing numbers were employed in urban occupations of commerce, craft and then industry, and the urban population increased from 5 to 25%. The industrial revolution created the concepts of unemployment and retirement, but also created national wealth and greatly enhanced the power of the state. At the same time, there was economic liberalisation which weakened social arrangements such as the old craft guilds. In many cases, old social systems were destroyed before new ones developed. This was partly an expression of conscious choice in a century of individualism and liberalism. The prevalent attitude was that each individual was responsible for the support of themselves and their relatives. If this became impossible, poor relief was a last-ditch alternative.

Ploug & Kvist (1996) used a Danish example to illustrate the changing circumstances and attitudes that led to the state intervening in social security. During the 1870s the price of corn fell in western Europe due to huge new supplies from Russia and the US. This caused a crisis in Danish agriculture and helped to accelerate agrarian reform and urbanisation. At the same time it was recognised that in a modern industrial society, the risk of poverty was no longer simply a question of individual behaviour but could result from economic forces over which the individual had no control. This helped to change understanding of the relationship between the individual and society and created the willingness for social reform.

In most European countries during the 19th century, amendments to the poor laws gradually passed responsibility to local government, but the poor laws remained in force until the passage of Social Security Acts in the last decade of the 19th and first decade of the 20th centuries. Up to that time, the poor laws provided very basic support, with severe social stigma, and were based on a distinction between the 'worthy poor' and those who were undeserving. The deserving got grudging charity; those who were judged to be 'unworthy' even if disabled could be warned out of town or subject to corporal punishment. America adopted the same poor-law approach.

In the 19th century in the UK, changed patterns of urbanisation and employment, coupled with the strong Victorian self-help ethic, led to the development of friendly societies, the co-operative movement and trade unions—the 'self-help movement'. The friendly societies were voluntary associations whose members paid dues in return for benefits to cover specific contingencies such as medical care and funeral expenses. Between 1815 and 1892, the membership of the friendly societies in the UK rose from under 1 million to 7 million— almost the entire working population. However, many of these workers could only afford minimal contributions and many received little more than death grants to provide a proper burial. This at least saved the victim's soul, even if it did little for him in this life. But the friendly societies could at best only deal with short-term adversity and did not have the resources to support long-term disability or retirement. By the turn of the 19th century, several UK friendly societies went bankrupt. Poverty remained widespread, particularly among the elderly. Against this background, private charity continued to play a major role. Indeed, in the latter half of the 19th century in London, private charity exceeded official poor relief. However, this Victorian charity carried strong moral messages about appropriate behaviour and that charity should really aim to create the power to self-help.

By the beginning of the 20th century, there was a strong movement against the form and spirit of the old poor laws which was expressed in the report of a UK Royal Commission on the Poor Laws and Relief of Distress (1909).

The second phase of development of the welfare state was made possible by rising national wealth, when welfare became concerned with assisting people to survive the vagaries of life and unexpected hardship and with trying to alleviate poverty (UK Government Green Paper 1998a). During this phase (Ploug & Kvist 1996), four core elements of social security were introduced—industrial injury insurance, sickness insurance, old-age pension and unemployment insurance, although there were striking national differences in the timing and relative priority given to these different elements (Table 1.10). Industrial injury benefits usually came first, old-age or sickness benefits came next, and unemployment benefits came

TABLE 1.10   Year of introduction of benefits in different EU countries

	Industrial injury	Sickness	Old age	Unemployment
UK	1897	1911	1908	1911
Sweden	1901	1891	1913	1934
Norway	1894	1909	1936	1906
Finland	1895	1963	1937	1907
Denmark	1898	1892	1891	1907
The Netherlands	1901	1929	1913	1916
France	1898	1898	1895	1905
Germany	1884	1883	1889	1927

Based on data from Ploug & Kvist (1996).

last. France had all four elements by 1905, Denmark by 1907 and the UK by 1911, but most other European countries did not introduce them all until the late 1920s or early 30s and Finland not until 1963. Although Germany had the first industrial injury, sickness and old-age benefits in the world, it did not introduce unemployment benefits until 1927.

Chancellor Bismarck in Germany introduced the first national system of social insurance to cover workers against the risks of occupational injury, illness and invalidity, and old age in the 1880s. This was quite different from earlier common law principles of employers' liability, but was a completely new social principle based on socialist philosophy. Frederick the Great gave official approval to the concept that 'it is the duty of the state to provide sustenance and support for those of its citizens who cannot provide it for themselves'. Yet the policy was introduced by the conservative Bismarck, who was no friend of the working man. Rather, it was an integral part of his *Socialpolitik* which aimed to develop a nation state, addressing the social situation of workers as a collective, bringing the industrial proletariat and employers together with the state as a third party. It was also a pragmatic, 'stick and carrot' political response to the emerging working class and the fledgling labour movement, designed to undermine the socialist opposition. The practical elements were one of the first efficient civil services, modern actuarial private insurance (setting premiums to cover compensation for specified risks) and the thriving 19th century German guilds which were run jointly by workers and employers to provide sickness, disability and death benefits. At the same time, German medicine led the world with a very biomedical model of disease. The combination produced what Hadler (1997) has described as the *Prussian paradigm* (Table 1.11). This was also a very moral

TABLE 1.11   Biomedical basis of the Prussian paradigm

Clinical and administrative decision	Criteria
Determine cause	Injury? Work-related?
Determine if permanent state reached	Can anything more be done to treat or rehabilitate?
Determine permanent (partial) disability	Based on objective evidence of pathology (impairment) (This now applies more in the US than in EU)

From Hadler (1997).

perspective, based on the western work ethic (Table 1.12). Who is more 'worthy' than the man who wants to work to support his family, who is working, and in the course of his work is injured, so that he is now permanently disabled and unable to support his family?

TABLE 1.12   Social application of the Prussian paradigm

Level of worthiness	Insurance fund	Indemnification
Work incapacity due to work injury	Workmen's Accident Insurance	Wage replacement until fit to return to work Medical care and rehabilitation Permanent partial awards
Work incapacity due to illness in a worker	Public Pension Insurance	Wage replacement for a finite period while under medical treatment and unfit for previous work Medical care and rehabilitation Some level of monetary transfer if disability persists
Sickness in a non-worker	Public Aid	Sustenance Medical care

From Hadler (1997).

In Germany, the combination of the western work ethic and the concept of the worthy poor led to Workers' Compensation in 1884, with Accident Insurance and Sickness Benefits for the employed, followed by the Disability and Old Age Insurance Act in 1891, and a comprehensive National Insurance Act in 1911. The Prussian model soon spread through Europe and served as a model for most of the industrialised countries. The first Workmen's (Compensation for Accidents) Act in Britain was in 1897 and made insurance compulsory for large groups of workers, regardless of fault. By 1906 it covered all workers and also included industrial disease as well as accident. One critical difference from the very beginning was that the Prussian welfare model directed considerable emphasis and resources to occupational health and rehabilitation, while the British model was confined to issues of financial support and made no provision for rehabilitation. The UK Liberal government from 1906 to 1916 continued these social reforms. The first real departure from the old poor laws was when retirement pensions were introduced in 1908, although these were designed for the 'respectable working class', for men only over the age of 70, and the benefits were modest and means tested. The first compulsory state insurance scheme to cover sickness and unemployment was introduced in 1911. From this time the state has provided a growing proportion of support for all sick and disabled, as in all European countries. The right to civil litigation for further compensation remains, but that is a bonus for a small minority and few sick or injured people now depend financially on civil litigation. The Unemployment Act of 1934 amalgamated issues of social support for unemployment and the old poor laws and introduced a national system of means-tested benefits for the unemployed, although the poor laws were not officially repealed until the 1946–1948 legislation which created a comprehensive National Health Service and Social Security system for all sickness.

However, North America was slow to follow the European example. The Progressive Party of Theodore Roosevelt and the American Association of Labor Legislation advocated Workers' Compensation at the end of the first decade of the 20th century, but federal legislation was considered to be unconstitutional and this first social insurance programme in the US was left to the individual states. The first legislation for Workers' Compensation was in New York State in 1910. By 1920, 45 states had enacted Workers' Compensation legislation but it was not until 1949 that all states had such legislation. (The US still does not have a universal system of health care and sickness benefits.) The first Workers' Compensation in Canada was introduced in Ontario in 1915, but it took another 60 years to be introduced to all the remaining provinces and territories. In Australia, in contrast, Workers' Compensation legislation was enacted in almost all states by the end of the first decade of the 20th century. In Canada, Australia and New Zealand, the introduction of compulsory, universal, no-fault, Workers' Compensation was conditional on workers giving up the right to civil litigation against their employer, unlike in the UK where common-law proceedings continue to this day in parallel with social security arrangements. In all of these countries, like Germany but in contrast to the UK, the Workers' Compensation legislation and systems made specific provision for medical and vocational rehabilitation.

The US National Commission on State Workers' Compensation Laws in 1972 (quoted by Barth 2000) identified five basic goals:

- The need for adequate and equitable benefits
- Broad coverage both of workers and of injuries and illnesses
- Full medical services
- A scheme that encouraged positive health and safety practices
- Efficient administration of the programme.

In the light of what has happened in more recent years, Barth (2000) added a sixth goal:

- The need to ensure that there is a long-term, productive return to work.

The process of democratisation and broadening the scope of the welfare state have tended to go together. Extension of the franchise to wider groups in society produced competition for votes and, consequently, gradual expansion of eligibility for social insurance schemes. The most evident change was the transition from employees' insurance to more all-encompassing social insurance of all members of society.

It is sometimes assumed, at least in the UK, that modern social security systems only began with the implementation of the Beveridge Report (1942) after World War II, but disability benefits and rehabilitation had already developed considerably during the first half of the 20th century (Bolderson 1991). Major social changes—two world wars, the shortage of manpower that arose in each and the resulting need to provide for disabled service men; developments in health care; the decline of mutual and provident societies; unemployment and the threat of social unrest; the growing strength of unions and their increasing concern with social policy affecting their members; political and democratic developments—all helped to shape policy for the disabled, as did the vested interests of employers and insurance companies. However, Bolderson (1991) suggested that social policy between the wars developed as a political response to these various pressures, rather than from any clear philosophy. In practice, most of the emphasis in the UK was again on providing financial support with very limited provision for rehabilitation services, except for wounded service men.

From Bismarck's initiative in 1884, no other single event had such a profound international impact on social security across the world as the Beveridge Report (1942) on *Social Insurance and Allied Services*. This was one of the earliest attempts by the UK wartime coalition to consider the post-war 'reconstruction' of society, set up in June 1941 and published in November 1942 during the darkest hours of the war. Experience of the 1930s depression and the World War II led to attitudes of national solidarity that had never existed before (or since).

Sir William Beveridge was a liberal civil servant who had been involved in welfare reform since the 1911 Acts. He attacked the inadequacies of the existing system and aimed to create an all-encompassing social safety net. He is sometimes described as a synthesizer rather than an innovator, who integrated a disparate series of different benefits into a unified system of social insurance which covered the entire population for all contingencies. But this fails to allow for his vision and inspiration in providing a social security rationale which has stood the test of time. Beveridge did not wish the UK to revert to pre-war class inequalities and there were political elements of social obligation, solidarity and redistribution of wealth. 'The common good' embodied a sense of values, a sense of responsibility and willingness to sacrifice that may seem idealistic and naive looking back through the money-driven, competitive, management-efficiency 1980s. Beveridge's aim was noble: 'The scheme as a whole will embrace, not certain occupations and income groups, but the entire population. Concrete expression is thus given to the solidarity and unity of the nation, which in war have been its bulwarks against aggression and in peace will be its guarantees of success in the fight against individual want and mischance'. The final paragraph of the report rang out: 'Freedom from want cannot be forced on a democracy or given to a democracy. It must be won by them. Winning it needs courage and faith and a sense of national unity: courage to face facts and difficulties and overcome them; faith in our future and in the ideals of fair-play and freedom for which century after century our forefathers were prepared to die; a sense of national unity over-riding the interests of any class or section. The Plan for Social Security in this report is submitted by one who believes that in this supreme crisis the British people will not be found wanting, of courage and faith and national unity, of material and spiritual power to play their part in achieving both social security and victory in justice among nations upon which security depends'.

Nor was this only a matter of social security: 'Want is one only of five giants on the road to reconstruction and in some ways the easiest to attack. The others are Disease, Ignorance, Squalor and Idleness'. In 1944 Beveridge published *Full Employment in a Free Society* and obviously felt there was an intimate relationship between social insurance and employment, and between work and welfare. Beveridge was close to the economist Keynes, and social insurance was considered to have a macro-economic function as an 'automatic stabiliser'.

One of Beveridge's first priorities was to examine the root causes of poverty amidst relative plenty—and how to prevent it. Beveridge (1942) stressed that social security could not be considered and would not be successful in isolation, but his plan assumed:

- 'The establishment of comprehensive health *and rehabilitation* [our italics] services for all citizens who need them'
- 'The maintenance of employment and avoidance of mass unemployment'. He recognised there would always be some structural unemployment, but also pointed out the costs of benefits and practical limitations of rehabilitating 'men by the million or the hundred thousand'.

It is often forgotten that Beveridge also stressed that the welfare state was not a complete replacement for individual effort: 'Social security must be achieved by co-operation between the State and the individual. The State should offer security for service and contribution. The State in organising security should not stifle incentive, opportunity, responsibility; in establishing a national minimum, it should leave room and encouragement for voluntary action by each individual to provide more than that minimum for himself and his family'.

A number of specific points in the Beveridge (1942) proposals are relevant to the present review.

Insurance for sickness and disability was only to be for those who were gainfully employed 'and not for persons who, since they have no earnings, do not lose income if sickness prevents them working'.

As a general principle, all benefits were to be at the same flat rate (with the exception of industrial injury benefit after the first 13 weeks). Beveridge laid out the case for a higher rate of industrial injury benefit (after the first 13 weeks):

- There should be extra compensation for workers because 'many industries vital to the community are also specially dangerous'
- Workers are injured while 'under orders'
- Provision of extra compensation for industrial injuries would facilitate the abolition of the old Workers' Compensation system, and make it possible to limit the employer's liability at Common Law 'to the actions for which he is responsible morally and in fact'.

(The argument for higher rates of benefit for occupational injury today is:

- Society's and national wealth is built on individuals' productive labour
- If this work exposes the individual to increased risk, they should receive increased compensation for any adverse consequences from their work.

However, if there is increasing evidence that the benefits of work outweigh the deleterious effects, this argument breaks down.)

Beveridge also argued that prolonged disability (or unemployment) required additional support:

- 'The income needs tend to increase rather than decrease; the other means at the disposal of the insured person become exhausted; expenditure on clothing and equipment which he may have been able to postpone become unavoidable, since they cannot be postponed indefinitely'

- 'Measures other than the provision of income become increasingly necessary, to prevent deterioration of morale and to encourage recovery.'

Beveridge paid little or no attention to the question of assessing sickness or incapacity for work. Perhaps, in the idealistic mood of the times and the Report, he assumed that only those who were truly sick and incapacitated would attempt to claim benefit. He may have taken for granted the ability of doctors to assess sickness and incapacity when issuing sick certificates. Alternatively, he may have been fully conscious of the potential difficulties but also the lack of any clear solution, so simply side-stepped what could have formed a major political and practical obstacle to his greater plan.

After the war, the Beveridge proposals for social security and parallel proposals for a National Health Service were implemented almost in their entirety in the 1946–48 legislation. The notable exception in the context of the present review was that no national rehabilitation service was ever established. The two other major weaknesses to Beveridge' proposals, revealed by subsequent developments, were the failure to deal with the question of assessment and the assumption that very few people would go on to chronic disability.

After Beveridge, international concepts shifted from the original German notion of social *insurance*, to the broader US New Deal concept of social *security* as part of the growth of citizenship. Marshall (1950) expressed the view that citizens in a modern western democracy have civil, political and social rights which include statutory social services. The emphasis shifted from the industrial worker to the citizen *per se*. Human and social rights are now enshrined in United Nations declaration and many national constitutions.

In Europe, concepts of the *welfare state* have increasingly embraced notions of universal support and solidarity as a fundamental social right; while in the US and Japan it is assumed that most people can arrange their own security through their employment and personal contract, and notions of *welfare* provided by the state have always remained a safety net associated with poverty and destitution, and the distinction between the deserving and the undeserving poor. However, the difference between Europe and the US should not be over-stated: there is the same debate about the role and impact of social security in Europe, and the recipients of social security in the US equally regard it as a right which is upheld by the courts. As the economic situation has changed and social security costs have risen during the last decade, most social security systems have also considered and experimented with alternative approaches. Nevertheless, there is a difference in philosophy which is reflected in the percentage of GDP spent on social security, social security legislation, entitlement, disability evaluation, and the levels and amounts of sickness and invalidity benefits. Interestingly, despite the historical legacy of Beveridge, the UK social security now falls somewhere between Europe and the US.

Ploug & Kvist (1996) pointed out that even though the political starting points for the construction and development of social security systems have differed considerably in each country, at least in the EU, they have all led to a broadly similar and comprehensive system.

No country has yet managed to produce the simple, just, user-friendly and cheap social security system that is so often sought in welfare debates.

Disability assessment medicine

Compensation and social security must always have depended on some form of assessment of disability, although as long as they were only for serious medical conditions this assessment was presumably obvious and could be carried out by caring physicians and lay people who administered the benefits. As the basis for compensation and social security was broadened, there was a need for more sophisticated and professional assessment. Expert evidence for civil litigation, compulsory medical examination for life-assurance policies and for compensation under the Workmen's Compensation Act in the 19th and early 20th centuries were really the start of disability assessment medicine. The introduction of Industrial Injury Disablement Benefit (IIDB) and Prescribed Diseases in 1948 was accompanied by the first statutory medical assessment in UK social security. Attendance Allowance (AA) in 1970 required a broader assessment of disability. Perhaps surprisingly, it was not until the 1980s in the UK that much attention was given to developing improved methods of assessing disability and capacity for work.

In the US, in contrast, the Workers' Compensation system and more active personal injury litigation led to greater professional interest and attempts to formalise assessment of impairment from a much earlier stage (AMA 1958, AAOS 1962).

Recent developments in disability assessment medicine as a speciality in its own right are described in the detailed review of social security in the UK (see p000). This is now producing greater links and cross-fertilisation between social security, insurance and under-writing, and occupational medicine.

Welfare state structures

Titmuss (1958), in an essay on *The Social Division of Welfare*, pointed out that statutory provisions for social well-being could include:

- Social security
- Fiscal policies, tax credits or tax deductions as well as cash benefits
- Occupational benefits, from fringe benefits at employment level to provisions through nationwide contracts negotiated by employers' organisations and trade unions
- Various types of voluntary assistance, charitable and mutual aid.

Social security must be considered within such a complete socio-economic context.

Olsson et al (1993) and Folkesson et al (1993) offered a Swedish overview of social security in various European countries in the early 1990s (Figure 1.5). Social security is now provided by various combinations of the public sector, the market and/or the family. Social security in Scandinavian countries is largely public sector: health care and social benefits are financed

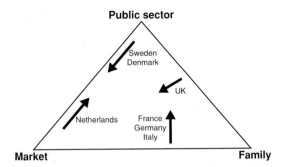

Figure 1.5 Seven European countries in the taxonomy of basic principles for health care and social services

Reproduced with permission from Folkesson *et al* (1993).

through taxes, to a large extent organised through the public sector, and distributed on equitable grounds, but there is a trend towards some market-like solutions. In the Netherlands, market-oriented solutions have always been stronger, such as private social security funds and private health care, but the government as the main funding agency is now taking an increasing regulatory role. In the UK, public-oriented systems of health care and parts of the social services are publicly financed, but some parts of the welfare system are still dependent on voluntary organisations, and there is some trend towards more market-like solutions. Finally, in countries like France, Italy and Germany, the long tradition of Catholic social teaching has encouraged family-oriented care and social support. However, the trend in these countries is towards increased public regulation, as in Germany where there has been a reaction against large increases of the cost of health care due to the growth of a previously almost unregulated market. Thus, there is some tendency for the social security systems in the various European countries to become more similar, which is not surprising in view of common EU membership and the trend of gradual harmonising of all national systems. In the US, in contrast, much social security and most health care is provided in the private sector, and the main role of the public sector is to provide a safety net for those who cannot afford to have private insurance.

Kingson & Schulz (1997) provided an overview of social insurance and social security. Governments in most advanced societies use some combination of six possible approaches to income support:

- Social insurance
- Employer mandate
- Individual mandate
- Voluntary (with or without fiscal encouragement, e.g. tax allowances)
- Means-tested programmes
- Universal programmes.

Social insurance is the largest single element and the foundation of the social welfare system in most industrial countries. There is no universal definition, but the characteristics of the social insurance approach include:

- Compulsory participation
- Government sponsorship and regulation
- Contributory financing
- Entitlement based on contributions
- Benefits laid down by legislation
- Level of benefits not directly related to level of contributions (i.e. some re-distribution)
- Separate accounting and explicit long-range financing.

Social welfare systems have two broad objectives (Kingson & Schulz 1997):

- To provide effective social protection to the population:
  - Treating individuals with dignity and respect
  - Comprehensive coverage. A social welfare system cannot provide effective protection for people it does not cover or does not reach
  - Equitable distribution of the costs and benefits. In particular, assuring that those with more limited economic resources are adequately protected
  - Efficient operation to minimise administrative costs and target resources to those in greatest need.
- To help promote a healthy economy:
  - Encouraging individual effort, work and thrift and avoid disincentives
  - Responsible government fiscal policies balancing social welfare with the other priorities of society
  - Supporting and facilitating the smooth operation of the economic and labour markets, particularly by minimising the social costs of economic change.

Kingson & Schulz (1997) provide an interesting evaluation of how well they considered the different approaches meet these objectives (Table 1.13).

Commonly, the key mechanism for targeting social security benefits on need is financial 'means testing'. Means tests are administratively complex and costly and have a number of weaknesses (Hill 1990):

- Under-claiming of entitlement
- The related problem of stigma
- The poverty trap.

TABLE 1.13   Impact of different social welfare approaches

	Social insurance	Universal cover	Means-tested 'welfare'
Treat people with dignity and respect	+[1]	+	−[2]
Comprehensive coverage	−	+	−
Equitable distribution of costs and benefits	+/−	+/−	+/−
Targeting on need	+/−	+	−
Administrative efficiency	+/−	+	−

[1]'Uplifting the human spirit'.
[2]'Corrosive effects of welfare on the human spirit create 'welfare dependency'.
Based on Kingson & Schulz (1997).

Political alternatives are either to seek ways of avoiding means tests or to try to produce more efficient means tests. Avoiding means tests tends to produce less effective targeting. The search for better means tests produces an inevitable tension between simplicity and accessibility and more effective targeting which increases complexity and administrative costs.

All EU countries have state-sponsored 'pay-as-you-go' social security systems (MISSOC 1995) with two broad aims:

- Social insurance against the traditional risks such as sickness, disability, old age and unemployment
- Social assistance to alleviate poverty, which often involves some degree of deliberate redistribution of wealth.

Disability policies in all countries have four main goals (Aarts et al 1996):

- Preventing disability
- Providing income support for those who are disabled
- Helping people to recover from disability and to restore capacity for work
- Re-integrating people with disability into society and employment.

The two key elements of social security are social insurance and social assistance. Social insurance aims to compensate to variable extent for economic losses in the event of specified social contingencies. Social assistance aims to support particular groups of the population in the event of a general social contingency. There are fundamental differences between these two elements, as seen in the social security systems of western Europe. There are generally considered to be three idealised welfare state models: the selective welfare state, the residual welfare state and the comprehensive welfare state, each with fundamentally different philosophy and methods (Table 1.14).

The selective model tries to insure that wage earners can maintain, at least to some extent, their previous living standards in the event of specified social contingencies, by entitlement to benefits that are a proportion of previous earnings. The residual model aims to provide subsistence benefits for those who are not otherwise entitled to any other form of social security and have no other family support. The comprehensive model tries to provide basic security for the entire population and at the same time income security for people who work. These different aims and methods produce different entitlements and levels of benefits. These models also represent different political ideologies about the role of the welfare state. Very broadly, the dominant ideology of the selective model is conservatism, while that of the residual model is liberalism. There may be a further distinction between political liberalism and economic liberalism: the former (à la Beveridge) supports legally-based minimum benefits in the form of either selective coverage through social assistance benefits or universal coverage through social insurance schemes; the latter, also known as laissez-faire or neo-classical liberalism, believes that the role of the state should be as limited as possible and the state should only provide for those in absolute need. The comprehensive model is based on a social democratic ideology, with re-distribution of income as well as providing social insurance for middle- and high-income groups of wage earners, although to an extent these goals are conflicting.

TABLE 1.14 Features of the three idealised welfare state models

Dimension	Selective	Residual	Comprehensive
Objectives	Guarantee previous living standards Promote the value of work, the state and the family Promotion of differences in status	Guarantee subsistence level Promotion of work ethics and efficiency Promotion of equal opportunities	Guarantee certain living standards Promotion of nationality and citizenship
Means	Compensation for economic loss	Relief of economic need	Prevention of economic need
Personal scope of application	People in work (e.g. trade)	People in need	All citizens
Allocation criteria	Selective rights	Means tested	Universal rights
Allocation entity	Social position (family, occupation, etc)	Individual	Individual
Criteria for calculating benefit levels	Earning- and contribution-related	Means tested	Flat rate and/or earnings-related
Administration	Social partners and the state	State institutions	State institutions
Sources of finance	Social insurance contributions	Taxes	Taxes
Method of financing	Funded (if possible, alongside pay-as-you-go)	Pay-as-you-go	Pay-as-you-go

Reproduced with permission from Ploug & Kvist (1996).

Different countries reflect the different welfare state models to varying degrees, although almost all are hybrid to some extent. Germany and now also France are closest to the selective model. Most Scandinavian countries are closer to the comprehensive model, although Norway and Sweden also now have some selective elements. The Netherlands is a combination of the selective and comprehensive models. The UK is a combination of the residual and the comprehensive models, although some European observers regard this as reflecting political rather than economic liberalism.

Social security structures and regulations in every country are complex because they must cover every possible entitlement and the legislation must be precise to withstand legal scrutiny. A Swedish review by Olsson et al (1993) considered that the social security systems in Sweden and the Netherlands had relatively clear principles: in Sweden 'the basic rate' (basbelopet) was fundamental to both taxation and benefits, while in the Netherlands benefits were mostly based on percentage wage replacement. The UK and Danish systems had mixed principles and many levels of benefits. The German system had multiple components, each covering a specific group of the population. With unification there were two systems in Germany, although the system in East Germany should gradually come into line with that in West Germany. France had a particularly complex social security bureaucracy. Most European countries apart from the Netherlands also provide special benefits for sickness due to work-related injury or occupational disease, although only Germany, Austria and Switzerland still provide any separate 'Workers' Compensation' services for health care or rehabilitation.

Bolderson et al (1997) provided one of the most recent comparisons of how social security benefits were actually delivered in Denmark, France, Germany, the Netherlands and the US compared with the UK. They considered how and where claims were made, the nature and treatment of any evidence required for the initial claims, decisions on claims, methods of payment, review of eligibility and entitlement, monitoring of the system and the routes to exit from benefit. They also looked at issues of decentralisation and devolution of the system. These five countries were selected because they were considered to have very different arrangements. In Denmark, nearly all benefits were administered by local authorities. Germany had numerous self-administered, independent or quasi-independent organisations in an institutionally fragmented but functionally integrated system. France had a relatively new social assistance benefit system which, unique in EU, was a central government scheme but with delivery by local and quasi-independent agencies. The Netherlands was in the process of undergoing change which appeared to have implications for the future role of the social partners, selected privatisation and market operations. The US had both national programmes with state and local initiatives that were likely to raise issues about guidelines and management of regional variation. Bolderson et al (1997) considered that none of these countries had the same central system of social security as the UK. They also considered how each country had responded to common problems such as pressure for cost-containment, prevention of error and fraud, and the potential to improve administrative efficiency using new information technology.

The Australian Heads of Workers' Compensation Authorities (1998) considered the principles, extent and boundaries of Workers' Compensation compared with social security (Table 1.15):

- Workers' Compensation is a *cause-based* system—for *occupationally-related* injury and illness. So entitlement depends on establishing causality. However, since a number of disabilities involve a combination of causal issues in addition to any occupational cause—genetic predisposition, life-style factors, ageing and degenerative factors, and psychosocial influences—there is an inherent tension about employer and Workers' Compensation liability
- Workers' Compensation is an *occupational disability* system
- Workers' Compensation is an all-or-nothing system: once entitlement is established the claimant gets the full range of benefits. Most Workers' Compensation schemes provide superior benefits to social security, so there is pressure from workers to be covered by Workers' Compensation and counter-pressure from the schemes to limit entitlement.

TABLE 1.15 Workers' Compensation compared with social security schemes for long-term disability due to work injury

Design element	Universal scheme	No-fault work injury scheme	Traditional Workers' Compensation scheme	Common law (pure fault model)	Personal insurance
Who is responsible	Government		Legislated responsibility		Personal responsibility
Who is covered	Universal	All workers	Workers defined by statute	Workers defined by common law	Individual
Basis of entitlement	Incapacity irrespective of causality	Occupational-related work incapacity (broadly defined) No fault	Work injury, tightly defined	Work injury + must prove negligence	Depends on defined risks in insurance contract
Basis of benefit	Need	Need	Need/compensation for loss	Compensation for loss	Insurance contract
Type of benefit	Flat rate	Flat rate	Earnings-related + damages	Common law damages	Depends on insurance contract
Who funds	Tax payers	Employers + employees	Employers	Employers	Individual
Interaction with social welfare	Same	Integrated	Ambiguous	Separate	None

Adapted from Heads of Workers' Compensation Authorities (1998).

The welfare debate

There is strong conceptual justification and public and political support for disability insurance, which Ball & Bethell (1997) considered the best example of what Abraham Lincoln described as the legitimate objective of government: 'to do for a community of people whatever they need to have done but cannot do at all or cannot do so well for themselves in their separate and individual capacities'. Mashaw (1997) attributed this universal support to fellow feeling rooted in our own sense of vulnerability to the risk of invalidity. 'To be born helpless and to spend some final portion of our lives coping with physical and mental infirmity is our common fate, but we would like to insure against the risk of such invalidity during the middle years of life when we expect to be economically productive.' Some form of disability insurance to provide wage replacement is the logical answer. However, disability raises other concerns in addition to the need for financial support:

● To promote improvement and return to as full and productive life as possible
● The impact on families—to support dependent children and enable them to overcome disadvantage
● Recognising the link between disability and poverty, to ameliorate poverty
● To recognise and overcome the aversion, prejudice and discrimination that disability may cause.

The multifaceted needs of people with disability and these multiple social goals inevitably lead to a complex set of social interventions: income replacement, financial compensation, health care, rehabilitation services, education and training, other social and personal support, adaptations to society and preventing discrimination, housing and employment. 'In short, in conceiving disability policies, we want to support, rehabilitate, motivate and mainstream persons with disabilities' (Mashaw 1997). Because of the very heterogeneous groups of claimants, the multiple goals, and the way social security systems have developed, disability policy is inevitably complex; it has never been possible to produce a system that is simple yet completely fair and just, that fulfils all the goals and at the same time avoids all the pitfalls. Despite the generally agreed principle, Mashaw (1997) described disability policy as 'complex, compromised and the source of almost continuous concern and reform' in almost every society. He listed these anxieties as:

● Actuarial uncertainty
● Perverse incentives
● Security of entitlement
● Legitimacy (definition and assessment of disability, targeting of benefits)
● Unmet needs
● Competing goals.

However, disability policy is not only a source of anxiety to social security administrators, policy makers and politicians but, perhaps even more, to disabled people who depend on these policies for essential support in their daily lives.

History shows that human society is in a constant state of flux. Halsey (2000) summarised the past 100 years of social change in four institutional systems which he categorised as:

production, population, power and communication. In the 20th century, Britain changed from being the dominant imperial power to having a much lesser position on the world stage, but nevertheless GDP per head of population increased 4.5-fold between 1900 and 1995. The share of wealth held by the richest 5% of the population fell from over four-fifths to a quarter, but nevertheless the century ended like it began with concerns about inequalities of wealth and the large minority of economically and socially disadvantaged. There were major changes in patterns of employment. The population changed after World War II, not so much in total numbers but in the age structure with massive increase in the number of older and retired people and the length of retirement; in family structure and the number of divorces and lone-parent families; and in ethnic structure and the number of immigrants. Halsey (2000) characterised all forms of power and authority (parents, politicians, priests, police and school teachers) as 'democratised early in the century and bureaucratised thereafter' and 'faltered in the second half of the century'. Communication expanded exponentially, particularly since World War II and not only in the current sense of informtion technology. Enlarging labour markets, the private motor car, air travel, radio, television, the telephone and now the mobile telephone, and the range of applications of the internet have had profound impact on patterns of finance, work, leisure, entertainment, politics and international relations, and the entire social structure.

So, the need for social security reform is not new or unusual but is the norm. Over the past 50 years all social security systems have had to adapt to these profound economic, social and political changes in society. Each generation over the past century has had to make decisions about major shifts in the direction of social security. The development from a system which simply attempted to replace lost income in certain adverse circumstances, to a system which also includes universal social and non-health-related benefits, put tremendous financial strain on the entire system. The big issue at each stage has been how best to meet the cost, and it is always necessary for the system to work as fairly and efficiently as possible. At the same time, the effects of social security changes are unpredictable and there is no permanent solution. The same problems of how to provide support, how to direct it to those in need, how to pay for it, and how to balance the needs and desires of the individual and society, have faced every stage of social security development. The challenge of welfare reform is how best to strike this balance in today's and tomorrow's circumstances (Ploug & Kvist 1994, 1996, UK Government Green Papers 1998a,b)—to find a way of marrying an open, competitive and successful economy with a just, decent and humane society (Grimshaw 1999).

Grimshaw (1999) described the welfare state as 'a central part of the post-war settlement, designed to provide free health care, decent housing and economic security for all. It was based on the assumption that the welfare of its people is the collective responsibility of the state, and the power of the state should be used to modify market forces. It was intended to operate in an environment of full employment, stable families, job security and retirement of short duration'. However, it has come under pressure due to radical social changes, including:

- Increased entry of women into the labour force
- Growth in lone-parent families
- Increased life-expectancy and increased duration of retirement
- Permanent rise in unemployment since the early–mid 1970s.

These pressures produced spiralling costs which led to political reaction and attempts at welfare retrenchment. Grimshaw (1999) considered that the Thatcher government which came into power in 1979 'saw the welfare state as one of the prime causes of poor economic performance. Its funding required high taxation, it discouraged work and investment, and encouraged welfare dependency. The cushioning effects of social programmes led workers to sustain unrealistic wage demands that destroyed competitiveness'.

Lazar & Stoyko (1998) provided a similar academic analysis of the welfare state from Canada. They considered that post-war welfare states in the advanced democracies were constructed on four social building blocks:

- Shared experience of the horrors of the Great Depression in the 1930s and World War II
- Political commitment to the idea of national or social solidarity and that citizenship gives rise to certain social rights
- Political development of national economic policy instruments
- Assumptions about underlying economic and social conditions, including strong traditional families and high employment. (Although not articulated at the time, it was also assumed that western societies would remain relatively homogeneous in ethnicity, language, culture and social mores.)

For the first few decades after World War II, economic growth was accompanied by some degree of greater equalisation of income. Lazar & Stoyko (1998) argued that over the past few decades technological, economic, social and political changes in society have undermined all of these original social building blocks. There is no longer the shared experience of adversity, but increasing diversity of social background and values. Social (and social security) rights and duties are no longer so closely linked. New technology is producing fundamental economic, social and cultural change. There is increasing urbanisation, ethnic mixing, political cross-fertilisation between countries, and globalisation of the economy. In recent years there has been a slow-down in economic growth (although the extent and timing varies in different countries). Labour force participation has increased, particularly among women, but unemployment and long-term unemployment have increased even more dramatically, particularly among the young and those approaching retirement. The number of people who are retired, the time they live on pensions and the cost of pensions have increased exponentially. There has been labour market polarisation, greater inequality in income distribution and increasing social exclusion. Social expenditure and fiscal deficits have risen, but some social security programmes have had unintended and undesirable side-effects. There has been erosion of faith in the state's ability to manage the economy and in traditional economic policy measures. Strongly socialist politics of the post-war years have tended to swing towards more conservative, market-based, economic politics. The traditional two-parent, one-earner family with two to four children of the 1940s has been replaced with more differentiated family structures. Affluent two-earner households, often with only one or two children, and lone-parent or no-earner households are more common. The social, employment and financial position and role of women, of young people and of pensioners has changed radically. The extended family all living close by and able to give mutual support has declined. These changes create tensions within society between growing needs for social security and social pressures to reduce social expenditure, while at the same time undermining the basic social assumptions of the welfare state.

Sullivan (2000) identified four challenges in the context of Workers' Compensation in Canada:

● There have been major changes in the nature of work, not only in the traditional sense of risk exposure but in work practices and demands and in the labour market
● Growing understanding of the social organisation of health, injury and illness has implications for prevention
● New evidence on the effectiveness of health-care interventions and on occupational health has implications for the timely treatment of injury and safe return to work
● It is now realised that psychosocial aspects of work may have a much more generalised and pervasive impact on health than traditional physical risks of injury.

Together, these challenges raise issues of entitlement, fairness and sustainability of Workers' Compensation in an era of liberalised trade arrangements.

Lazar & Stoyko (1998) compared trends in different countries and suggested that although most western countries have been moving towards more flexible, less re-distributive and leaner social security systems in recent years, they are still as far apart in their generosity as they were two or three decades ago. Those countries that have been most effective at controlling unemployment have also had the greatest increases in income inequality. Taxation has been shifting from the corporate tax base to the income tax base and from income taxation to the taxation of consumption, and this has reduced the redistribution of wealth. At least from a North American perspective, the economic role of the state relative to market forces has been reducing.

Ploug & Kvist (1996) pointed out that when the present social security systems were established and extended during the period after World War II up to the mid 1970s, it was assumed that only a small proportion of the population would need or claim social support at any one time, and only during transitional periods from one position of self-support to another. One of the main expectations of all of the original welfare systems was that public support would be and should be of limited duration. At this time, there were fewer elderly people, most people only survived a few years after retirement, economic growth was considerably higher than today and the unemployment rate considerably lower. Today, however, far more people than originally envisaged are now receiving cash benefits and depending on them for longer periods. Most members of society now receive some form of social security benefits at some time in their lives and social security has become a source of prolonged support for a large minority of the population. The economic situation is no longer improving so rapidly, the demand on social security has risen greatly, and the accumulated public sector deficit may now account for half or more of GDP, with interest and repayments limiting the amount of funding available. In other words, the economic foundation upon which the welfare system rests has altered fundamentally while social security systems themselves have remained basically unchanged.

Lonsdale (1993) looked at trends in long-term invalidity benefits in the UK, Ireland, the Netherlands, Sweden, Germany, the US and Australia (Table 1.16). In most of these countries, the main increases occurred during the 1970s, whereas in Britain they occurred in the 1980s. During the 1980s, in most of these countries the growth in long-term invalidity benefits had slowed down and Germany actually managed to reverse it. The majority of recipients of these benefits in all of these countries were men, but the number of female recipients rose faster in all countries apart from Australia. However, in most countries by 1990, men on benefits still out-numbered women by approximately 2:1, except in Sweden where women actually out-numbered men. Lonsdale (1993) could not obtain accurate figures for Germany but suggested that the same trend in female recipients did not occur there because of a policy change in 1985 which disproportionately curtailed the entry of women into disability pensions. Overall, the changing female pattern appeared to be related to changing patterns of female employment and increasing entitlement to these benefits. Lonsdale (1993) pointed out that among older recipients of long-term sickness and invalidity benefits it was often difficult to distinguish those who should be regarded as part of the labour force and those who should really be regarded as pensioners.

TABLE 1.16   Percentage increase in numbers of people on long-term invalidity benefits in selected countries 1970–1990

	1970–1980	1980–1990
UK	53	91
Sweden	87	34
The Netherlands	142	32
Germany	19	−7
US	92	20
Australia	83	48

Based on data from Lonsdale (1993).

Lonsdale (1993) pointed out that the increase in the number of people receiving long-term sickness or disability benefits had occurred in countries with very different benefit systems, ranging from those with liberal criteria for benefits, such as the Netherlands and Sweden (although that had now changed to at least some extent), to those where benefits depended on insurance contributions or recent employment history, such as the UK, US and Germany, to those with a means-tested system of benefits, such as Australia. In some countries the increase was due to more people claiming benefits, as in Sweden and the US. In most countries, including the UK, however, it was also due to an increase in the duration of benefits and in the number of people who remained on benefits.

Lonsdale (1993) suggested that during the 1970s and 80s the function of these benefits had changed from being a form of support for employees who developed a long-term or permanent sickness or disability to being a benefit increasingly used by people who might otherwise be defined as unemployed. In some countries, at this time particularly the Netherlands, Sweden and Germany, these benefits also appeared to have become an institutionalised way in which older members of the work force could get early withdrawal from the labour force as an alternative to unemployment. For the claimant, long-term sickness or invalidity benefits might be a better system of income maintenance than unemployment benefits. The controls were usually less onerous, and it was arguably easier to obtain medical certification from a doctor than to prove to social security adjudicators that one was genuinely looking for employment. Sickness and disability benefits were usually perceived as less stigmatising than unemployment benefits. They were often more generous, if not in the basic rate then in the linked eligibility for additional benefits and in taxation status. They also generally continued indefinitely until receipt of retirement pension, while unemployment benefits might be time limited.

Against this background, it is not surprising that the welfare state and social security systems enjoy such a high priority on the political agenda in most western European countries and have been the recurring subject of debate since World War II. Now that the labour market has become so volatile and fragile, there is increasing sensitivity to the complex interaction between the social security system and the labour market (ISSA 1996). Despite this, it is still uncertain how these interactions work or their magnitude. This makes many of the social security reforms and interventions experimental. Nevertheless, the political debate can be described as the battle between those who believe that the best way of securing welfare is to provide optimal circumstances for economic growth, and those who believe that the state should intervene in order to secure stable economic growth without huge deviations and with more equitable distribution of wealth as well as opportunities for individual development. The first group argues that social protection is a disincentive that holds back society economically. The latter argues that social protection is important for social cohesion, political stability, and an efficient labour market. A high level of social protection is only possible in a relatively wealthy society, but strong social protection may be an investment which aids labour flexibility and upgrading to launch and sustain economic growth. Despite the conflict of philosophy between these two points of view, almost all political parties in western European countries have contributed to the growth and development of the welfare state.

Ploug & Kvist (1994) reviewed this debate and pointed out that the 'crisis' of the welfare state has been an issue for many years. At the end of the 1960s and the beginning of the 70s, the debate was about disillusionment—the collapse of the idealistic view that the welfare state would create well-being, social cohesion and content. By the mid 70s the debate was on the legitimacy of devoting so much GDP to a public welfare system which was seen as over-administered and bureaucratic. The system seemed to be incapable of solving the problems, not least the problems of unemployment, and the appearance of anti-tax parties in Denmark and Norway demonstrated the strength of such concerns. There seemed to be a mismatch between welfare expenditure and what it actually achieved. In the early 90s, the debate was whether Europe could afford the welfare state and whether it created structures and barriers that prevented a return to full employment. Some neo-liberal approaches in Europe questioned whether the two principles of solidarity and insurance could be separated, providing at least some aspects of social security through private insurance under state legislation or compulsion. However, the fundamental limitation was that those who are most in need of welfare spending are generally least able to pay for private insurance, which raises political issues of re-distribution of wealth. By the mid–late 90s, two crucial areas were seen to be incentives and competitiveness. Incentive problems concern how or to what extent social security may influence people's inclination to work and to contribute to the creation of GDP. This includes some specific economic questions. Does increased tax pressure and a relatively high marginal level of taxation mean that people will want to work less as their personal economic benefit decreases? Do improved social security benefits mean that to some extent people will be less willing to work and instead come to rely on these benefits?

Ploug & Kvist (1994) summarised three basic arguments against the welfare state:

1. It destroys people's incentives to support themselves and their relatives
2. It does not change social conditions but simply disguises fundamental imbalances in society
3. It is too expensive.

In a world of increasing international trade and competition from the US, Asia and Eastern Europe, which do not have similar social security systems, it may be questioned whether western European countries can sustain the present type of welfare state or whether more fundamental changes are required. Low economic growth and high unemployment rates also raise the question of whether the European welfare systems may have contributed to these current economic and social problems. However, Hoskins (1996) pointed out that there is little empirical evidence that social security expenditure affects competitiveness. Some countries with high social expenditure are nevertheless highly competitive (e.g. Germany) while others are not (e.g. Norway). Some countries with low social expenditure are competitive (e.g. Japan) while others are not (e.g. at that time, the UK).

During the 1980s and early 90s, there was a general public and political perception in Europe that welfare costs were rising, or might in the future rise, and that there was a danger they may get out of control. As long as economic times were good, society could afford welfare, but whenever the national economy stagnated, with fears of falling tax revenue and increased social costs of unemployment, this perception grew more acute. By the early 90s, there was a growing debate throughout Europe about this financial 'welfare crisis' and an apocalyptic fear that the welfare state might not survive, at least in its present form (Nachemson 1991, Olsson et al 1993, MISSOC 1994, Ploug & Kvist 1994, 1996). Average public expenditure in Europe did rise by about 10% of GDP between the mid 70s and mid 80s, but then remained more or less constant until 1991, and then rose another 2–3% between 1991 and 1993. Average social security expenditure rose by about 4–5% of

GDP between the early 70s and mid 80s, remained static up to 1991, and then increased another 3% by 1995 (Waddell & Norlund 2000). In most countries, sickness benefit costs, at least to the state, were actually falling and invalidity benefits remained about the same. So to some extent this welfare crisis was more a perception than a reality, although it may be argued that the social pressures and potential for much greater increases were always present and only forestalled by legislative or administrative checks.

MISSOC (1998) reviewed social policy development in Europe and suggested that it was not a high priority during the early years of the EC. In the early 1970s the Commission proposed a Social Action Programme of community legislation for employment law, equal opportunities, health and safety at work and a European Social Fund. The launch of the single market in 1985 then led to a consensus that social legislation needed to be improved, culminating in the Social Chapter in 1989 (signed by all EU countries except the UK). The Charter contained 47 initiatives, nearly two-thirds of which have now been adopted. The Commission then had a second social action programme largely directed to employment conditions. In November 1993, the Commission published a consultative green paper on the future of European social policy. The key messages were that there was a distinctive European social model based on democracy and individual rights, free collective bargaining, a market economy, the need for equality of opportunity for all and the importance of social welfare and solidarity. In July 1994, the Commission published a white paper which argued the balance of social and economic policy, and the fundamental need to deal with unemployment as an underlying structural problem. In April 1995, the Commission adopted its third social action programme with three main messages: the extent of socio-economic change required a dynamic and flexible European vision; social policy was at the heart of European integration; economic, employment and social policy were interdependent and needed to be more closely aligned. It proposed ambitious plans for employment, equality of opportunity for women, the idea that society belongs to all its citizens, and the need for studies and research in the social area.

By 1994–1995, MISSOC (1995) reported that the economic situation was beginning to improve, with rising output and falling unemployment in most European countries. More people were contributing to the mandatory social security schemes, and although the funding of many schemes was still not in balance, they considered the worst was over. 'State-sponsored pay-as-you-go social security has survived its most severe test since the 1930s.'

By 1996, recovery was still slow and uneven, unemployment remained high, and the rising cost of social security remained a concern for Europe (MISSOC 1996). Nevertheless, after some years of emphasis on the negative economic and social effects of social security, MISSOC (1996) considered that this was now balanced by increasing realisation of its positive benefits. There was now little argument that social security was a fundamental and essential part of a modern society, and that it would survive in some form or other for the foreseeable future. There was increasing acceptance that adequate social protection is important for social cohesion, political stability, an efficient labour market and economic progress. The debate now focused more on exactly what social security could and should aim to achieve, and how to structure the social security system to achieve these goals (Commission of the European Communities 1995).

Recent developments in disability benefits

Since about the 1970s, all countries have been attempting to control the growth and costs of long-term disability and incapacity benefits (Lonsdale 1993). Nevertheless, Ploug & Kvist (1994) concluded that up to about 1992 there had been no fundamental changes in the social security systems in most European countries. Most earlier changes simply adjusted benefit formulas and levels to the current economic situation, and did not involve any fundamental modification of the welfare state blueprint. However, by about 1992, many EU countries appeared to be questioning whether the state should in future play a lesser role in providing cash benefits and whether people themselves should play a greater role in providing for their own welfare and choosing their own welfare blend. In Finland, there was a desire to preserve basic social security but the severe economic situation might mean that little else could be afforded. In Germany, demographic and unemployment trends raised the possibility that there might need to be future cuts but 'it should always be kept in mind that a minimum subsistence must be guaranteed for everyone'. In the Netherlands, there seemed to be a lack of any fundamental debate about the future of the welfare state and cash benefit systems and a fear that crucial changes would be made without any underlying philosophy. In the UK, there was at this time a much more radical political attempt to question the established welfare system. In Sweden, there was a similar, although less radical, questioning of the future role of the welfare state.

Ploug & Kvist (1996) posed the fundamental questions: Who should receive cash benefits and how much should they receive? Who should pay for social security? Who should administer the social security system?

In an earlier report, Ploug & Kvist (1994) expanded on elements of the welfare state's crisis:

- Increasing expectations of improved social benefits
- Increasing costs
- Ineffectiveness—the welfare state was originally developed to serve the middle class, and did not provide answers to new kinds of social need such as social exclusion, poverty and homelessness which had increased in several European countries in recent years despite economic prosperity
- Unintended side-effects: lack of control, disincentives, economic impact, social marginalisation.

A UK Government Green Paper (1998a), *New Ambitions for our Country: A New Contract for Welfare* identified three similar problems to the present UK social security system:

- Inequality and social exclusion are worsening, especially among children and pensioners, despite rising spending on social security
- People face a series of barriers to paid work, including financial disincentives
- There is abuse of the system which takes money away from those in real need.

The MISSOC (1995) review of trends in social security systems in the EU summarised several recent approaches to meeting these problems:

- Cutting benefit costs, either through direct cuts or by restricting access to benefits, or to a lesser extent by attempting to make the schemes more efficient
- Privatisation, or partnership with the private sector, shifting some of the costs from government to the employer or private insurance schemes
- Targeting social security benefits to the most needy or deserving, and then it might be possible to improve benefits for some very selected groups, which the private sector often has difficulty covering
- Re-structuring the contributions to widen the financial basis of statutory schemes and re-structuring both contributions and benefits to remove some of their more negative effects.

Lonsdale (1993) summarised various methods of putting this into practice for invalidity benefits:

- Reducing benefit levels and tax differentials compared with other social security benefits
- Tighter medical criteria for disability
- Abolishing labour market considerations
- Introduction of rehabilitation and employment programmes for disabled people
- Stopping early retirement pension options
- Regular reviews of recipients.

However, the US experience shows, and most countries agree anecdotally, that if long-term disability and incapacity benefits are stopped, many of the recipients simply move to other social security programmes (Lonsdale 1993). This suggests that stopping disability and incapacity benefits for these people without dealing with their employment needs may simply mean that they move to another part of the social security system. Any policy attempts to curb incapacity benefits will have little effect unless there is a simultaneous policy to promote employment and re-integration into the labour force. This must focus not only on helping the individual to return to work, but also encouraging employers to re-employ them.

MISSOC (1996) also considered the background to recent trends and policy changes in invalidity pensions. They suggested that there was a general tendency for the number of invalidity pensions to increase, and that in a worsening economic and employment situation, employers become more selective. Unemployed people with any form of sickness or disability appeared to give up hope of re-employment and preferred to claim invalidity benefit which was generally financially better and also less restrictive than unemployment benefit. This was closely linked to the tendency to earlier retirement. MISSOC (1996) considered this had all been encouraged by governments and social security authorities, either tacitly or overtly, to improve job vacancies for young people. By 1996, there were deliberate attempts to reverse this policy throughout Europe. All member states were trying to disentangle the medical and employment criteria which had become intertwined in the assessment of disability. The aim was to return to the original concept in which incapacity for work is measured purely on medical grounds without reference to actual employment possibilities. Invalidity pensions should also no longer be seen as a permanent exit from the labour force. Instead, the new emphasis was on review of invalidity status, rehabilitation and return to work.

In some countries, particularly Sweden and the Netherlands, the use of labour market considerations in assessing incapacity was explicit policy. In most others, it became more or less accepted practice. Lonsdale (1993) concluded: 'the difficulty of disentangling the different factors affecting employment such as physical or mental impairment, low levels of skill, age, and employer prejudice against older and disabled workers remains, however, and may well turn out to frustrate rehabilitation policies as much as it does social security policy'. By 1996, one of the most interesting developments was the extension of wage subsidies to people moving from social security benefit into employment.

By 1996, the structural emphasis turned to administrative and managerial reforms, tighter financial control and the fight against fraud (ISSA 1996). A sudden and nearly simultaneous assault on fraud in social security systems was launched right across Europe and at first sight appears somewhat surprising. There was little evidence that there had been a sudden EU-upsurge in deceit in so many different settings. Political anxiety may be more infectious. Assaults on fraud also become tempting when other forms of cost saving become limited and they raise less political contention than most other actions in this highly contentious field. Technology is another route for cost savings, if properly managed, and offers new weapons to control costs and fight fraud. Political convergence may be slow but the spread of technology is rapid.

By 1996, there was particular awareness of the problem of a rising trend of early retirement, and the policy of using state disability and pension schemes to remove older workers from the labour market was now being reversed throughout the EU (ISSA 1996). The previous readiness to use disability pensions as a permanent exit from the labour market was out of favour, with a new emphasis instead on review and rehabilitation. These observations were valid for nearly all EU countries and this common concern was striking. For example, disability benefit had been re-named Rehabilitation Benefit in Finland. In Austria, all disability pensions were to expire after 2 years and would not be renewed unless rehabilitation efforts could be shown to have been unsuccessful. Spain adopted a new system of assessing disability benefit claims which no longer relied on the decision of a single doctor but on a multidisciplinary panel provided by the National Social Security Institute. Denmark was in the process of reviewing its Anticipatory Pension Scheme, which covered all long-term benefits awarded before the normal retirement age, with particular attention to rehabilitation. Most of these measures were directed at the lower levels of disability, where there was still some potential for re-employment, given the right conditions, incentives and assistance.

In general, most eastern European countries were tending, at varying speeds, towards western European systems of social security, although this was often constrained by their economic situation. After 5 years of political, economic and social transition, these countries still faced serious challenges to the development of viable and sustainable health and social security programmes (MISSOC 1996). There were major problems to collecting contributions and taxes from both employers and employees, massive deficits in social security funds, and inefficiency in social security administration. Many individuals might only be eligible for the most basic social assistance schemes which were neither cost-effective nor efficient.

ISSA (1996) suggested that following a number of years of 'wait and see' many social security systems in western Europe were now undergoing radical reforms of their structure. These reforms included the privatisation of public pension schemes, wide-scale reductions in benefits, and questioning the role of the public sector in administering social programmes. In some instances, economic and market priorities had taken precedence over social protection and improvements:

- Make access to benefits more selective
- Although the principle of basic social protection provided and guaranteed by the state had generally not been seriously questioned, actual delivery of that promise in practice had been reduced to varying degrees.

As already stated, social security schemes have always been subject to frequent adjustments to their methods of financing, eligibility requirements and benefits, to meet changing social needs and economic conditions. However, what is striking is the growing consensus that new and more fundamental changes are now required. There is increasing agreement across the world that the future of social security can no longer be ensured merely by increasing contribution rates or adjusting benefit entitlements and that such technical adjustments are no longer enough.

Olsson et al (1993) suggested that the structural problems and reform strategies were largely common to many European countries—but not in the way that is commonly thought. Social securities that are closer to market insurance principles have the traditional problems of market failures: creaming of good risk categories, unfair premium differences, inefficient competition, cost expansion, lower labour mobility and funding safety. In these systems, structural forms tended towards more public system principles, such as risk sharing, fixed budgets and public control. Unified, tax-financed public social security insurance systems have other structural problems, such as lack of effectiveness, unbalanced budgets and problems with incentives. Here, policy changes were towards more market mechanisms like premium systems, defined contributions systems and capital funding, self-risks and freedom of choice. Corporate insurance systems based on collective agreements had some of the problems of market failures, such as creaming of good risk categories, poor cost control and lack of incentives, and also the rigidity typical of public systems. In addition, these systems probably tended to optimise internal efficiency while increasing external costs. In corporate systems, reforms tended to introduce both more public system features like better control, and more market-like features such as freedom of choice.

Olsson et al (1993) made three tentative conclusions. First, writing in the early 1990s, they foresaw increasing harmonisation of social security systems within the EU.

Second, contrary to this tendency to harmonisation, the social security systems in most countries tend to retain their unique cultural heritage, even when the growing needs and problems of the system necessitate structural reform. Ploug & Kvist (1994) considered that although in almost all other socio-economic fields life was becoming more international, there were some indications that common approaches and provisions of social security were unlikely to emerge in the near future. Increasing diffusion of ideas and desire for harmonisation within Europe might lead to the risk of hasty import of methods from other systems and these might not work in the same way when applied in a completely different system in another country. They might cure some problems but lead to other undesirable effects.

Third, and perhaps most important, social security systems and any proposed structural reforms could potentially have a major effect on the level of marginalisation and social exclusion. In the early 1990s, in many European countries, this was regarded as the most dangerous, most complex, and most costly, long-term social problem. Increased marginalisation causes increased social expenditure, taking a larger proportion of GDP and increasing taxation. There are many social forces feeding into this process, but Olsson *et al* (1993) considered that social security incentives were probably as important as wages and taxation. High wage replacement rates and little loss of disposable income reduce the individual's incentive to work. If the risk of unemployment rises and social benefits are lower, individuals and trade unions may apply political pressure to improve incapacity and early retirement benefits rather than relying on more uncertain income from work and low unemployment benefits. If employers try to control overheads by hiring young and healthy workers, this may support individual preference. If employers and trade unions also control profits and insurance systems by excluding unhealthy workers, this will effectively stop rehabilitation and add to social exclusion.

Welfare state institutions originally developed with their major focus on workers in permanent, full-time employment. However, welfare problems also arise, and nowadays often to a greater extent, in members of society who do not have such firm attachment to the labour market due to changing jobs, part-time work, casual work or unemployment. The financial problem is that if an increasing proportion of the population becomes more loosely attached to the labour market, this produces less revenue from taxation and increased demand on social security. This raises issues of entitlement to benefits and social rights. In most European countries, such people receive relatively low social assistance benefits, which might increase the pressure on sickness and invalidity benefits.

In a report to the 25th General Assembly of ISSA in November 1995 (Hoskins 1996), the Secretary General reviewed the social imperatives of change:

- Despite increased life-expectancy, earlier retirement may reduce social security contributions and entitlement
- Increased part-time and black market work may reduce social security contributions and entitlement
- Increasing numbers of young unemployed who do not join the labour force may reduce social security contributions and entitlement

- Increasing poverty, marginalisation and exclusion may reduce social security contributions and entitlement
- Increasing numbers of working women and increasing gender equality—who will look after the frail elderly?

He identified the major challenges facing social security as:

- Social security now serves primarily to facilitate exit from the labour force (retirement, disability, unemployment, etc). To what extent does it encourage dependence rather than re-employment of the young, the disabled and the older unemployed?
- In a time of rising prosperity, social security should do a better job of caring for the most vulnerable and needy members of society, as envisaged by the founders of post-World War II welfare society. Instead, at the end of the 20th century, there is some tendency to return to the *laissez-faire* approach of the 19th century and means-tested welfare
- There is poor public understanding and debate about the real issues. The debate is often more emotional than intellectual.

He agreed that technical adjustments to contribution rates or benefit entitlements were no longer sufficient, and supported the increasing consensus from social security organisations around the world about the need for new and fundamental re-considerations of social security policy. Improvements in the administrative structure of the social security system and privatisation of elements of it might produce some degree of improved efficiency but the effects are finite and do not resolve the underlying problems and questions. The underlying problems will not be solved by the next improvement in the economic cycle. Instead, there is a need to reconsider the fundamental aims, principles and structures, although change and reform do not mean dismantlement. He suggested that reform was most likely to succeed if it returned to basic principles:

- Insurance
- 'Welfare'
- Redistribution of wealth.

To some extent these aims may conflict. Increased emphasis on insurance may penalise the poor, the inactive and the needy. Increased emphasis on welfare may be questioned or resisted by working tax payers. There must be a balance between these aims, and the system must be seen by all to be fair and efficient. Social security planning must consider not only financial and budgetary issues, but must be balanced by questions of social policy objectives and social justice. Social security must be integrated with both economic and social planning.

Intertwined with these practical issues, there has been also been political and philosophical debate in the EU about the future of social protection. The European Council Recommendations (1992) on the *Convergence of Social Protection Objectives and Policies* again confirmed that responsibility for the organisation and financing of social protection systems was in the hands of member states. The European Commission Communication (1995) launched the debate on *The Future of Social Protection: A Framework for a European Debate*. There was then an EU Social Action Programme 1998–2000.

A further European Commission Communication (1997) reviewed the background to *Modernising and Improving Social Protection in the European Union*. Social protection systems provide the bulk of expenditure on social support, health care and pensions and now account for 28% of EU GDP, although that varies from 16 to 35% in different countries. They are considered to have played a fundamental role in ensuring income redistribution and cohesion, maintaining political stability and economic progress in the EU. The objectives, financial and operative structures of most systems were established even before the EU, and the basic needs remain unchanged, but the social and economic conditions have changed and the social protection systems must adapt accordingly:

- The changing nature of work, where a new interplay is called for between policies designed to improve flexibility and those designed to provide security
- Change in the gender balance in working life, where equal opportunities bring new issues and requirements in terms of social protection
- The ageing of the population, where the rapid growth in the dependent population is creating new needs as well as forcing the pace of pension reform
- The need to reform the co-ordination of national security schemes for people moving within the EU.

This Communication tried to indicate the routes along which modernisation could be pursued and to present proposals for European-level support. It presumed that there was a common understanding that:

- Each member state is responsible for organising and financing its own social protection system
- The EU is responsible for the co-ordination of national social security schemes in cases where citizens exercise their rights of free movement within the EU
- The EU also serves as a forum for promoting better mutual understanding of long-term perspectives and for identifying common challenges facing member states.

Against that background, it proposed an agenda of issues for further analysis, debate and action:

- Social protection as a productive factor
- Making social security systems more employment friendly
- Adapting social security systems to an ageing population
- Adapting social security systems to the new gender balance at work
- Reforming the system of social security co-ordination for people moving within the EU.

The fundamental beliefs throughout this Communication were that good social protection and successful economic performance are mutually supporting and also that increasing co-ordination of European social protection systems is inevitable.

MISSOC (1998) summarised the challenges:

- Unemployment remains stubbornly high
- The world of work is changing rapidly
- Poverty and social exclusion exist side by side with rising prosperity and wealth.

Social policy is the mechanism that helps to ensure that economic progress and European integration benefits all citizens. European surveys suggest that most people want a cohesive and inclusive society, based on solidarity and equality, as well as a high quality of life and health. Public policies can help achieve this by boosting employment, developing and maintaining the capacity of people through their working life, promoting income redistribution and alleviating poverty, providing a safety net for those genuinely in need, and by combating discrimination and inequality. The considerable expenditure involved reflects the shared conviction that social protection underpins economic growth and social progress.

A European Commission Communication (1999), *A Concerted Strategy for Modernising Social Protection*, again started from the conviction that: 'Social protection systems have an important role to play throughout the EU, in the lives of individuals and families and in underpinning the development of society and the economy'. It concluded that in the EU there is now 'a recognition that strong social protection systems are an integral part of the European Social Model which is based on the conviction and evidence that economic and social progress go hand in hand and are mutually reinforcing factors'. Gone are the days of doubt about the survival of the welfare state! It proposed four key objectives:

- To make work pay and provide secure income
- To make pensions safe and pension systems sustainable
- To promote social inclusion
- To ensure high quality and sustainable health care.

The new context included:

- Deepening of economic integration in the EU, with the internal market and the single currency
- The agreements to develop a European Employment Strategy
- The enlargement of the EU.

Central to the development of the European Employment Strategy is the recognition that employment and social protection policies are closely linked. Against the above-noted background of demographic, social and economic change, work and family life must be reconciled. The provision of guaranteed income 'protection' against the traditional risks of sickness, disability, old age and unemployment is no longer enough. Adapting to these changed conditions calls for striking a new balance between security and flexibility as well as between rights and responsibilities.

Particularly relevant to the current review, this Communication also stressed that tax and benefit systems must provide *incentives* for work, and that *activation measures* must focus on the needs of the individual and require strong links between the benefits and employment systems. 'It may also require a review of conditions governing benefits to ensure that the appropriate balance is struck between an individual's entitlement to benefit and their availability for training or other measures.'

Within the European Commission there is now some political commitment to a common European approach to social policy (Vandenbroucke 2000). Current ideas for the next year or two would probably take the form of 'soft law' with comparative studies and co-operation on 'best practice' and the setting of 'standards of excellence' or 'benchmarks'.

The *Report on Social Protection in Europe 1999* was adopted by the European Commission (2000) and backed by the European Parliament in February–March 2000. This had a different format from earlier MISSOC annual reports but, as previously, reviewed recent developments in social protection expenditure and receipts. It once again emphasised the major demographic, economic and social changes over the past 20–25 years which had profound implications for social protection systems. However, it presented the four major trends in slightly different combination and balance:

- The ageing of the population in all member states and the expected increase in the rate of growth in the number of elderly people from 2010 onwards
- The growing participation of women in the labour force and the changing gender balance
- The persistence of long-term unemployment, especially among older workers, and the trend towards earlier retirement
- The increase in the number of households with people living alone or with no-one in work.

In this Report (European Commission 2000), pensions accounted for 43% of social protection expenditure across the EU, health care for 22% and disability benefits for just over 8%, which was about equal to unemployment benefits, although in 9 out of 15 member states expenditure on disability benefits exceeded unemployment benefits. Despite the ageing of the population, the main change in social protection expenditure in the EU from 1990 to 1996 was not on old-age pensions or health care. Rather, the greatest relative increase was in disability and housing benefits and social exclusion. Since 1990, the main fall in state social protection expenditure had been on sickness benefits (which had increasingly been transferred to employers).

Under the broad objective 'to make work pay and provide secure income' this Report (European Commission 2000) noted that a prominent feature of policy across the EU in the past few years had been a widespread re-examination of conditions for benefit payments. As a result, many member states had tightened the qualifying conditions for eligibility to benefits. This included but was not confined to unemployment benefits and increased activation of the unemployed to find a job. There had also been changes in disability and early retirement schemes to reduce their use as a more generous substitute for unemployment benefits. Several countries had also introduced flexible retirement schemes.

Since the election of a New Labour government in 1997, there have been various attempts to consider welfare reform in the UK. Earlier, Bradshaw (1992) had concluded that Thatcher policies were ineffective in practice and confirmed three hypotheses about social security:

- Social security is deeply impervious to change. It is ingrained in our culture, economy and system of exchange to such an extent that governments can only succeed in tampering at the margins

- The reason is that social security is recognised by a substantial body of opinion (the electorate—those who stand to benefit but also those who do not, MPs of all parties and the House of Lords) as essential to a civilised society
- For a radical government seeking to make reforms to the social security system, HM Treasury has a devastatingly unhelpful influence. It is made up of short-term thinkers, focused on current expenditure and incapable of long-term planning or strategy.

A UK Government Green Paper (1998a) laid out some basic principles. It suggested that welfare should be based on the three core values of work, security and opportunity. The key philosophy was to encourage work for those who can and provide security for those who cannot work.

- The new welfare state should help and encourage people of working age to work where they are capable of doing so
- The public and private sectors should work in partnership to ensure that, wherever possible, people are insured against foreseeable risks and make provision for their retirement
- The new welfare state should provide public services of high quality to the whole community, as well as cash benefits
- Those who are disabled should get the support they need to lead a fulfilling life with dignity
- The system should support families and children, as well as tackling the scourge of child poverty
- There should be specific action to attack social exclusion and help those in poverty
- The system should encourage openness and honesty and the gateways to benefit should be clear and enforceable
- The system of delivering modern welfare should be flexible, efficient and easy for people to use.

The UK Government Green Paper (1998a) proposed a new welfare contract between the government and the individual, based on responsibilities and rights (Table 1.17).

Conclusion

Ploug & Kvist (1996) concluded that the European welfare state had not only survived 20 years of economic crisis but had been a success. Material poverty and gross deprivation have generally been eliminated throughout Europe. There is an enormous difference between the economic situation of those unemployed today and those who were unemployed during the depression of the 1930s. The goal of providing social security against income loss has generally been achieved. There has been a general reduction in income differentials in many west European countries since World War II, even if more recently this trend has been reversed in some countries. There have also been tremendous advances in other public services such as education and health care. Steuerle & Bakija (1997) similarly concluded that the US Social Security system had made tremendous achievements in providing financial support and health care for the elderly and disabled, removing millions

TABLE 1.17 A new welfare contract

Duty of government	Duty of individual
Provide people with the assistance they need to find work Make work pay	Seek training or work where able to do so
Support those unable to work so that they can lead a life of dignity and security	Take up the opportunity to be independent if able to do so
Assist parents with the cost of raising their children	Give support, financial or otherwise, to their children and other family members
Regulate effectively so that people can be confident that private pensions and insurance products are secure	Save for retirement where possible
Relieve poverty in old age where savings are inadequate	Not to defraud the tax payer
Devise a system that is transparent and open and gets money to those in need	

Duty of us all

To help all individuals and families to realise their full potential and live a dignified life, by promoting economic independence through work, by relieving poverty where it cannot be prevented and by building a strong and cohesive society where rights are matched by responsibilities

From UK Government Green Paper (1998a).

from conditions of poverty and giving the elderly the means to live their last years with dignity. However, expectations have also now risen greatly and there is increasing concern across Europe about current levels of marginalisation and social exclusion. There is also concern across the world about whether these expectations and demands on the social security system may exceed taxation revenue or what society is prepared to pay.

Despite continuing debate, a majority of the populations in all European countries is proud of its welfare system, which seems to form an important part of the culture of each country (Ploug & Kvist 1996). All US surveys also show strong public support, even if there is concern that benefits may be inadequate or unfair (Kingson & Schulz 1997). It is easy to find critics of the welfare state, but when all is said and done every population seems to agree that its welfare state is the best in the world. There is a general political satisfaction with the welfare system—the problem may be that at present we can only afford an austere version.

Some independent observers, however, are less self-congratulatory. Hill (1990) suggested that there are now three 'social welfare classes' in Britain, which presumably applies to most of the countries in this review. The first class are people who are in relatively well paid and secure employment, and their welfare does not really depend on the social security system, even though they pay contributions and draw benefits when they are entitled. When sick they receive employment-related sick pay which may provide full salary, and when they retire they have generous employment pensions. Unemployment is relatively rare and short-lived (although this is less true now than previously) and usually cushioned by generous redundancy and early retirement provisions. Some women in this class, however, may be dependent on their male partner's entitlement and may be vulnerable to marital breakdown. The second class are the traditional working class for whom the social security system was originally designed and for whom it still has considerable validity. When sick they receive some form of Statutory Sick Pay (SSP) and then invalidity and related benefits which can provide a reasonable income even for long-term and severe disability, *provided they have built up sufficient entitlement*. Between redundancy payments and Unemployment Benefit they have some cover for short-term unemployment. When they retire they receive a state pension, possibly with some employment-related supplement. However, women in this class may be much less adequately covered, particularly if they are in part-time or low paid jobs, and long-term sickness or unemployment may 'demote' both men and women to the third class. The combination of social security benefits and some employment-related entitlement works reasonably well for many members of this class, but some 'fall through the cracks in the system' and are easily demoted to the third class. The third class are the socially disadvantaged, with low education and skills, a poor and low-paid employment record, limited financial resources and more sickness (Acheson 1998). When sick, they get the minimum SSP and their employment is likely to be terminated. They may have built up limited entitlement to social insurance benefits. When they are sick or unemployed, it is more likely to be prolonged. When they retire, they will receive the basic state retirement pension or less if their employment record is poor. The original Beveridge vision of social security funded by insurance contributions fails for this class and instead many of them are dependent on the means-tested 'safety net' to stave off poverty, both when they are out of work and sometimes even when they are in work. People in the first and especially the second class may fall into this third class as a result of prolonged unemployment or sickness, but people in the third class face many barriers and vicious circles that trap them there.

Lazar & Stoyko (1998) took a more balanced, academic approach to the future of the welfare state, although they admitted they had no simple answer. They concluded that, whatever its problems and weaknesses, the welfare state is remarkably resilient and its record demonstrates its great social and economic value. As Ball & Bethell (1997) commented: 'a system that has never missed a payday in 60 years of existence is soundly bottomed on principles that, as polls continue to show, have broad appeal for Americans. A system founded and funded on such principles has every reason to endure—and I believe it will, in much the same form and based on the same principles'. There is no substitute for the state as the guarantor of last resort for the most disadvantaged members of society, and this inevitably involves taxation of those who are better off and some degree of re-distribution of income. At the same time, social security provisions must recognise and deal with the increasing diversity of society, the increasing demand for personal choice, and the need for cost-efficiency. Social, employment and economic policies are inextricably linked, and increasingly act within a global market place. It is tempting to argue that the solution to increasing demands on social security and increasing taxation needs is economic growth, but economic growth over the last four decades has not solved the social security conundrum. Perhaps the need is to include more members of society in that economic prosperity. Ultimately, Lazar & Stoyko (1998) submitted that the effectiveness of the welfare state must be judged not by how generously it protects against adversity, but by the extent to which it helps individuals to achieve the greater goals of self-sufficiency and self-determination.

Workers' Compensation

[Adapted and expanded with permission from Waddell G (1998), which provides a more comprehensive review of the biopsychosocial model of LBP and disability.]

Before going any further, it is important to stress that true malingering, or the complete fabrication of symptoms that do not exist, is rare. Most workers have entirely 'genuine' physical pain, although reasonable people may reasonably disagree about the degree of recovery, the appropriate duration of sickness absence, and the level of (in)capacity for work.

Few issues around back pain have given rise to more controversy than the question of compensation and secondary gain. *Secondary gain* is a vague term which suggests the person is somehow rewarded economically, physically or emotionally as, a result of their injury or illness (Fishbain 1994, Fishbain *et al* 1995).

All illness involves some secondary gains. Illness may provide a reason for avoiding different kinds of activities and entitle the person to various forms of social support. For some people, it may provide an emotional crutch to deal with life's problems. Some people simply do not have the emotional and social resources to deal with life, particularly in times of adversity. Some people are passive and dependent, and health professionals offer a ready source of support. There is another group of people who have always coped remarkably well, but when illness does strike they never manage to return to their previous hyperactive state. They then have difficulty adjusting and 'never seem to get over it'. This does not mean that any of these people consciously contrive their situation. They are not malingering. They have genuine symptoms. It is just that they are unable to cope with them well and may continue to varying degrees in the sick role.

Too often, however, discussions about secondary gain focus on money and imply malingering. Any perceived gain such as disability payments then casts suspicion on the legitimacy of the patient's symptoms. If treatment fails, secondary gain makes a good excuse. This is all a very circular argument, which may say more about the bias of the observer than the motivation of the patient. No one raises questions of secondary gain about the disabled patient with a stroke.

These discussions also forget that secondary gains are usually balanced by secondary losses (Fishbain 1994). Money is only one part of the secondary gains and losses of stopping work and going sick, and not necessarily the most important. Loss of all the other social benefits of working, loss of financial and social status, and the major change from a working role to a sick role are probably all more important. For most patients they greatly outweigh any emotional gains. Even if the argument is confined to money, the value of compensation should not be over-estimated. Danson (1993) showed that the mean wage-replacement rate for temporary total disability under US Workers' Compensation ranged from 63.9% in 1960 to 67.9% in 1985. Nagi & Hadley (1972) showed that 82% of disabled people in the US were worse off financially than when they were working, 17% had little change, and only 1.5% were better off. This has not changed. In a personal series, only 5% of our patients with back pain were financially better off sick than working, and these few were generally part-time or very poorly paid workers whose wages were so low that they gave little financial incentive to work in the first place. Looking at their whole social situation, the vast majority of people off work with back pain are much worse off in many ways. Social security or Workers' Compensation benefits are a very inadequate replacement.

Against this background, however, financial gain is unquestionably a major motivating force in a material society. Everyone responds to financial incentives and disincentives. Indeed, it should be recognised that many health professionals and social security employees make much greater secondary gains from back pain than any patient ever did.

Compensation must be assessed in the context of injury, of work-related injury or disability, of Workers' Compensation and of disability pensions.

Turk & Okifuji (1996) showed that the injury event may have a lasting psychological effect. They compared traumatic and non-traumatic onset of chronic pain in patients attending a specialised pain centre: 29% had LBP, 21% leg pain and 22% pain at multiple sites. Those receiving any form of financial compensation had similar physical findings but reported more severe pain, more emotional distress, greater disability and greater life interference than those not receiving compensation. However, separate analysis of patients not receiving any compensation showed that those who attributed their pain to a specific trauma also reported more severe pain, more emotional distress and greater life interference. It is possible that 'injury' may have lasting effect, with altered perceptions about work, fear of (re-)injury, fear-avoidance beliefs and different coping strategies, and act as an obstacle to return to work (Waddell 1998, Main & Spanswick 2000).

Several studies show that injuries which occur at work lead to significantly longer work loss than comparable non-work injuries. Sander & Meyers (1986) studied US railroad workers who lost time from work and returned to work with restrictions after a back injury. They found that the average time off work after a work injury was 14.2 months compared with 4.9 months for a comparable non-work injury. The pattern was the same for those who had a lumbosacral sprain/strain and for those who had back surgery, even if different in magnitude. Leavitt (1990) studied patients from US orthopaedic office practices and compared 1373 who had a back injury sustained at work with 417 who had a non-work injury: 23.7% of those injured at work were off longer than 12 months compared with 13.2% of those with a non-work injury. However, work-related injury is not quite the same thing as receipt of Workers' Compensation.

Most of the evidence about the impact of compensation is based on studies of modern Workers' Compensation systems in the US and to a lesser extent in Canada and Australia. As background, Elgie (1995) and Sullivan (2000) reviewed the history of Workers' Compensation systems in Canada. The Meredith Commission in Ontario laid out the key principles of workers' compensation, in line with the German social insurance model and the emerging Workers' Compensation system in the US:

- Compensation based on work-relatedness rather than fault
- Earnings-related benefits for as long as disability lasts
- In lieu of damages under common law tort
- Fairness.

The first Workers' Compensation Board (WCB) in Ontario in 1915 provided compensation for wage loss, but made no allowance for non-economic loss. At an early stage, this was considered to be unfair, and additional allowance was soon made for permanent partial disability even if the worker was still able to work. With or without specific legislation, and partly for administrative convenience to prevent litigation, almost all WCBs moved to making permanent partial disability awards based on tables of permanent impairment. From then to the late 1960s, Workers' Compensation systems were 'fine-tuned' and benefit levels rose to about 75% gross wage replacement. In the mid 1960s the definition of an accident was extended to ensure entitlement to compensation even when there was no obvious chance event. Workers' Compensation was also extended to cover conditions which developed over time even if there had been no accident, provided it could be proved that they were 'work-related'. Between the 1970s and early 1990s, most WCBs provided an earnings loss system, usually providing 90% net wage replacement, with an additional award for permanent impairment. Several WCBs also introduced legislation which provided a time-limited right to return to work so long as the injured worker was able to perform the essential duties of the job or was able to perform some other suitable work. Injured workers are most likely to return successfully to their original work, and this legislation supported the worker's attachment to his or her work place and the employer's obligation to his workers. Different appeal structures were developed, usually independent of the main WCB. The structure of the WCBs also changed, and most now have an independent Board of Directors representing workers, employers and the public.

Margoshes & Webster (1999) reviewed studies which showed unanimously that medical costs are higher in Workers' Compensation than in non-compensation systems and concluded the cost differences were due to service utilisation rather than price discrimination.

Miller (1976) was one of the first to calculate that benefits of more than about 50–55% of wages were associated with an increase in the days of disability claimed by insured persons, and his report to the US House of Representatives, Committee on Ways and Means, is still quoted. There have been many such studies since this time, reviewed and analysed by Loeser et al (1995). The evidence is not entirely consistent, and not all studies show any effect. However, their best available literature synthesis suggested that a 10% increase in Workers' Compensation benefits is associated with a 1–11% increase in the number of claims and a 2–11% increase in the average duration of claims. This is an average increase of 2–5 days off work with back pain. These findings are similar for 'verifiable' injuries like fractures as well as more subjective, soft tissue injuries. Gardner (1989) made a comparable, earlier review for the Workers' Compensation Research Institute, which included over 100 studies on the impact of incentives on claims and return to work.

Kreuger (1990) analysed US Population Survey data on Workers' Compensation. He found that a 10% increase in benefits was associated with about a 7% increase in claim rate. The waiting period to qualify for claims (at that time 7 days or less in all states) had a substantial negative relationship to the claim rate. Time-series analysis showed that the growth in claims during the 1970s corresponded reasonably well to the growth in real benefits over this period.

Ruser (1993) analysed a longitudinal data set from 2798 manufacturing establishments. He found that increased Workers' Compensation benefits were associated with increased frequency of most non-fatal injury claims, although there was no change in the frequency of fatal injuries. Higher benefits were also more likely to be associated with any time off work after an injury.

Galizzi & Boden (1996) studied 118,965 workers in Wisconsin who lost time off work in 1989–1990 and followed them until 1994. A 10% decrease in benefits was associated with 0.8 days shorter absence from work. For those off work for more than a month, the incentive effect of return to a better paid job appeared stronger than the effects of lower benefits.

Baldwin et al (1996) analysed first return to work and subsequent work loss in 8690 WCB patients in Ontario, Canada. All else being equal, a higher wage-replacement rate was associated with longer first absence in women but not in men. However, the chances of successfully returning to work, subsequent absences and eventually giving up work were all unrelated to the wage-replacement rate in both men and women.

Meyer et al (1995) reported a natural experiment when two states increased the maximum weekly benefit under Workers' Compensation by approximately 50%. Effectively, benefits were only increased for high-earning workers but there was no change in benefits for low-earning workers. For all injuries, duration of work loss increased for those eligible for the higher benefits but remained unchanged for those whose benefits did not change. For back pain, one of the states showed a highly significant change, but the other showed no change.

Hadler et al (1995) made one of the most detailed comparisons of 505 Workers' Compensation patients and 861 non-compensation workers who sought health care for an acute episode of LBP. The compensation patients described their jobs as physically more demanding and were more likely to have taken time off work in the month before seeking health care. The compensation patients had slower subjective recovery, but there was no significant difference in recovery of function or return to work. This delay was independent of the severity of their back pain, perception of job demand, or type of health care.

Several studies have looked at the nature rather than the amount of compensation payments.

Carron et al (1985) compared patients at multidisciplinary pain clinics in the US and New Zealand and commented on the different compensation systems in these two countries. However, the highly selected nature of the patients and different local referral patterns makes it impossible to draw any general conclusions.

Jamison et al (1988a,b) in Tennessee looked at patients with chronic LBP attending a pain control centre, and compared those receiving time-limited Workers' Compensation and unlimited disability payments. Time-limited payments were generally received during the initial period that a patient was receiving medical treatment following an accident. Once maximum medical outcome was achieved, there was settlement and no further benefits were given. Unlimited compensation was regular financial disability benefits for an indefinite period until the worker returned to work. This study showed that patients with unlimited compensation took more analgesics, showed more pain behaviour and physician-rated symptom dramatisation, and were less likely to return to work. However, these were two completely different groups of patients: those on unlimited benefits were older and had been off work 18 months longer. The two groups of patients were not comparable and it is not possible to draw any conclusions about the effect of the two types of payment.

There is very little evidence on the effect of lump-sum settlements. Lump-sum awards for partial permanent disability are an actuarial manoeuvre that makes two assumptions (Hadler 1986):

- The potential of a lump-sum payment will not alter illness behaviour or the course of the illness
- The potential of a lump-sum payment will not alter the claim rate.

Both these assumptions may not be true. There is conflicting evidence on whether the possibility of a lump-sum payment may encourage claims. Alternatively, the payment of a lump sum and then stopping further benefits may encourage return to work, although this assumes that there are no alternative benefits then available and that there is no appeal. All of these possible effects may vary with the size of the lump-sum payment (compare Japan, Australian and US Workers' Compensation, and civil litigation).

Greenough & Fraser (1989) looked at lump-sum settlements under the South Australian Workers' Compensation scheme. This study had major strengths and major weaknesses. The strengths were careful control for clinical factors and injury severity, and 96% follow-up at 4 years. However, the weaknesses were that this was a selected group of patients referred to a single surgeon's practice, the authors did not allow for any of the other work-related factors that might influence return to work (see below), or perform any kind of multivariate analysis. On univariate analysis they found that in men, only 49% of compensation patients returned to work compared with 89% of non-compensation patients. For women the corresponding figures were 54 and 93%. More importantly to the present discussion, they looked at the effect of lump-sum payments, wherein liability for any one incident could be commuted either at the initiation of the worker or indirectly by the insurance company. They found that a much lower proportion of Workers' Compensation patients who received lump-sum payments returned to work (men 35%, women 46%) than those who received continued, regular payments (men 85%, women 80%). However, they again did not make any allowance for other work- or injury-related factors that might influence return to work. The authors also pointed out that those on regular payments were a different group of patients, with a higher incidence of previous claims, dispute concerning their injury, and disputed claims that had been stopped unilaterally by the insurance company. These all imply differences in the nature of the claim, the disability and/or the worker. Any conclusions from this particular Australian Workers' Compensation situation cannot be extrapolated more generally.

Wood et al (1993) made one of the most detailed mathematical analyses of the method of settlement of 8232 Workers' Compensation claims in Western Australia, and found that lump-sum settlement was associated with substantially higher costs. In particular, lump-sum settlement of a common law action was associated with a 4-fold increase in costs. Various forms of lump-sum settlement of the Workers' Compensation claim were also associated with increased costs, although not to the same degree. However, eligibility for lump-sum settlement depended on the type of injury, recurrent history and the nature of the claim. Once again, it is not possible to separate the effect of the method of payment from these associated factors, or to extrapolate this from the particular Australian Workers' Compensation situation. (This study covered all injuries and not only back injuries.)

Thornton (1998) speculated that lump-sum payments might be used to finance job search activities but conversely might support exit from the labour market. In the New Zealand Accident Corporation system, lump-sum payments for pain and suffering have now been abolished and replaced by an Independent Living Allowance to assist with the additional costs of disability.

Thomason (1993) analysed the transition from temporary to permanent disability under the Workers' Compensation system in New York State. He suggested that claimants exercise some discretion in the pursuit of a permanent disability claim. He found that the higher the financial benefits of permanent disability status and the lower the uncertainty of achieving it, the more likely claimants were to pursue and achieve permanent disability status.

Worrall et al (1993) also made a highly·mathematical analysis of the transition from temporary to permanent disability under the Workers' Compensation system in Massachusetts and Illinois. They again found that the structure of benefits and increase in financial benefits could be associated with a sizeable increase in permanent disability claims.

Clinical studies of Workers' Compensation in the literature show a striking dichotomy. At one extreme, some pain clinic studies and experts say that there is no clinical difference between compensation and non-compensation patients. At the other extreme, some medico-legal experts, who are mainly orthopaedic surgeons, imply that many of the claimants they see are little short of frank malingerers. The difference seems to be a combination of case selection and observer bias, in both directions.

Rohling et al (1995) made the most careful review of this literature, although they cautioned that most studies were in pain clinic settings and the results may not apply to more routine compensation patients. They found 32 studies that gave usable data on 3802 compensated and 3849 non-compensated patients. Compensation patients consistently reported more pain, although the difference was quite small—about 6%. Rohling et al (1995) and another review by Walsh & Dumitru (1988) concluded that compensation does seem to be associated with delayed clinical recovery: the outcomes of conservative treatment, back surgery and chronic pain rehabilitation programmes are consistently poorer in compensation patients. However, there is conflicting evidence on the magnitude of this effect, with estimates ranging from 0 to 30%. Tito (2000) also pointed out there is no evidence whether compensation delays return to work or the lack of compensation pressures patients into returning to work, or which of these is medically ideal. Many studies show that there is little difference in the physical findings and levels of distress in compensation patients. Some studies suggest that compensation patients are more depressed. To put this all in context, 75–90% of compensation patients do respond well to health care, and do recover and return to work rapidly. It is only a small proportion of cases who go on to long-term disability and high costs.

Most of these findings are based on retrospective studies and cross-sectional analysis, but they are confirmed by several recent, prospective, longitudinal studies. Atlas et al (2000) looked at long-term disability and return to work among patients with sciatica, who generally had a clearly defined physical pathology. Those receiving Workers' Compensation at baseline were more likely to be younger, male, less educated, smokers and in physically-demanding jobs. On multivariate analysis, Workers' Compensation status was an independent predictor of less improvement in symptoms, quality of life and functional status, and of still receiving disability benefits at 4-year follow-up (27% compared with 7%; OR 3.5 95% $p = <0.001$). Nonetheless, most patients returned to work regardless of their initial disability status. Patients receiving Workers' Compensation at baseline were only slightly less likely to be working at 4-year follow-up (80% compared with 87%), and on multivariate analysis this difference was not significant.

Taylor et al (2000) examined a wide range of socio-demographic, clinical and biomedical factors in a prospective cohort study of 281 patients in Washington State undergoing surgery for degenerative back problems. On multivariate analysis, compensation status was significantly predictive of very bothersome LBP, very restricted physical activity and less improvement in quality of life at 1-year follow-up. (Other predictors of poorer outcomes included older age, previous low back surgery and litigation.)

Rainville et al (1997) made a prospective study of patients with chronic LBP referred to a spinal rehabilitation centre. Patients with any form of financial compensation (Workers' Compensation, social security, private disability benefits or personal injury litigation) were again younger, less educated and did heavier labour. They reported more pain, depression and disability, even after controlling for baseline differences. Compensation status did not influence compliance with the rehabilitation programme. After completing the programme, physical improvements were similar in compensation and non-compensation patients. Both groups showed improvement in depression and disability, but this was significantly less in the compensation patients. At 12-month follow-up, the non-compensation patients had improved pain scores but the compensation patients reported no improvement. The authors suggested that compensation had little or no impact on physical outcomes of rehabilitation but did influence self-reported complaints.

The above findings are not unique to back pain. Binder & Rohling (1996) showed a similar effect in mild head injury. Their meta-analysis of 17 studies with 2353 patients showed that patients with financial incentives reported more symptoms and disability, with a moderate effect size of 0.47.

Economists often play down the role of health care and psychosocial factors in their studies, just as health-care providers often overlook economic and administrative issues. Yet disability, health care and compensation are closely linked. There are no hard data on the influence of health care and its providers on the submission and duration of claims, although clinical decisions certainly have a major impact on health-care costs, and compensation duration and costs. However, this relationship works both ways. Gardner & Butler (1996) extended their analysis of 'moral hazard' to show the impact of Workers' Compensation on health care. Simmonds & Kumar (1996) made an experimental study of 69 physical therapists who each viewed three videotaped assessments of patients with LBP. Knowledge of the patients' Workers' Compensation status did not influence their assessment of the physical findings but did influence their judgement of prognosis, which might bias their approach to the patient and clinical management. Taylor et al (1996) suggested and the findings of Atlas et al (2000) also appear to show that compensation status may even influence patients' and professionals' decisions about back surgery. Before passing moral judgement on how compensation incentives influence workers, consideration should also be given to how they influence employers, health professionals and lawyers.

It is also too easy to assume that this is all a direct effect of compensation, but this does not allow for other differences in these patients. Leavitt (1992) pointed out that Workers' Compensation patients are a very different occupational, economic and social group. They usually have heavier physical jobs, and are generally younger, male, less educated, of lower social class, and often include more immigrants. As noted above, they differ in the traumatic onset of symptoms, the fact that this is work-related, and in their patterns of referral and clinical management. These differences may have more direct and much greater impact on their clinical progress and return to work than compensation itself. However, there is conflicting evidence from multivariate analyses. Dworkin et al (1985) found that employment status was most strongly related to pre-injury employment status and the outcome of pain management, and compensation or litigation did not add anything. Leavitt (1992) showed the importance of job demands, but found that work-related injury and compensation was associated with more prolonged disability, even after allowing for job demands. Sanderson et al (1995) found that both unemployment and compensation were related to disability, but employment status was most important. Non-compensation and compensation patients who became unemployed because of their injuries showed similar outcomes. Rainville et al (1997) found that compensation patients reported more pain, depression and disability and had poorer clinical outcomes, even after controlling for baseline differences. Atlas et al (2000) found that after allowing for other influences, compensation status still predicted subjective outcomes but no longer had a significant effect on return to work.

Most Workers' Compensation studies report that the average duration of back injury claims is longer than non-back injury claims. However, Galizzi & Boden (1996) suggested there were actually two rather different types of back injuries. Those with minor back injuries did relatively well: looking at workers who returned to work within 1 month, they found that those with back injuries actually returned faster than those with non-back injuries. However, those with more severe injuries did relatively badly: looking at longer duration claims, they found that workers with back injuries returned more slowly than those with non-back injuries. Nagi & Hadley (1972) hypothesised that in patients with more severe physical injuries, social factors were less important, but in those with less severe injuries, higher education, higher income, greater loss of income and more dependents seemed to be associated with higher motivation to return to work. This is supported by some of the studies quoted above. Burns et al (1995) also provided empirical evidence to support this. Workers' Compensation patients with no previous back surgery and low levels of pain responded as well to a multidisciplinary pain programme as non-compensation patients. It was the sub-group of Workers' Compensation patients with previous surgery and high pain levels who had poor results. They also suggested that moderating and mediating factors are more important than compensation itself.

Overall, the level of compensation is probably a very small factor in the decision to stop work, and only one factor in maintaining the sick role (Table 1.18). As already noted, there have been great changes in attitudes to work and disability and compensation over recent decades. There is rapid change in conditions of employment, with much more unemployment, job insecurity and job turn-over. The average job tenure in the US is now <3 years. This has inevitably changed attitudes to work, employers and unemployment. These changes are all probably much more important than the level of compensation.

TABLE 1.18 Socio-economic issues around Workers' Compensation

- Work demands
- Work environment
- Availability of modified work
- Income
- Job security
- Advancement/career potential
- Pension
- Natural job attrition
- Job availability
- Compensation

Tito (2000) pointed out this is all a very 'professional' perspective on Workers' Compensation. The 'system' is concerned mainly with the small proportion of people who go on to long-term disability and high costs, but most injured workers either do not lose any time off work or return to work rapidly. Compensation statistics and financial data tell one story that is important to policy makers and society, but they fail to acknowledge the personal experiences of the injured worker and his or her family. When a previously healthy worker is suddenly injured or disabled, and especially if they do not recover rapidly and get back to work, they may find themselves in a very strange, frightening and difficult situation. Tito painted a graphic picture of confusion and alarm, of disempowerment, of anger and frustration; of health-care systems which often do not deliver best practice care; of administrative systems which give injured people mixed messages; and of compensation arrangements which create systematic barriers to early recovery. The lack of expected correlation between apparently relatively minor (often musculoskeletal) injury and duration of time off may lead to suspicion and mistrust. The 'system' explicitly or implicitly questions the injured worker's veracity or motivation, who in turn adopts defensive behaviours. But most injured workers want to work and only a small minority deliberately abuse the system. Strategies are too often designed to discourage or punish the injured worker, but these are ineffective and may be counter-productive. 'The interface between health care and compensation is intimate and complex: a marriage of convenience out of different cultures, with all the conflict, tension and interest that this can create.' There is a lack of hard data and of real understanding about which elements in compensation, administrative, benefit or funding arrangements contribute to positive health outcomes. 'A crucial challenge for health professionals and compensation administrators is how to minimise the additional disabling impact of compensation processes themselves, so that all injured people have to deal with is the original injury.'

Conclusion

Most of this evidence is on Workers' Compensation in the US, and to a lesser extent Canada and Australia, and may not apply equally to other sickness benefit systems.

There is very little data on gender issues and most of these Workers' Compensation studies are largely of male workers.

There is no evidence that Workers' Compensation causes back pain or changes the condition of anyone's back. There is little doubt that Workers' Compensation does affect what individuals do when they have back pain, but it does not cause the pain or create the situation these patients are in. It is only one, and probably one of the less powerful, social influences on whether they get into this situation and what they do to get out of it. The best available literature synthesis suggests that a 10% increase in Workers' Compensation benefits is associated with a 1–11% increase in the number of claims and a 2–11% increase in the average duration of claims. There is insufficient evidence to draw any conclusions about the type of benefit payments, and in particular about regular payments or lump-sum settlements. Compensation patients consistently report more pain, although the difference is quite small—about 6%. Most studies show that there is very little difference in the physical findings and levels of distress in compensation patients. The outcomes of conservative treatment, back surgery and chronic pain rehabilitation programmes are consistently poorer in compensation patients, but there is conflicting evidence on the magnitude of this effect, with estimates ranging from 0 to 30%. All of this evidence deals with statistical associations in groups of patients, which is quite different from attributing motives or judging the individual patient. To put it in context, 75–90% of compensation patients do respond well to health care, and do recover and return to work rapidly, while secondary losses usually greatly outweigh secondary gains (Table 1.19).

TABLE 1.19 Relationship of Workers' Compensation to low back pain and disability

Relationship of compensation level to claims:
- There is no evidence that Workers' Compensation changes the actual injury rate
- A 10% increase in compensation level is associated with a 1–11% increase in claims rate
- A 10% increase in compensation level is associated with a 2–11% increase in duration of disability
- This affects 'verifiable' injuries like fractures as much as more subjective, soft-tissue injuries

Relationship of Workers' Compensation to surgical outcome:
- Workers' Compensation patients are less likely to have a good result from back surgery
- These findings have been criticised because: these men often have heavier physical jobs, and they may get over-aggressive surgical intervention
- Despite this, >75% of Workers' Compensation patients do return to their previous work after primary surgery for a well-defined disc prolapse

Relationship of Workers' Compensation to rehabilitation outcome:
- Workers' Compensation patients respond less well to pain management and rehabilitation
- These findings have been criticised because: there are methodological flaws in many of these studies—they are often small samples of highly selected patients with poor diagnostic criteria, follow-up is poor, and there is failure to allow for other factors such as job demands; differences are small
- Despite this, many Workers' Compensation patients do benefit

It is also too easy to assume that this is all a direct effect of compensation, but this does not allow for other differences in these patients. Workers' Compensation patients usually have heavier physical jobs, and are generally younger, male, less educated, of lower social class, and include more immigrants. They form a very different occupational, economic and social group and their selection and referral patterns are quite different. These differences may have more direct and much greater relationship to their clinical progress and return to work than compensation itself.

The following reviews are suggested as a starting point for more detailed reading of differing views about compensation: Brena & Chapman (1984), Mendelson (1988, 1992), Weighill & Buglass (1989), Fishbain (1994), Fishbain et al (1995), Butler et al (1996), Boden (1996), Loeser & Sullivan (1997), Bellamy (1997).

2 Comparison of sickness and disability arrangements in various countries

Table 2.1 lists the countries included in this review.

TABLE 2.1 Countries reviewed

UK
Ireland
Sweden
Norway
Finland
Denmark
The Netherlands
Belgium
France
Germany
US
Australia
New Zealand

Social security benefits

Social security now provides various forms of benefits for those who are unable to work because of injury or illness. In general, sick pay and sickness benefits aim to provide replacement income for those who are temporarily unable to work because of sickness. This is basically short term, in expectation of recovery and return to work. Long-term or permanent incapacity is covered by invalidity benefits, which may alternatively be regarded as a form of disability pension for those who have not reached pension age. Most countries also make special arrangements for sickness due to work-related injury or occupational disease. In the UK, all Department of Social Services (DSS) sickness and invalidity benefits are now combined in *Incapacity Benefit* (IB). Statutory Sick Pay (SSP) is provided by the employer, while various levels of IB provide short-term cover for sickness for those who are not eligible for SSP and longer-term cover for invalidity after SSP finishes.

The Social Security Administration (SSA 1999) characterised the structure of social security programmes in the countries being reviewed (Table 2.2).

The sickness and disability benefit systems in different countries developed from different cultural and historical traditions, and also different welfare goals, which is reflected in the rules of eligibility and entitlement. In some countries the focus is social security for all

TABLE 2.2 Types of social security programmes

Country	Type of social security programme
UK	Dual social insurance and social assistance (means-tested) system
Ireland	Dual social insurance and social assistance (means-tested) system
Sweden	Dual universal and social insurance systems (old system)
	Unified social insurance plus mandatory private accounts (new system from 1999)
Norway	Dual universal and social insurance systems
Finland	Universal pension programme and statutory earnings-related pension programme
Denmark	Dual universal and social insurance systems
The Netherlands	Social insurance system
Belgium	Social insurance system
France	Social insurance system and mandatory supplementary pension systems
Germany	Social insurance system
US	Social insurance system
Australia	Dual social security (means tested) and mandatory occupational pension (earnings based)
New Zealand	Dual universal and social assistance systems
Japan	Social insurance system

From SSA (1999).

citizens, while in others it is more income replacement for employees. There are also marked differences in the ease or difficulty of getting benefits. Claimants do not need to meet any prior conditions for entitlement to benefits in Finland and the Netherlands, while most other countries require a minimum period of work and/or contributions. The requirements for medical certification of sickness vary greatly, from none in the Netherlands, to strict medical certification from the first day in Belgium. The UK and Sweden take an intermediate position, with self-certification up to 7 days, and medical certification required thereafter. There are no waiting days before starting benefits in Denmark and Germany, employers in the Netherlands have the option of applying up to 2 days, most countries have 1–3 days, while Finland has 9 days, although in some countries these waiting days may then be paid retrospectively.

Tables 2.2–2.5 provide more detailed comparisons of the main characteristics of the social security benefits for sickness, disability and work-related injury in the EU countries being reviewed, although it should be remembered that these descriptions are only of the basic social insurance arrangements.

Sickness benefits

Tables 2.3 and 2.4 show the basic sickness benefit arrangements in various European countries.

Invalidity and long-term incapacity benefits

Table 2.5 shows the arrangements for longer-term and incapacity invalidity benefits in various European countries. In almost every country the method of calculating the various possible

TABLE 2.3   Sickness benefit arrangements in European countries on 1 January 2000

	Eligible	Qualifying conditions	Sick certification	Waiting period
UK	Employees: Statutory Sick Pay Various other groups: Incapacity Benefit Others: lower Disability Living Allowances	Sufficient contributions (approx. 2 years)	Self-certificate first 7 days, then family doctor certificate	3 days
Ireland	Employees aged over 16	39 weeks contributions	Family doctor's certificate from start	3 days
Sweden	Employees and self-employed aged over 16 Unemployed also eligible	No work period, but minimum income level (ECU 614 per year)	Self-certificate first 7 days, then (family) doctor certificate	1 day
Norway	Employees and self-employed aged over 16 Unemployed also eligible	14 days of employment or self-employment	Self-certificate first 3 days, then family doctor certificate	None
Finland	All residents aged 15–64 Unemployed also eligible	Residence in country No work period	Doctor's certificate from day 1	9 days
Denmark	Employees and self-employed Unemployed also eligible	Worked 120 hours in 13 weeks	Medical certification from 4th day	None
The Netherlands	All persons aged <65 in paid employment	Membership in approved sickness fund No work period	No medical certification Notify insurance officer	None
Belgium	All workers with contract Voluntary affiliation for unemployed	6 months employment and contributions	Notify sickness fund doctor within 2 days	1 day (none if unemployed)
France	All residents	Sufficient contributions (approx. 6 months work)	Doctor's certificate	3 days
Germany	All persons in paid employment Unemployed also eligible	Membership in sickness fund No work period	Doctor's certificate	None[1]

[1] No waiting period in Germany if due to work injury or disease or if hospital treatment required.
From MISSOC (2000); see also SSA (1999).

TABLE 2.4   Benefits paid in European countries on 1 January 2000

	Amount of benefits (January 1 2000)	Duration	Benefits taxed
UK	Statutory Sick Pay: basic ECU95 per week Incapacity Benefit: basic ECU81 and 95 per week Estimated median 80–90% of earnings Complex ceiling approx. ECU500 per week	Statutory Sick Pay for 4 days to 28 weeks Short-term Incapacity Benefit for further 52 weeks	Most liable
Ireland	ECU 95 per week Allowances for dependents	Unlimited (if worked 5 years)	Fully liable
Sweden	80% of earnings Ceiling ECU500 per week	No formal limit (but converted to disability pension 'if the illness continues for an extended period of time')	Fully liable
Norway	100% of covered earnings Self-employed and temporarily employed: 65% of assessed earnings after 14-day waiting period Ceiling ECU700 per week	52 weeks Then disability pension or rehabilitation allowance	Fully liable
Finland	Complex formula on earnings: Approx. 70% of earnings Ceiling ECU730 per week	50 weeks in 2 years for same illness	Fully liable
Denmark	100% of basic hourly earnings Ceiling ECU357 per week Unemployed = previous benefits	52 weeks in 18 months	Fully liable
The Netherlands	70% of daily wage Ceiling ECU725 per week	1 year	Generally fully liable to tax
Belgium	60% of earnings Ceiling ECU470 per week	1 year	Fully liable
France	50% of earnings Ceiling ECU185 per week	1 year but 3 years for 'protracted sickness'	80–90% of benefits taxable
Germany	70% of normal earnings, but not exceeding 90% of net earnings	78 weeks over 3 years After 1 year adjusted as pension	Tax free

From MISSOC (2000).

elements of benefits paid is so complex that it is not possible to provide any typical estimate of the amount of benefit paid, what wage replacement level this represents or any ceiling.

The practical arrangements for invalidity benefit vary greatly between countries. For example, either the employee or the employer may need to apply, or the change from sickness to invalidity benefit may be made automatically by the social security agency. Different countries

TABLE 2.5   Invalidity and long-term incapacity benefit arrangements in European countries on 1 January 2000

	Minimum level of incapacity	Start	Initiate claim	Degrees of invalidity	Duration
UK	'Incapable of all work'[1]	After 52 weeks incapacity	Employer	1	Men: to age 65 Women: 60
Ireland	'Incapable of all work'	After 1 year of sickness benefits	DSS/claimant	1	To death; no upper age limit
Sweden	25%	When fulfil conditions	Claimant	4	To age 66
Norway	50%	When fulfil conditions	Claimant	2	To age 65
Finland	Disability pension 60% Partial disability pension 40% Early retirement age 58+[2]	After 1 year of sickness benefits	DSS	3	To age 65
Denmark	50%	When accept permanent incapacity	Claimant	3	To age 67
The Netherlands	15 or 25%	After 1 year of sickness benefits	Claimant	7	To age 65
Belgium	66.7%	After 1 year of sickness benefits	Employer	2	Male age 65 Female 61
France	66.7%	After 3 years of sickness benefits or when fulfil conditions	DSS	3	To age 60
Germany	Occupational 50% General 100%	When fulfil conditions	Employer	1	To age 65

[1] Operationalised as a relatively modest score on the *All Work Test* (see p 154). No real % equivalent
[2] Early retirement age 58+ in Finland if: 'incapable of continuing present employment because of work-related stress and fatigue and other factors'. No %
From MISSOC (2000), Prins *et al* (1998), SSA (1999).

set different minimum levels of disability or loss of earning capacity, e.g. the Netherlands accepts 15% and Sweden 25% partial disability, most countries set the level at 50–67%, while the UK requires 'incapacity for all work'. The type of pension also differs in the extent to which it is earnings related or flat rate, e.g. earnings related in the Netherlands, Belgium and Germany, flat-rate in the UK, and mixed in Sweden and Denmark. Every country except Germany applies an earnings ceiling to entitlement, although the level can vary greatly. As a whole, the arrangements in Germany, Belgium and the Netherlands are generally regarded as the most favourable.

In the UK, the Netherlands, Belgium and Finland, sickness benefits and invalidity benefits are linked. Once claimants reach the end of their entitlement to SSP or sickness benefits, they more or less automatically receive long-term Invalidity Benefit (IVB) (or in the UK move between the various levels of IB). In other countries invalidity pensions are quite separate, at least in principle. The legislation in Sweden allows sickness benefits to continue indefinitely, and in France for several years. However, claimants in Sweden, Denmark, France and Germany may change to an invalidity pension at any time, as soon as their incapacity is considered to be permanent. Depending on how invalidity benefits are applied in practice, they may be viewed either as extended sick pay, or as a means of exit from the labour force because of permanent disability. At least theoretically, this may determine the emphasis laid upon rehabilitation and attempts at return to work, although in practice under every social security system once someone is on long-term invalidity benefit the chances of return to work are now low.

Industrial injury benefits

Almost all countries, with the exception of the Netherlands since 1967, make special benefit arrangements for work-related, 'industrial' injuries and occupational diseases. As part of the current social reform process, almost all Central and East European countries have passed or are preparing new legislation on accident insurance, against the advice of international agencies such as the World Bank and the International Monetary Fund (IMF). Even in the Netherlands, there is some discussion about re-introducing some arrangement for industrial injuries, at least one reason being that employers feel this might help limit their financial liability (Sokoll 2000). Industrial injury benefits are almost always more generous than the corresponding sickness and invalidity benefits, following the original Prussian paradigm of the 'deserving' worker. They generally have no qualifying conditions apart from being employed, no waiting period, higher benefit levels, no time limit, and various supplementary benefits and allowances. Table 2.6 summarises the arrangements for industrial injury benefits.

Tables 2.4–2.6 only show the basic benefit arrangements and are over-simplified, so they may give a false impression of what people who are incapacitated with back pain actually receive. Most of the apparently generous wage-replacement rates have a ceiling which means that higher paid workers do not receive anything like this level of replacement. Conversely, as in the UK, claimants may be eligible for more than one type of benefit, with differing criteria for entitlement. Certain benefits lead to additional entitlement to various 'top-up' housing, child and other benefits. Nor does this basic description allow for benefits in kind and municipal spending in some countries.

It is also important to emphasise that only the basic state benefit arrangements are shown. Many groups of workers and unions have negotiated more generous terms, both for short-term sickness and disability pension arrangements. In most European countries, most salaried public sector employees such as health-care workers, civil servants, education workers and the police receive relatively generous sickness benefits, usually with no waiting period and with full salary for periods of up to 6 months or more. Permanent invalidity is considered

TABLE 2.6 Benefits for industrial injuries and occupational diseases in different European countries on 1 January 2000

	Temporary incapacity		Permanent incapacity	
	Basic wages continued	Benefit level (% of earnings)	Minimum loss of earning capacity	Pension (% of gross earnings)
UK[1]	No	Flat-rate supplement to other benefits	14% disablement	Flat rate
Ireland	No	Flat rate = sickness benefits	1%	Flat rate
Sweden	No	Sickness benefits	1/15	100% (ceiling ECU31,000 per annum)
Norway		100% of covered earnings	15%	100% of base amount (ECU4700), then reducing %
Finland	No	Sickness benefits for 4 weeks, then 100% of earnings	Working capacity 10% + loss of earnings 5%	Up to 85% 70% after age 65
Denmark	No	Up to 100%	15%	Up to 80% (ceiling ECU33,263 per annum)
The Netherlands	No special arrangements: standard sickness and invalidity benefits			
Belgium	30 days	Up to 90% basic earnings	No minimum	2–100% (ceiling ECU23,671 per annum)
France	No	60% for 28 days then 80%	No minimum	Up to 100% (ceiling ECU113,000 per annum)
Germany	78 weeks	100% basic earnings	20%	Up to 67% (ceiling ECU44,000–73,000 per annum)

[1]In the UK, Industrial Injury Disablement Benefit is paid *in addition to* rather than as an alternative to sickness and invalidity benefits
From MISSOC (1998, 2000), Prins et al (1998), SSA (1999).

as compulsory early retirement and the benefits form part of the employment pension scheme. In Sweden, Denmark and the Netherlands, employees in the public sector have very much the same arrangements as in the private sector. However, in Germany and the UK about 50% of public employees do not have any special cover, and simply fall under the basic state benefit system.

Sick certification, adjudication and appeals procedures

Emanuel (1994) considered methods of controlling the number of people joining and staying on social security programmes and the associated social security costs. One obvious approach is to lower the level of benefits, which directly reduces expenditure and is also likely to lower demand, and the duration of benefits. However, this affects those who are really disabled and unable to work, which limits its social and political acceptability. Another approach is to encourage employers to employ disabled workers, either by incentives to continue to employ or even to take on disabled workers, or disincentives against dismissing existing workers who become disabled. However, there are many loopholes to such an approach and little proof that it is effective. Emanuel (1994) concluded that efforts to improve direct controls were likely to be more productive:

- The definition and operationalisation of criteria for admission to and continuing on benefits
- Efforts to return people to the work force
- Separating the administrators of the benefits system from conflicting interests
- Improving administrative efficiency.

Setting the criteria for admission to benefits is the most fundamental and critical issue in directing benefits to those in 'real' need, who deserve social support from the tax payer. Unfortunately, there has been considerable difficulty in practice trying to agree concepts and definitions of incapacity to work because of sickness and disability, as seen in most social security legislation.

Bloch (1994a,b), from a US perspective, compared the claim-processing and appeals procedures for disability pension in the US, Canada, the UK, Sweden, the Netherlands and Germany in 1992–1993. All countries used similar procedures to make initial disability assessments, although the exact details of the process varied and assessments might be carried out by social security or outside physicians. There was continuing debate on whether an internal administrative review of eligibility decisions was of any value. All countries had at least one level of appeal on factual and legal issues, although the procedure varied. Perhaps surprisingly, there was no clear evidence on how these various systems influenced the number of claims, the process of claims, the numbers of claims accepted, the number of appeals, or the final outcome of appeals.

Rehabilitation and return to work

The US National Academy of Social Insurance (Mashaw & Reno 1996) suggested that the primary goal of national disability policy should be the integration of people with disabilities into American society. All governments support this goal. For example, the UK Government Green Papers (1998a,b) suggested that 'those who are disabled should get the support they need to live a fulfilling life with dignity' by:

- Introducing effective civil rights for disabled people
- Removing barriers to work and giving active help to disabled people who wish to work
- Fundamentally reforming IB for future claimants
- Ensuring the welfare system recognises the extra costs faced by disabled people.

However, there is often some confusion in such discussions. Much of the debate, many of the principles and the common examples are about people with severe, life-time handicaps such as blindness, amputations or confinement to wheelchairs. But these are now a minority of disabled people on social security benefits. Some of the discussion and principles are equally applicable to the rehabilitation and re-integration into society of people with more common forms of sickness and incapacity such as back pain, but in other ways these people present a completely different problem.

Nocon & Baldwin (1998) briefly summarised the rehabilitation literature. Rehabilitation had its roots in several separate developments since World War I, which are still reflected in the continuing debate about its aims and nature. Modern rehabilitation is not a purely medical process but also includes social, psychological and work-related components. Nocon & Baldwin (1998) considered there is an emerging consensus that:

- The primary objective of rehabilitation involves restoration (to the maximum degree possible) either of function (physical or mental) or role (within the family, social network or work force)
- Rehabilitation will usually require a mixture of clinical, therapeutic and social interventions that also address issues relevant to a person's physical *and* social environment
- Effective rehabilitation needs to be responsive to users' needs and wishes, purposeful, involve a number of agencies and disciplines and be available when required.

They pointed out that rehabilitation is often a function of services, not necessarily a service in its own right.

The TUC (2000) also adopted the broadest possible description of rehabilitation to cover 'any method by which people with a condition resulting from sickness or injury which interferes with their ability to work to their normal or full capacity can be returned to work. This can involve medical or other treatment, vocational rehabilitation or retraining, adaptations to the work environment or working patterns'. They emphasised this is not purely a medical matter, that no profession has a monopoly for the provision of good rehabilitation and that a multidisciplinary approach will almost always be useful.

Table 2.7 compares statutory arrangements for rehabilitation in European countries.

Social security and compensation systems may modify the behaviour of sick and disabled workers and of their employers and so influence whether they are likely to retain or leave their job. Statutory or negotiated sick pay can help to maintain the employer–worker relationship, and the costs may provide an incentive to employers to support return to work. In Sweden and the Netherlands, SSP is linked to a statutory obligation on employers to follow up absent workers and plan their return to work. However, once SSP finishes, this may reduce the employer's incentive to do anything further. In Germany, the US, Canada and New Zealand there are separate workers' compensation schemes for those injured at work, which all have a rehabilitation component and provide greater statutory protection of employment. Issues of wage-replacement levels, benefit traps, return to work with partial benefits, the 'all-or-nothing' assessment of work incapacity and the assumption that these benefits are permanent, may all influence the chances of returning to work and of retaining or leaving employment. Sweden, Germany, France and Canada all have arrangements in at least some circumstances to pay additional benefits during rehabilitation.

TABLE 2.7   Statutory arrangements for rehabilitation in European countries as at 1 July 1996[1]

UK	Medical therapy and rehabilitation supplied by the NHS
	Vocational assessment and rehabilitation and supported employment provided through the Department of Employment and Education
	Allowances payable during rehabilitation and retraining
Ireland	Medical therapy and rehabilitation supplied by the health service
	Support in returning to work provided through the Department of Social, Community and Family Affairs
Sweden	Rehabilitation programmes for ages 16–64 provided by local sickness benefit insurance office. Rehabilitation benefits as sickness benefits
	Appliances and aids provided for ages <65 by local health authorities and for >65 by local municipal authorities
Finland	Pension institutions provide rehabilitation services, which have to ensure the applicant's prospects of rehabilitation have been investigated before making a disability pension determination. A rehabilitation allowance is payable for the period of rehabilitation
Denmark	Measures to lessen effect of invalidity: assistance for special medical care, maintenance allowance for vocational rehabilitation, appliances and aids supplied by local authority
The Netherlands	*Law of 11 Dec 1975:* Possibility for the person concerned of measures to maintain, restore or improve his or her capacity for work, such as rehabilitation, training or retraining. Measures may also be taken to improve his or her living conditions
Belgium	Functional and occupational retraining, in accordance with decision of panel of doctors, in specialised establishments
France	Vocational retraining in specialised vocational retraining centres or establishments, subject to psycho-technical examination, with the social security funds contributing to the costs
	Pensions or part of pensions are continued
Germany	Medical benefits and occupational training as well as other measures including transitional benefits

[1]See reviews of individual countries in Chapter 4 for numerous, more recent developments.
From MISSOC (1996).

One of the obstacles to returning to work is uncertainty and apprehension (in both the worker and the employer) about ability to cope, which may be resolved by trial work periods. In Sweden workers may retain sickness benefits during such a trial work period without formal time limit. In Germany, there is an arrangement for gradual return to work or 'step-wise rehabilitation'. Both public and private insurance-based incentives, such as experience rating, are increasingly used to influence employers to retain workers who become sick and disabled.

Rehabilitation and employment support services include a wide range of personal support services to prevent sickness developing into disability, help recover working capacity and support re-adjustment to work. This may include a wide range of public services, but these are often very fragmented and unco-ordinated. In most countries, the main rehabilitation services for workers who are injured or become sick is part of the social insurance system (e.g. Sweden, the Netherlands and Germany) or the workers' or accident compensation system (e.g. the US, Canada, Australia and New Zealand). Thornton et al (1997) and Thornton (1998) compared the arrangements to support and assist disabled people to return to work in various countries and identified three main models:

- The employer is responsible for monitoring sickness absence, planning rehabilitation and providing support in the work place, while the insurance or compensation system purchases external rehabilitation, e.g. the Netherlands and US
- The employer identifies the need for rehabilitation and contacts the insurance or compensation system case-manager who takes responsibility for care planning and service co-ordination, e.g. New Zealand
- The employer notifies sickness absence to the insurance or compensation system which contacts the absent worker to assess the need for (vocational) rehabilitation and provides or co-ordinates services, e.g. Germany.

The balance of advantage to the worker and employer may vary. If the employer has total responsibility and bears the costs, minimising sickness absence costs may take priority over rehabilitation. Rehabilitation efforts may also be decided by the likely cost–benefits, and be directed to younger and more productive workers. Even in highly regulated systems, there may be little monitoring of rehabilitation efforts and sanctions against employers who fail to meet their statutory requirements are rarely applied. In practice, most systems appear to leave at least initial rehabilitation efforts to the health-care system, although in some countries there is also strong occupational health involvement, e.g. the Netherlands. Thornton (1998) pointed out that in every country in practice there are major medical, administrative and even legal obstacles to early interventions designed to promote return to work. Assessment for rehabilitation is still dominated by medical issues and most clinicians' lack of knowledge, awareness or even interest about occupational and rehabilitation issues. There are often long delays of months for assessment. There are limited facilities for rehabilitation. Often, workers have lost their jobs before they actually receive any active rehabilitation. There is often insufficient, fragmented and reduced state financing, multiple providers, and competing philosophies and policy aims.

Thornton (1998) suggested that there is a need for a more coherent and co-ordinated policy towards rehabilitation and return to work, that this should be less medically oriented, and that it is becoming more work-place focused, with public agencies enabling rather than substituting for work-based efforts. There are now many innovative and experimental early intervention schemes, although little conclusive evidence on their effectiveness.

Thornton et al (1997) showed that most countries in their review made some arrangements for partial incapacity and that benefits could be combined to some extent with income, but the scope for this was generally limited and variable and there was little evidence of their impact.

There is also increasing recognition of the need to adjust the work place as far as is reasonable to meet the needs of individuals to enable them to overcome their disabilities. The UK and US now have Disability Discrimination Acts, while the building regulations in

New Zealand demand provision for disabled people. Health and Safety at work regulations may oblige employers to improve working conditions both generally and for disabled people, e.g. Sweden, the Netherlands and the US. Efforts to increase productivity may include improved ergonomics in the work place, e.g. Germany and Canada. Equal employment opportunity legislation may include the disabled; Canada, New Zealand, Sweden and the US were said to provide particularly good technical advice and assistance to businesses for improving the work place.

Ultimately, business cultures, philosophies and strategies about sickness and disability may be most important, although these are not well documented. They inevitably depend to some extent on labour market and economic conditions, and also reflect employer–worker relationships. They may be modified by business incentives, e.g. to control the costs of workers' or accident compensation in the US or New Zealand. Strategic approaches include 'disability management in the work place' and efforts to reduce sickness absenteeism. Disability management is most advanced in North America, where a large enterprise may assume control and responsibility for prevention, monitoring, early intervention and re-integration of injured and disabled workers. The National Institute of Disability Management and Research (2000) released Canada's first *Code of Practice for Disability Management* which was designed to provide a framework within which employers, unions, legislators, insurers and health providers could work together to support return to work for workers with disabilities. The major aim of the Code was to identify and offer guidelines, criteria and benchmarks on the management practices and policies which facilitate work retention and return to work, and lay out the roles and responsibilities of the major participants. The Canadian Code will form part of the basis for current efforts by the International Labour Organisation to develop an international code of practice for disability management. In Europe, however, the greatest emphasis has generally been on monitoring and controlling absence, while other efforts are less common and there is rarely a co-ordinated approach. European research suggests that the best approach to sickness and disability is very similar to good management practice to promote industrial relations.

However fine the statutory requirements and strategies of rehabilitation are in principle, the real question is the level of resources, their co-ordination and the delivery of services to the individual. Aarts et al (1996) compared expenditure on labour market measures for the disabled (Table 2.8).

TABLE 2.8 Public expenditure on labour market measures for the disabled

Country	Vocational rehabilitation (%GDP 1991)	Direct job subsidies (%GDP 1991)
UK	0.01	0.02
Sweden	0.10	0.68
The Netherlands	<0.01	0.64
Germany	0.13	0.09
US	0.05	<0.01

From Aarts et al (1996).

Berkowitz *et al* (1987) and Berkowitz (1990) reviewed rehabilitation arrangements in Sweden, Belgium, the Netherlands, France, Germany and Israel in the late 1980s from a US perspective, while the ISSA Report XII (1995b) compared rehabilitation schemes in Germany, the US, Australia and Israel in 1993–1995. Berkowitz focused on the relationship between the disability benefit systems and rehabilitation programmes, rather than the disability benefits systems themselves, while the ISSA Report XII studied the quality, effectiveness and efficiency of rehabilitation programmes, using an in-depth case-study approach to specific examples.

Berkowitz considered that in some countries, such as Belgium and the US, the benefits system and rehabilitation programme were administratively and in practice quite separate. It was usually left to the health-care system to initiate rehabilitation. In other countries, such as the Netherlands and Israel, rehabilitation specialists were an integral part of the disability assessment team. In these countries, the social security system did not leave the initiative to the individual or the health-care system. Instead, the social security system automatically assessed the rehabilitation potential and needs of all disability benefit claimants and refusal to accept rehabilitation could lead to reduction in benefits.

Sweden had the advantage of one of the first completely integrated benefits systems with readily accessible information and Berkowitz considered it could offer lessons on providing efficient rehabilitation. Rehabilitation resources are finite and require rational planning for the maximum effectiveness and cost-effectiveness. There must be early identification of those in need of rehabilitation and accurate assessment of rehabilitation potential. Sweden had made a particular effort to co-ordinate medical, social, psychological and occupational resources to provide more holistic rehabilitation.

The unique feature of rehabilitation in the Netherlands was that the same agencies organised the entire short-term sickness benefits, long-term disability benefits and rehabilitation systems. Disability assessment personnel were intimately involved in rehabilitation evaluation and re-employment, with a common assessment system in both processes.

In Belgium, rehabilitation services were quite separate from the benefits system, and the latter was not directly concerned with the details of rehabilitation. However, all agencies used a common disability rating system, the *Bareme Officiel Belge des Invalidites*. The worker had to take the initiative in applying for rehabilitation to the National Fund for the Social Resettlement of the Disabled. This Fund co-ordinated the usual range of rehabilitation services to the individual and subsidised rehabilitation providers for capital improvements and maintenance of facilities. A major portion of the subsidies went to collective workshops, although since the mid 1980s there had been increasing effort to integrate disabled workers into normal employment. There had been experiments with special apprenticeship programmes for the disabled, which were provided by private employers under government contract. There were also programmes of limited-duration, wage subsidies to disabled workers, and subsidies to employers to make up for the lower productivity of disabled workers. From the description, however, it appears that much of this discussion about Belgium related to the permanently handicapped, rather than healthy workers who became sick and disabled.

France had a complex arrangement of organisations and arrangements for rehabilitation. A medical consultant to the social security agency and occupational physicians continuously monitored each case and the clinical decision process, and the goal from the outset was to return to work as rapidly as possible. Various sections of the social security agency evaluated working capacity and any residual handicap, and provided vocational training or short-term training programmes with employers. They also provided various forms of protected employment. There was an extensive system of incentives for employers to encourage them to hire disabled persons.

In Germany, rehabilitation programmes were decentralised, and each social insurance agency provided rehabilitation benefits for people entitled to that particular benefit (ISSA 1995b). Berkowitz (1987) and Berkowitz et al (1990) considered the German system to offer many potential innovations. It had a strong, basic philosophy which placed rehabilitation before pension, with an effective system of early identification and prevention of long-term disability leading to permanent pension. Although in principle the individual had voluntarily to request rehabilitation before it could begin, the caring physician had a statutory duty to inform the Social Security Agency after a worker had 6 weeks' sickness absence. The agency then had to decide whether the individual could be expected to recover unaided, if they required continued monitoring, or if they should be referred for rehabilitation. There was a distinction between medical and vocational rehabilitation. In practice, about one-quarter of claimants received 'rehabilitation' without losing time from work, and another 40% received medical rehabilitation within 3 months of sickness absence. There were extensive facilities for vocational training and retraining, usually lasting 6–12 months but sometimes up to 2 years. Germany had a wide range of wage subsidies, job modifications, technical aids, transportation allowances and aids, all designed to help re-integrate the worker into the labour force. ISSA (1995b) found this system managed to re-integrate about 60% of patients with a considerable level of impairment due to paraplegia, cardiac disease or mental illness back into work, although it did not publish any separate data on back pain.

In the US, there is a large 'health industry' of vocational rehabilitation and case-management with an extensive medical literature, even if it may be argued that the scientific evidence for its effectiveness and cost-effectiveness is limited and inconsistent (Waddell & Burton 2000). This is outwith the scope of the present review which focuses specifically on the evidence for vocational rehabilitation and case-management in SSA disability benefit recipients. Rehabilitation is not the responsibility of any one agency or provider, so it depends on the individual's insurance and the nature of their condition or injury, and is fragmented and variable (ISSA 1995b). Most health insurance covers 'medical' rehabilitation but does not make any provision for vocational rehabilitation. In contrast, Workers' Compensation and an increasing number of employer's collective insurance plans for work-related injury or illness do provide for some vocational rehabilitation. The Rehabilitation Services Administration comes under the Department of Education, which is separate from the SSA. The primary responsibility of the state vocational rehabilitation agencies is to identify those who need rehabilitation, but they then usually assign them to public and private service providers who do the actual evaluation and training. Access to vocational rehabilitation is very dependent on referral patterns, on eligibility and on rehabilitation potential. It is therefore not surprising that in 1991–1993 only about 6000 people per annum in the US successfully completed a vocational rehabilitation programme and returned to gainful employment (ISSA 1995b).

Dean & Dolan (1991) reviewed the US Vocational Rehabilitation (VR) Program which was a federal/state partnership providing services to help people with disabilities return to work. However, although the programme spent $1.5 billion per annum, between 1975 and 1985 it declined from 6 to 3.9% of total federal expenditure on people with disabilities. Dean & Dolan (1991) were generally positive, but considered that assessment methods were crude, it was difficult to assess the effectiveness or cost-effectiveness of the programme, and assessment methods needed to be improved.

There is a series of papers from the New Beneficiary Follow-up Survey of disabled workers receiving SSA disability benefits (www.ssa.gov/pub/statistics/nbds/nbs). Hennessey (1996) reported that 12% of those receiving Social Security Disability Insurance (SSDI) benefits returned to work after an average of 3.4 years, but half of them stopped work again for health reasons. Hennessey & Müller (1995) found that male gender, younger age, higher level of education, and the absence of a spouse were associated with higher rates of return to work. Vocational rehabilitation efforts (in the form of physical therapy, vocational training, general education and job placement) seemed to have a positive impact on return to work. However, certain work-incentive provisions in the SSDI programme (particularly trial work periods, extended period of eligibility and extended Medicare cover) could actually function as disincentives to return to work. Schechter (1997) found that most of those who returned to work did so because of financial need and not because of any improvement in their health. They were more likely to be younger and to have higher education levels. The likelihood of return to work was broadly comparable across disabling conditions: there were no published data on musculoskeletal or back conditions, although of those with 'arthritis, rheumatism' 8.5% returned to work. Most of those who did return to work, did so with a different employer, less physical exertion, fewer hours and lower pay than they had in their pre-benefit work. Hennessey (1997) focused on the ability to sustain successful return to work. Those beneficiaries who had physiotherapy were more likely to return to work and less likely to stop work again; those who had general education or vocational training were more likely to return to work but these interventions did not lead to sustained return to work. Once again, the work incentive provisions in the SSDI programme could actually function as disincentives to return to work.

Broader statistics suggest that only about 0.5–3% of US Social Security disability recipients return to work each year (ISSA 1995b). The US General Accounting Office (1996) considered how the SSA Disability Program might be re-designed to encourage more benefit recipients to return to work. It identified a number of fundamental problems including rising numbers of older recipients and those with mental impairments, both of whom had less prospect of returning to work. It considered that about 50% of claimants might be realistic candidates for return to work. It pointed out that there were major difficulties in assessing capacity for work, particularly when it must be 'either/or' total incapacity or fit for work and fails to allow for partial capacity and incapacity. Nevertheless, it considered that weaknesses in the design and implementation of the programme and its focus on disabilities limited its ability to identify and assist potential abilities. Of particular value, they identified a number of disincentives in the current SSA programme which may be of more general relevance:

- The disability determination process encourages work incapacity
- The benefit structure provides disincentive to low-wage work
- Work incentives are ineffective in motivating people to work
- Different programmes provide different benefit protection and work incentives
- The design of work incentives reduces their effectiveness
- Beneficiaries fear losing medical cover
- Beneficiaries who return to work risk losing other federal and state assistance
- Work incentives are poorly implemented in practice
- Beneficiaries are generally unaware of work incentive provisions
- Beneficiaries generally do not understand complex work incentives.

They also identified a number of barriers to vocational rehabilitation (VR) in the disability programmes that may again be of more general relevance:

- Access to VR through SSA is limited
- Restrictive state policies limit VR referrals
- SSA does not routinely monitor the referral process
- SSA beneficiaries are perceived as less attractive VR candidates
- SSA reimbursement is insufficient to motivate state VR agencies
- Beneficiaries are unaware of VR services and are not encouraged to use them
- There is a lack of evidence on the effectiveness of VR services for SSA beneficiaries
- Timing of referrals for VR can limit its effectiveness
- The overall service delivery structure may limit the quality and effectiveness of VR services.

They concluded that weaknesses in the design and implementation of the SSA programmes meant that little was done in practice to identify and help those recipients who might benefit from rehabilitation and assistance to return to work. They recommended that the SSA programmes must place greater priority on return to work. The SSA should design more effective methods of identifying and developing recipients' work capacities. There should be better implementation of existing return to work mechanisms. There was also a need to develop an integrated approach to put this into practice. They cited three specific practices as showing most promise for returning the disabled to work:

- Intervening as soon as possible after a disabling event to promote and facilitate return to work
- Identifying and providing necessary return to work assistance and managing cases to achieve return to work goals
- Structuring cash and health benefits to encourage people with disabilities to return to work.

Sim (1999) examined the General Accounting Office recommendations and particularly their citing of arrangements in Germany, Sweden and the private sector. She pointed to major differences in Germany and Sweden compared with the US. For SSA benefits, disability had to be total and was based on impairment. Both Germany and Sweden allowed for partial disability or incapacity. Germany focused on the social rights of the disabled. Sweden's disability policy had political, economic and social goals of full participation and equality for all citizens, and recognised that disability depended on interaction between the individual and their situation. Both countries had universal health cover independent of employment and much more comprehensive rehabilitation services—Germany spent 2- and Sweden 2.6-fold more on vocational rehabilitation. At that time there were no reliable statistics to compare the effectiveness of vocational rehabilitation in the three countries. There was general agreement in both Germany and Sweden about the importance of the three specific principles proposed by the General Accounting Office, but little evidence for their effectiveness in practice. In conclusion, Sim (1999) cautioned against attempting to 'borrow' practices from other countries without taking full account of the unique economic, social and political differences.

In 1991, the SSA set up Project Network to test case-management to assist SSDI and SSI recipients return to work; Kornfeld & Rupp (2000) summarised the results. Participation was voluntary, but only about 5% of benefit recipients participated and they were generally more 'work ready'. The design was experimental with random allocation to case-management or a control group of routine management. The case-management intervention did not have any significant impact on coming off benefits and returning to work for either SSDI or SSI recipients. For those who did return to work, case-management produced a $200 per annum increase in earnings for the first 2 years after return to work but this effect disappeared by the third year. Overall, Project Network was not cost-effective.

In Australia, most 'medical' rehabilitation is provided by the health-care system, but the Department of Human Services and Health also provides a completely separate Commonwealth Rehabilitation Service (CRS) for tertiary vocational and social rehabilitation after medical treatment is complete (ISSA 1995b). A Disability Reform Package in 1990 set up an administrative mechanism to co-ordinate social security, CRS and Department of Employment, Education and Training services. The CRS has over 160 community-based regional units and provides rehabilitation for those who are of working age (14–65 years), have substantially reduced capacity to work and are likely to benefit from a rehabilitation programme. A large percentage self-refer to the CRS. In 1994 24,000 people attended a CRS programme, 70% completed the programme and about two-thirds of them successfully obtained employment (ISSA 1995b).

The International Labour Organisation published the first results of an *International Research Project on Job Retention and Return to Work Strategies for Disabled Workers* (Thornton 1998). The preliminary study examined policies and practices in the UK, Sweden, the Netherlands, France, Germany, the US, Canada, Australia and New Zealand. Reports were prepared on each individual country and used to prepare a *Key Issues* paper (Thornton 1998) which:

- Identified policies, programmes and practices which can support job retention and return to work and considered their effectiveness in national contexts
- Identified barriers and facilitators to effective national policies and practice
- Considered the potential for transferring these policies and programmes between countries
- Attempted to develop efficient and equitable strategies for job retention and return to work.

This project provided the best analysis and overview of public and firms' policies and also uniquely focused on job retention, rather than simply returning people to work after they had lost their job. A national system contains many elements: policies (laws, regulations, operating principles), programmes (structures for organisation and funding), practices (operating processes) and players (policy makers, agencies, representative bodies, service providers, consumers and their representatives). The research was organised around five themes:

- Public policies to promote employment of disabled people
- Benefit and compensation systems
- Rehabilitation and employment support and systems
- Adaptation of work and the work place
- Enterprise strategies.

Each element was judged on activity, effectiveness, efficiency and equity.

This project defined 'disabled' to include all workers who became disabled, injured or ill, whose health condition affected, was likely to affect or might create discrimination about their working capacity or prospects of continuing or advancing employment. Because of this very broad definition, the review tried to cover and did not always distinguish policies, programmes and practices for those with severe disablement and those with more minor incapacities. As with many reviews, however, the examples and discussion focused more on those with severe, long-standing disablement rather than those with long-term sickness.

Changes in the labour market and conditions of employment have tended to increase firms' autonomy and reduce the job opportunities and security of disabled workers, and all eight countries in this review now have policies that influence employment practices for workers with disabilities. All the mainland European countries have large and expanding sheltered employment sectors for the severely disabled. There is a 'quota-levy' system in which employers must either employ a target percentage of disabled people or pay a levy to a central fund. In contrast, the four English-speaking countries now have human rights and anti-discrimination legislation. Much of this legislation is designed primarily to promote the interests of people with severe, long-standing disabilities, although it is usually framed in such a way that it includes workers who become disabled, and they are usually now the majority of the beneficiaries. For those who become sick, there are more specific public policies:

- Maintaining the connection with the employer during sickness absence and medical treatment:

- linking employment protection to social insurance benefits, e.g. Sweden, the Netherlands
- linking employment protection to injury and accident compensation, e.g. Germany, the US, Canada, New Zealand
- 'disability leave', e.g. the US
- Preventing dismissal on grounds of disability:
  - automatic protection until negotiated dismissal, e.g. Germany
  - Disability Discrimination Acts also protect against dismissal, e.g. the UK, the US
  - building disability into employment security law, e.g. Sweden.

Although some of these measures are undoubtedly effective, there is little data to measure the magnitude of their effect, and measures to promote job retention can sometimes have a perverse effect of discouraging employers from taking on workers at risk of long-term disability.

Prins & Meijerink (1997) and Prins et al (1998) compared return-to-work strategies in selected EU countries. They obtained information from personal contacts in each country on:

- Quota arrangements for employers to hire or retain a certain percentage of workers with disabilities
- Compulsory employers' rehabilitation or re-integration plans for sick or injured workers
- Personal rehabilitation budgets, which enable workers to chose vocational rehabilitation measures or providers
- Financial incentives to employers, both to retain and employ disabled workers
- Diagnosis-related work-resumption strategies, including modified or progressive return to work.

Quota arrangements

Table 2.9 shows the quota arrangements in selected countries, although in contrast the Scandinavian countries and Switzerland have never had quota arrangements because they are considered to create different classes of worker and stigmatise disabled workers. Prins & Maijering (1997) concluded that there are major problems to quota systems: with the possible exception of France and Germany they do not seem to work effectively; definitions, criteria and administration of these schemes are complicated; in none of these countries

TABLE 2.9 Quota arrangements for employment of disabled workers in selected EU countries

Country	Number of employees	% Work force	Legal sanctions
UK (Up to 1995)	>35	3	No
Belgium	>20	3	No
France	>10	6	Yes
Germany	>15	6	Yes
Italy	>35	15	No

Prins & Meijerink (1997).

do employers actually meet the quotas; sanctions are rarely applied; and in some countries some disabled workers oppose the system because they feel the stigma actually reduces rather than improves their chance of work. The German scheme was considered the most effective: people classed as disabled are employed as 4.3% of the work force and the penalties for failing to meet the full target also finances the rehabilitation fund.

Compulsory employers' rehabilitation or re-integration plans

Only in Sweden and the Netherlands is there any statutory obligation on employers to develop a rehabilitation or re-integration plan for sick or injured workers. Since 1999 in Sweden, a re-integration plan must be prepared when a worker has been sick for 4 weeks, and submitted to the social security office once the worker has been sick for 8 weeks. Since 1994 in the Netherlands, a rehabilitation plan must be prepared when a worker is sick for 13 weeks. There is some doubt about how fully these obligations are being implemented and no data are available on whether they have had any impact.

Personal rehabilitation budgets

These are described in the US section of Chapter 4 (see p 240) but despite some debate have not been implemented in any EU country.

Financial incentives to employers

Many countries offer financial incentives to employers to retain or employ disabled workers, most commonly including subsidies, grants, tax or social security contribution allowances. The largest and most comprehensive range of measures is in Germany. In most countries there seems to be little information on the uptake of these schemes and no information on whether they have any impact on the employment of disabled workers.

Diagnosis-related work-resumption strategies

Germany has a number of schemes of part-time, progressive or 'step-wise' return to work over periods of up to 7 weeks. Such schemes depend on co-operation from the treating and occupational health physician, the worker, the employer and the social security agency, which may create barriers and result in relatively low uptake. There is also limited and conflicting data on whether these schemes do actually succeed in returning workers to full duties.

Prins et al (1998) concluded that most EU countries have some statutory arrangements to encourage the retention or employment of disabled workers, of which the most common are medical rehabilitation, training and re-training, financial incentives to employers and the creation of subsidised jobs. However, there appear to be major barriers and limited uptake of these schemes. There is very little data and it is not possible to reach any firm conclusions on whether or how much impact they have on the retention or employment of disabled workers. Moreover, almost all the schemes are designed primarily for the long-term severely disabled and there are no data on how effectively they deal with a chronic sickness or disability such as back pain.

The ISSA study

The recently published ISSA study, *Who Returns to Work and Why?* (Bloch & Prins 2001), collected data on what actually happened to cohorts of claimants from Denmark, Germany, Israel, the Netherlands, Sweden and the US who had been on social security benefits for back pain for at least 3 months. The main questions addressed were:

1. Do the various interventions of the health-care system, social security system and employers make a difference to health status and work resumption patterns of those suffering from back pain?
2. If so, what are the best interventions?
3. How is the process towards re-integration into the labour force influenced by health status, living conditions, social conditions, job requirements, working conditions, the labour market, incentives, disincentives and the social security system?

Tables 2.10 and 2.11 show the variation in medical consultations and interventions received. In general, there was a high level of 'medical' consultation and investigation, and 'passive' therapies. On regression analysis, there was rarely any statistically significant and no consistent relationship between any modality of conservative treatment and change in pain intensity or back function over 1 year (Hansson & Hansson 2001). None of the medical interventions made any material difference to work resumption within 1 year, with the sole exception of surgery during the first year in Sweden (which also had the lowest surgery rate, presumably reflecting the most selective use of surgery). There were, however, a number of demographic and job-related characteristics which did have a significant impact (Table 2.12).

Table 2.13 gives the rehabilitation and vocational interventions received. On any of these measures, Germany actually delivered (one of) the lowest levels of all interventions designed to assist workers in returning to work (with the exception of receiving physiotherapy within the first 3 months of sickness absence where Germany was about average).

Table 2.14 gives the final outcome measures of return to work within 1 and 2 years. (These rates appear very low because they are for patients in the selected high-risk group who were already off work for 3 months: these are not total return to work rates.) Germany and Denmark had by far the lowest return to work rates and at 2 years Germany had

TABLE 2.10 Medical consultations (% of cohort) in different countries

	Denmark	Germany	Israel	The Netherlands	Sweden	US
Consult GP within 90 days	95	72	74	97	74	34
Consult GP within 1 year	98	85	96	97	86	77
See company doctor within 1 year	4	15	17	97	27	15
See specialist within 1 year	83	87	99	88	73	84

Data from Bloch & Prins (2001).

TABLE 2.11   Treatment received (% of cohort) in different countries

	Denmark	Germany	Israel	The Netherlands	Sweden	US
X-ray within 90 days	64	35	92	74	58	75
Average time of X-ray from stopping work	Day 27	—	Day 32	Day 48	Day 25	Day 67
X-ray, CT, MRI within 1 year[1]	86	72	99	86	81	94
Bed rest within 90 days	23	0	84	51	7	48
Hospitalisation within 90 days	21	19	25	32	11	31
Hospitalisation within 1 year	31	29	38	49	24	45
Surgery within 90 days	11	9	10	18	6	32
Surgery within 1 year	15	15	18	31	17	41
Heat or cold within 365 days	56	45	75	36	43	84
TENS, ultrasound, SWD within 365 days	53	53	68	70	62	71
Manipulation, etc within 365 days	59	34	54	29	44	66
'Active' physical activities, back school, etc within 90 days	47	54	14	61	42	55
'Active' physical activities, back school, etc within 365 days	66	75	34	84	63	86

[1]There are no separate data published on CT and MRI.

Data from Block & Prins (2001)

SWD = Short wave diathermy; CT = computed tomography; MRI = magnetic resonance imaging; TENS = transcutaneous electrical nerve stimulators

TABLE 2.12   Magnitude (%) of improvement in return to work at 1 year from significant demographic, job-related and medical predictors (based on logistic regression)

	Denmark	Germany	Israel	The Netherlands	Sweden	US
Each year lower age	4	4		4		5
Male	76	72				
No treatment before sick-listing	52					54
Lower psychological demands of work		42				
Higher decision latitude at work	64			135		
Lower physical demands of work	41	89	113	67	79	140
Surgery					113	

Data from Hansson & Hansson (2001).

the highest rate of early retirement. The German cohort were significantly older (38% >55 years of age), less educated (70% primary education only) and included more blue-collar workers than any of the other countries. Although 32% of the German cohort predicted at 3 months they would never be able to return to work (higher than for any other country), German return to work rates were still lower even for comparable age groups and education levels.

Most return to work occurred within the first year, although an additional 10% did return in the second year (and conversely about 10% stopped work again). In the Netherlands, Sweden and Germany, 82–94% of those who returned to work returned to their previous

TABLE 2.13   Rehabilitation and return to work interventions received (% of cohort) in different countries

	Denmark	Germany	Israel	The Netherlands	Sweden	US
Physiotherapy within 90 days	61	68	70	75	63	52
Physiotherapy within 1 year	79	74	88	95	90	77
Rehabilitation plan	58	41	6	50	66	21
Test of vocational capacity	23	7	8	7	17	18
Vocational rehabilitation and job training	20	9	7	8	26	15
Work accommodations (% of those who returned to work):						
Adaptation of workplace	24	14	15	31	24	23
Adaptation of working hours	45	20	59	62	31	43
Job redesign/change of workplace	61	19	65	46	28	40

Data from Bloch & Prins (2001).

TABLE 2.14   Return to work rates in different countries (% of those off work for at least 3 months)

	Denmark	Germany	Israel	The Netherlands	Sweden	US
Working at 1 year (from stopping work)	32	41	49	73	53	63
Working at 2 years (from stopping work)	40	35	60	72	63	62

From Bloch & Prins (2001).

employer, while in the US more than one-third and in Denmark and Israel more than one-half returned to new employers. The best predictors of return to work were demographic, baseline health, personal expectations and still having a job available. Medical interventions had little or no impact. Non-medical and vocational interventions were difficult to assess: only work-place accommodations and therapeutic work resumption appeared to have a consistent effect in various countries; disability assessment had a negative effect (presumably reflecting moves towards termination of employment or disability pension); case management also had a negative effect (which may reflect case selection).

Long-term incapacity and return to work

The major concern in every system is that once anyone has been off work and on long-term benefits for >6–12 months they have a very low chance of returning to work. There is very little evidence that any system is particularly effective at preventing or overcoming this. Until very recently the UK has probably put least effort and resources into any rehabilitation or re-employment arrangements or services to tackle this problem. Even now, there are some good intentions and commitments, but little evidence that effective interventions have actually been developed and implemented on any scale.

Rowlingson & Berthoud (1996) pointed out that physical or mental capacity to perform certain tasks is only one aspect of finding and keeping a job. [Although their study was of Disability Working Allowance (DWA), the discussion is relevant to all forms of incapacity and benefits.] Capacity and incapacity for work depend on complex interactions between the worker's medical condition and physical capabilities, ergonomic demands of the job and psychosocial factors. The factors that influence stopping work may be different from those that influence staying off work and different again from those that influence going back to work. The social process of becoming sick and incapacitated probably usually occurs insidiously and unconsciously rather than as a conscious decision. Obtaining and returning to work may be a completely different process and not just a reversal of the original process of stopping work.

Back pain illustrates the complexity of the relations between sickness, incapacity for work, sick certification and social security benefits. CSAG (1994a) considered three possible scenarios:

- Back pain might be the direct cause of incapacity, sickness absence and job loss, leading directly to sick certification and social security benefits
- The physical, psychological and social ill effects of unemployment might interact with and aggravate back pain and incapacity
- People with back pain who lose their job (for whatever reason) might be more likely to receive sick certification and sickness and invalidity benefits.

These corresponded broadly to the three routes of entry to and exit from invalidity benefits identified in a DSS study by Ritchie & Snape (1993):

- *Condition-led entry:* the nature and severity of the illness and loss of faculty lead to long-term or permanent incapacity. Coming off benefits depends on the nature of the incapacity and treatment received and the availability of employment
- *Employment-led entry:* restricted employment opportunities combined with illness/disability (and often also age) cause loss of employment or inability to gain work and hence the start of benefits. The main barriers to coming off benefits are employment opportunities, availability of rehabilitation or retraining, and age
- *Self-directed entry:* some interaction between the individual's medical condition, employment opportunities and motivation to continue or gain employment result in sickness and invalidity benefits being seen as a possible option. This could be either with the support of the family doctor or negotiated with the family doctor. The main barriers to coming off benefits are age, low motivation and restricted employment opportunities, often related to their condition. Coming off benefits largely depends on external triggers, which are usually independent medical review by the DSS or the family doctor's decision to stop sick certification.

Chew & May (1997) made a qualitative study of how UK family doctors dealt with this situation and suggested that they faced a dilemma. They further suggested that back pain might form a social resource for some patients, and this had major implications for how both patient and doctor approach the consultation:

- Chronic low back pain (LBP) permitted withdrawal from normal social obligations
- These patients recognised that their doctor was unable to help, but viewed the doctor as a resource through which their social and economic inactivity could be legitimised
- These patients did recognise the relation between psychosocial factors and pain
- Chronic LBP involved both the patient and the doctor negotiating conflicting roles.

Rowlingson & Berthoud (1996) also studied the barriers to and needs of disabled people returning to work. (Although published in 1996, this research was actually carried out on 1992–1994 claimants under the previous system of Invalidity Benefit.) They found that the 1.6 million adults of working age on the four main disability benefits in 1993 had a very low level of economic activity and expectation. Two-thirds did not expect to work again in the future and only about a quarter (425,000) showed any attachment to work (Table 2.15). The rate of movement off disability benefits and into work was very low: only 2% of all disability and incapacity benefit recipients had moved into work in the 18 months before they were interviewed. Movement into work was strongly related to the severity of impairment and health condition but in addition younger people, single men and women with working partners were more likely to move off benefits and into work. Women whose partners were also out of work had particularly low expectations of ever working again.

TABLE 2.15 Expectation of working again among those on Invalidity Benefit and related benefits

Age	18–29 (n=803) (%)	30–39 (n=1055) (%)	40–49 (n=1685) (%)	50+ (n=2929) (%)	All workers (n=6619) (%)
Have a job to go back to	2	2	1	1	1
Looking for work	11	5	6	2	4
Hoping to look for work	19	17	10	4	9
Would need help or training before work	25	24	16	7	14
Do not expect to work again	38	47	64	82	67

From Rowlingson & Berthoud (1996).

Those surveyed considered working preferable to being on benefits because it provided a social identity, meaning and interesting activity, social contact and financial independence from the state. They felt that the main attractions of particular jobs were good wages, job security and good relations with employers. Flexible or short hours were not major attractions but those surveyed did value the ability to take time off when required. Those with a strong labour market position, e.g. those who were younger, better qualified, with recent work experience and less severe impairments, were more likely to be looking for work. However, even in these groups few people actually managed to obtain work. Most of those who were out of work when they were surveyed in 1993 and again a year later in 1994 were still looking for work. About a quarter had become less active and 16% more active in their search for work. Those surveyed considered that the main barriers to work were the general lack of jobs, the limitations imposed by impairments and employers' views of the disabled. People generally managed to get into work either when their condition improved, when they found a job which accommodated their condition or when they had a sympathetic employer.

Rowlingson & Berthoud (1996) looked at the types of incapacities reported by those surveyed who were in or on the margins of work. The average number of incapacities reported was 3.3. The most common were walking (62%), exhaustion/pain (61%) and depression/mental illness (46%). Interestingly, and particularly relevant to back pain and the present review, Rowlingson & Berthoud (1996) appeared simply to assume that 'some disabled people may be completely incapable of any work task if they have conditions involving pain or extreme tiredness', although they did qualify this—'most disabled people are probably capable of some productive tasks in certain conditions even if productivity is very low'. They highlighted the general problem of total or partial incapacity. Most social security benefits were based on total incapacity, but many sick and disabled people were not totally capable or totally incapable of work. A substantial proportion of disabled people could be considered, or considered themselves, as 'partially (in)capable of work' but prior to the introduction of DWA in 1992 there was no 'partial incapacity benefit' in the UK. They might be able to perform a particular task but might only be able to do it for a limited length of time and not for a complete working day or every day. Some disabled people might need continuing treatment. A major concern of many of these people was that even if their symptoms were not too bad at present, they might become worse if they returned to work. They might have difficulty travelling to and from work. Few employers might be willing to provide the right conditions and pay for those tasks that they could do. Getting work was also highly competitive and disabled people inevitably faced some degree of disadvantage and a lower chance of successfully gaining and keeping employment.

These partially incapacitated people might then find themselves in a difficult situation. The dilemma was that they had to demonstrate what they *could not do* for the social security system in order to obtain benefits but at the same time demonstrate what they *could do* for employers in order to obtain work. Willingness to work did not in theory affect entitlement to incapacity benefits, but claimants might feel that if they showed too much ability and willingness to work they might be taken off their current benefits and forced to accept other benefits at a lower rate. Many of those surveyed felt that neither the benefit system, the labour market nor society in general recognised 'partial incapacity' and that they were forced to be either totally incapacitated or would be treated as if there was nothing really wrong with them.

Rowlingson & Berthoud (1996) also found that disabled people believed that employer discrimination against them was widespread and it was interesting to see how some of them managed to overcome it. Some disabled people managed to find sympathetic employers, although they counted themselves very lucky to have done so. Others did not tell prospective employers that they were disabled. Others had some trial period in which they could prove to the employer that they could do the job. Trial employment schemes were suggested as being most honest, and let both the disabled person and the employer find out if they could manage the job adequately.

Berthoud (1998) offered further discussion on return to work. He suggested British labour market policy had been based on the false premise that economic (dis)incentives are the major determinant of whether people work or not. However, he pointed out the effects of incentives vary in different social groups. Men tend to work whether their incentives are high or not, mainly because they expect and are expected to. Pensioners do not work, whatever the incentives, mainly because they do not expect and no one expects them to. From this argument, married women have most freedom to chose and are most sensitive to incentives. Berthoud concluded that labour market policies are likely to be more important than changing incentives in enabling disabled people to return to work.

Wemyss-Gorman (1999) independently studied barriers to return to work in 133 UK chronic pain patients who had completed a Pain Management Programme; 41 of these patients had given up work because of pain. After the programme, 21 of them tried to return to work but only nine were successful. The most common reasons given for being unsuccessful were employers' reluctance to take on people with a history of back pain, lack of retraining opportunities, and employers being unwilling to make adjustments or concessions. Wemyss-Gorman (1999) suggested this was contrary to the 1995 Disability Discrimination Act and argued that health professionals in the pain field should lobby politicians 'to exert maximum pressure on the government to implement their expressed good intentions'.

3   International comparison of social security trends

When considering benefit trends it is important to distinguish the number of new cases (claims and awards), the number of people currently on benefits at each point in time, and the total benefits paid over time, e.g. per annum. These may each show very different patterns, although they are obviously inter-related. For example, there may be no change in the number of new cases, but if more people stay on benefit longer and fewer come off benefit, then the number currently on benefits and the total benefits paid may rise dramatically. Or the number of new cases may fall substantially but if those already on benefit remain on benefit over many years, then any change in the number currently on benefit and the total benefits paid will be delayed and much more gradual. Each kind of data provides a different perspective on what is happening. Total benefits paid may be the best measure of total societal impact and costs. Epidemiologically and clinically, the number currently receiving benefits may be most relevant. The number of new cases is likely to be the earliest and most sensitive measure of change. The ratio of awards/claims, duration on benefits and patterns of coming off benefit may be the process measures which help to understand the mechanisms of change.

Most of the tabulated data comparing different countries in this section is from official Eurostat, MISSOC or OECD sources. In addition, the AS/tri Research and Consultancy Institute in the Netherlands provided an independent cross-check. Its data are based on official statistics, but are generally obtained through personal contacts in each country, and the data are then adjusted for various factors such as gender, age, etc. Prins *et al* (1992) and Einerhand *et al* (1995) provided detailed methodology. However, many of the more recent AS/tri reports provide insufficient methodological detail or data to check how the final figures have been reached.

Comparison of prevalence of disability

Eurostat (1995) (Table 3.2) suggests that the number of people with self-reported disability is comparable in most EU countries. However, this comparison suggests that there is considerable variation in the number of adults of working age who receive a disability pension, with the UK being by far the lowest and the Netherlands and Denmark being highest (although this may depend on the definition of a 'disabled person'). The percentage receiving a disability pension is much lower than the number of people with a disability because:

- The rate of disability refers to the whole population and is much higher in the older age group, while the number receiving disability pensions is for those under age 60. (The rate of disability in persons under age 60 varies between 6 and 8%)

- Receiving benefits for disability depends on a certain minimum level of disability and on eligibility and entitlement.

Eurostat (1995, 2000) gave data on self-reported health (Table 3.1) and the prevalence of disability (Table 3.2) in different EU countries.

TABLE 3.1   Self-reported health and restrictions for adults aged over 16 years (1994)

	Perceived health very good or good (%)	Activities restricted in past 2 weeks for physical or mental reasons (%)	Hampered in daily activities due to chronic conditions (%)
UK	74.7	14.6	0.7
Ireland	79.7	9.7	18.1
Denmark	52.6	15.4	20.1
The Netherlands	74.2	16.4	25.3
Belgium	73.5	9.0	21.0
France	64.0	—	19.3
Germany	69.4	15.1	24.4
Mean EU12	67.4	11.6	21.8

From Eurostat (2000).

TABLE 3.2   Prevalence of disability in different EU countries (1991–1992)

	Persons with a disability (%)	Disabled persons <60 years old receiving disability pensions (%)
UK	11.9	2.8
Ireland	—	4.2
Denmark	12.5	6.5
The Netherlands	12.2	6.4
Belgium	11.9	5.5
France	10.3	4.4
Germany	12.5	4.5

From Eurostat (1995).

Comparison of incapacity benefits

AS/tri provided an independent comparison of incapacity benefits in six European countries (Table 3.3) (Prins et al 1992, 1998, Einerhand et al 1995). Its most recent data were for 1995, although because of the changes in the UK benefits scheme in 1994–1995, 1996 UK data were used instead (Table 3.4).

Most of these six countries show very similar rates of total social security benefits for incapacity, with very little change between 1990 and 1995. The main exception is the Netherlands with nearly double the average rate. The UK was slightly below average and Sweden slightly above average in 1990, but both had come closer to the average by 1995. Denmark was about average in 1990, but had risen slightly above average by 1995.

TABLE 3.3 1990 total incapacity benefits (sickness, industrial injury and invalidity), standardised for age (as % of labour force)

	Men			Women		
	Temporary	Long-term	Total	Temporary	Long-term	Total
UK	2.3	3.3	5.6	2.8	3.0	5.9
Sweden	5.3	3.4	8.7	7.0	3.1	10.1
Denmark	3.7	3.7	7.4	5.4	3.5	8.9
The Netherlands	6.4	8.8	15.2	7.9	7.5	15.5
Belgium	3.1	4.0	7.0	4.8	4.3	9.0
Germany	5.2	3.3	8.5	4.5	2.4	6.9

From Einerhand et al (1995).

TABLE 3.4 1995 total incapacity benefits (sickness, industrial injury and invalidity), standardised for age (as % of labour force)

	Men			Women		
	Temporary	Long-term	Total	Temporary	Long-term	Total
UK	3.1	4.8	7.9	4.0	4.2	8.2
Sweden	3.3	3.7	7.0	4.3	3.5	7.8
Denmark	5.0	4.1	9.1	7.5	3.8	11.2
The Netherlands	4.4	7.6	12.0	6.1	7.0	13.1
Belgium	3.0	4.1	7.1	3.9	4.4	8.3
Germany	4.6	3.1	7.6	4.2	2.4	6.6

From Prins et al (1998).

Prins & Veerman (1998) estimated the numbers of disability benefit recipients in a wider range of countries (Table 3.5) and suggested that the UK was closer to the EU average for men, although lower for women. In all the AS/tri data, the Netherlands had by far the highest rates of long-term incapacity benefits.

TABLE 3.5 International comparison of the numbers of disability benefit recipients per 1000 insured (1996)

	Number of new disability recipients per annum		Total disability recipients	
	Men	Women	Men	Women
US	4.9	6.4	37.5	28.8
Sweden	5.3	5.8	54.6	64.2
Denmark	5.7	7.7	55.4	43.8
UK	7.3	4.6	60.4	28.3
Belgium	7.3	8.0	62.0	59.4
Norway	8.1	9.4	64.8	93.2
Germany	9.8	7.8	72.0	96.1
The Netherlands	9.9	16.3	131.9	121.8

From Prins & Veerman (1998).

Trends

Aarts et al (1996), from the Foundation for International Studies on Social Security in the Netherlands, found dramatic differences in trends of disability benefit from 1970 to 1994 in several countries (Table 3.6). [Note that these tables are not disability rates per 1000, but *ratios* of those on disability benefits to those who are actively working. Hence they are not directly comparable to the data above.] Over the past 25 years, almost all OECD countries have seen increasing numbers of people available for work due to the baby boom after World War II and increasing female participation in the labour force. Most countries have also seen decreasing participation in the active labour force by older men (and more recently older women also), increasing availability and generosity of sickness and incapacity benefits, and increasing numbers of workers receiving disability benefits and retiring early on disability benefits. Aarts et al (1996) again found the Netherlands had by far the highest growth in the numbers on long-term incapacity benefits, rising from about average in 1970 to double the level in any country in the world by 1980. They suggested that the Netherlands differed from the other countries in that it had deliberately and vigorously used disability benefits to reduce unemployment even for younger workers (although other data show that the numbers receiving unemployment benefits were little different from other countries). The UK, Sweden and Germany did not do this for younger workers, but relaxed eligibility criteria did permit increasing numbers of older workers to receive disability benefits for a combination of economic as well as health reasons. The US initially showed a similar trend, but started to tighten eligibility criteria at the end of the 1970s, and disability benefit rates remained low and steady until about 1990. Only the recession of the 1990s produced a significant rise in the US and Sweden. Germany also introduced much tighter eligibility criteria in 1985, and actually reduced the total disability rate to the pre-1980 level where it has remained steady since. However, this low total rate in Germany hides a particular problem in older workers (Table 3.7).

Prins et al (1998) also analysed and compared trends in incapacity benefits in the UK, Sweden, Denmark, the Netherlands, Belgium and Germany from 1980 to 1995. This was prepared as a private report for The Swedish Council on Technology Assessment in Health Care (SBU), although the main findings were published in Waddell & Norlund (2000). Unfortunately, the data were all 'normalised' to an initial 1980 base of 100 so it is very difficult to check or interpret them in absolute terms.

TABLE 3.6 Ratio of disability benefit recipients per 1000 active labour force participants aged 15–64, 1970–1994

	1970	1975	1980	1985	1990	1994
UK	29	28	31	56	68	—
Sweden	49	67	68	74	78	97
The Netherlands	55	84	138	142	152	151
Germany	51	54	59	72	55	54
US	27	42	41	41	43	62

From Aarts et al (1996).

TABLE 3.7   Ratio of disability benefit recipients per 1000 active labour force participants aged 60–64, 1970–1994

	1970	1975	1980	1985	1990	1994
UK	219	195	209	357	413	—
Sweden	229	382	382	512	577	658
The Netherlands	299	437	1033	1283	1987	1911
Germany	419	688	1348	1291	1109	1064
US	154	265	285	254	250	294

From Aarts et al (1996).

Prins et al (1998) suggested that the number currently on short-term spells of sickness benefit stayed more or less constant or fell slightly in most of these countries over this particular period, with the exception of Sweden which had a rise of about 50% in the late 1980s before falling markedly in the early 1990s. However, these data related solely to social security sickness benefits and probably bear little relationship to actual sickness absence from work. The apparent falls in the UK in 1982–1984, Sweden in 1992 and the Netherlands in 1993–1994 correspond to legislation which shifted an increasing proportion of sick pay to the employers and so excluded it from social security statistics.

Prins et al (1998) found more variation in the incidence of new awards of long-term invalidity benefits. In Sweden and Denmark the incidence grew steadily over this period, although in Sweden it fell rapidly after 1993 to just below the 1980 level. The Belgian incidence gradually fell slightly without any dramatic change. The UK, Sweden, the Netherlands and Germany each showed a sharp drop at different times. The UK incidence fell in the early 1980s when there was a substantial change in the complete benefits system. The German incidence fell in the mid 1980s when some categories of insured were excluded from benefits. The incidence in Sweden and the Netherlands fell in the early 1990s when stricter eligibility criteria and assessment methods were introduced.

The total numbers currently receiving long-term invalidity benefits showed a very different pattern. For most countries the rate per 100 insured remained more or less constant or gradually increased slightly over this period. The one exception was the UK where the rate more or less doubled (although Table 3.6 shows this was mainly a matter of 'catching up'). However, the major exception was Germany where there was a gradual fall from 1984 to 1992, which had been attributed to changed eligibility and the alternative possibility of early old-age pensions. This levelled out following German re-unification in 1992.

Prins et al (1998) also analysed trends in social security expenditures on sickness and invalidity benefits from 1980 to 1993 as a percentage of GDP. In most countries the cost of sickness benefits paid by the state fell by 10–45% over this period, although in many countries this again simply reflected a shift of costs to employers. The major exception was Sweden, where the rapid rise in costs in the late 1980s and sharp fall in the early 1990s reflected the number of spells of sickness benefits. Four of the six countries showed virtually no change in expenditure on long-term invalidity benefits over this period. In the UK, however, expenditure almost doubled (although as noted above this was largely a matter of 'catching up'), while in Sweden it increased about 50%, which largely reflected the numbers currently receiving long-term invalidity benefit. The rise in expenditure relative to GDP in Sweden was also partly because Swedish GDP fell for 3 years while benefits were maintained relative to rising salaries.

Prins et al (1998) gave little data on individual causes of sickness or invalidity, but did point out that in most countries three main diagnostic groups accounted for the large majority of people receiving long-term invalidity benefits: musculoskeletal disorders, cardiovascular disorders and mental disorders. They had no separate data on back pain but did analyse the number of new awards of invalidity benefits accounted for by musculoskeletal disorders. Most countries showed a gradual rise of 10–50% between the early–mid 1980s and the early 1990s, and a levelling or slight fall from about 1992–1993, although most were still about 20–40% higher by 1995. Only the Netherlands maintained a much steadier proportion and then fell below the 1980 level by 1995. The marked exception to this overall trend was the UK, where Prins et al (1998) suggested the proportion of new awards of invalidity benefits for musculoskeletal disorders more than doubled from 1980 to 1995. This is consistent with UK data on back pain and other musculoskeletal disorders up to 1991–1992, analysed independently in Table 4.38. There is no obvious explanation why the pattern of musculoskeletal disorders should be so different in the UK. This difference from other EU countries implies that the exponential increase in DSS benefits paid for back pain in the UK is not representative of other EU countries.

Beljaars & Prins (2000) updated their graph comparing the numbers of disability beneficiaries per 1000 insured in the Netherlands, Belgium and Germany from 1968 to 1997. This showed that in 1968 the Netherlands occupied an intermediate position, with the German rate slightly higher and the Belgian rate slightly lower. The German rate remained roughly constant throughout with a minor peak about 1986. The Belgian rate gradually caught up, has remained more or less steady since the mid 1980s and now equals the German rate. The Dutch rate increased dramatically between 1968 and 1977, rose more gradually to a peak in 1985 and then fell gradually, although it still remains nearly double the rate in the other countries.

Siegelier & Prins (2000) updated their comparison of the number of people on disability pensions in various European countries (Table 3.8).

TABLE 3.8 Number of people on disability pensions in different European countries in 1998

	As % population aged 14–64	As % active population
UK	4.7	6.2
Sweden	5.8	7.5
Denmark	4.3	5.4
The Netherlands	6.3	8.6
Germany	3.6	5.0

Based on data from Siegelier & Prins (2000).

The major limitations of the As/tri data by Prins and colleagues are that much of the data are apparently based on personal sources, there is inadequate description of exactly how they are obtained and 'adjusted', and it is impossible to check their accuracy.

Eurostat (1995) provided separate data on the numbers receiving benefits for occupational injury or disease. There appear to be marked differences in the number of occupational accident pensions awarded in different countries (Table 3.9). The UK, Ireland and Spain have very low rates, Germany pays three times as many, Belgium and Italy seven times as many, and France about 13 times as many. Trends over time also differ (Table 3.10), with the UK showing no change, while France, Belgium and Ireland show an increase of 10–60% between 1980 and 1991. The Danish data are not comparable because they only relate to new awards each year, while all the other data relate to the total number of pensions paid.

TABLE 3.9   Social security occupational injury and disability pensions paid in different countries (1991)

	Population (millions)	Number of occupational injury or disease pensions (thousands)	Number of occupational disability pensions per 1000 population
UK	58	186	3.2
Ireland	3.6	9.7	2.7
Belgium	10	205	20.5
France	58	2249	38.8
Germany	81	763	9.4
Italy	57	1273	22.3
Spain	39	121	3.1

From Eurostat (1995).

Table 3.11 shows trends in social security expenditure since 1960 in the countries under comparison. Average European expenditure on social security rose from 9.7 to 17.7% between 1960 and 1985, and since this time has risen slightly to about 20%. US expenditure was about half the average European level throughout, which reflects the greater US reliance on individual provision for security, but showed the same trend rising from 5.1 to 10.8% between 1960 and 1985 and then to 13.1% by 1995. Australian and Japanese levels were very similar to those in the US throughout. However, there is considerable variation between different European countries. In 1960, social security spending ranged from 5.1% in Finland to 13.5% in France, while by 1995 it ranged from about 15–16% in the UK and Norway, 18.6% in Germany, and 23–25% in all the other European countries. Although all European countries show the same rising trend, the increase has occurred at different times in different countries. The Netherlands, Belgium and France had all reached a high level by 1985, and since then have had very little further change in percentage of GDP spent on social security. The UK and Germany have always been lower than the EU average and somewhat closer to the pattern in the US and Japan, but since 1985 there has been a further rise of about 2–3%. During the same period there has been a rise of 4–5% in Sweden, Norway and Denmark and a more recent rise of nearly 10% in Finland with its severe economic crisis.

TABLE 3.10 Social security occupational accident pensions in different EU countries (thousands), 1980–1991

	Population (million)	Data type	1980	1981	1982	1983	1984	1985	1986	1987	1988	1989	1990	1991
UK	58	(3)	196	192	189	186	184	188	184	186	189	185	185	186
Ireland	3.6	(1)	—	6.1	7.5	8.1	8.6	9.2	9.5	8.5	8.5	9.1	9.6	9.7
Denmark	5	(2)	5.2	5.2	5.4	5.7	5.9	7.1	7.6	6.1	4.7	2.2	—	—
Belgium	10	(1)	91.3	85.5	80.2	83.8	86.1	91.0	96.9	102.3	106.5	111.7	116.8	121.6
France	58	(1)	2048	2077	2092	2114	—	2117	2139	2161	2183	2205	2227	2249

1. Persons drawing occupational accident pensions
2. New occupational accident allowances
3. Persons drawing Industrial Disablement Benefits (for occupational injury or disease)

From Eurostat (1995).

TABLE 3.11 Social security transfers as a percentage of GDP, 1960–1999

	1960	1968	1974	1985	1990	1991	1992	1993	1994	1995	1996	1997	1998	1999
UK	6.8	8.7	9.2	13.5	11.9	14.0	15.6	16.0	15.7	15.4	14.9	14.4	13.7	13.5
Ireland	5.5	6.5	11.4	16.5	11.3	12.0	12.4	12.2	12.1	11.3	11.0	10.5	9.8	9.6
Sweden	8.0	10.6	14.3	18.2	19.5	21.1	23.4	23.3	22.8	21.3	20.3	19.6	19.3	18.9
Norway	7.6	10.5	13.3	11.8	15.9	16.4	17.1	16.9	16.4	15.8	15.2	14.7	15.5	15.5
Finland	5.1	7.5	7.6	14.8	14.9	18.6	22.5	24.0	23.8	22.2	21.5	19.9	18.4	17.9
Denmark	7.4	10.8	12.0	16.3	17.9	18.4	18.9	19.8	21.2	20.4	19.8	18.9	18.2	17.3
The Netherlands	—	16.2	20.7	26.2	25.8	26.0	26.4	26.6	25.4	15.3	14.8	13.9	13.0	12.6
Belgium	11.5	14.2	18.0	—	16.2	16.6	16.7	17.1	16.8	16.6	16.6	16.3	16.0	15.7
France	13.5	17.0	15.5	—	16.9	17.3	17.7	18.5	18.4	18.5	18.7	18.8	18.4	18.4
Germany	12.0	13.7	14.6	16.2	15.2	15.7	16.3	17.4	17.7	18.1	19.3	19.3	18.9	18.9
Mean EU15	9.7	12.4	13.3	17.7	16.1	16.8	17.7	18.3	18.2	17.6	17.4	17.3	16.8	16.8
US	5.1	6.4	9.6	10.8	11.1	12.2	12.9	13.0	12.8	13.0	12.9	12.6	—	—
Australia	5.5	5.1	7.1	9.5	7.3	8.3	8.5	8.8	8.6	8.6	8.2	8.0	—	—
Japan	3.8	4.5	6.2	10.9	11.4	10.8	11.3	11.9	12.5	13.4	13.5	13.7	14.6	—

No data for New Zealand.
From OECD Historical Statistics (1997, 2000)—these give completely different figures for the same years in some countries (including the UK), which casts doubt on their accuracy.

The UK and Ireland spend the lowest percentage of GDP in Europe on total social security expenditure (Table 3.11), social security expenditure for sickness/invalidity/occupational accidents (Table 3.12), and the relative percentage total social security expenditure spent on sickness/invalidity/occupational accidents (Table 3.13).

TABLE 3.12 Sickness, invalidity and occupational injury benefits as %GDP, 1980–1994

	1980	1990	1993	1994
UK	6.8	7.1	8.4	—
Ireland	8.5	6.8	7.6	7.4
Denmark	10.0	8.4	9.1	8.8
The Netherlands	14.1	13.7	14.2	13.5
Belgium	9.2	8.8	8.9	9.2
France	8.5	9.2	10.0	9.8
Germany	—	—	11.4	11.5
Mean EU12	8.7	8.8	9.4	—

From Eurostat (2000).

TABLE 3.13 Sickness, invalidity and occupational injury benefits as % of all social protection benefits, 1980–1994

	1980	1990	1993	1994
UK	32.9	32.9	31.3	—
Ireland	43.4	36.6	37.1	36.8
Denmark	35.8	29.2	28.1	27.0
The Netherlands	48.5	44.3	44.5	43.6
Belgium	34.6	34.5	34.5	35.4
France	35.6	34.9	34.1	34.0
Germany	—	—	38.4	38.8
Mean EU12	—	—	35.2	—

From Eurostat (2000).

Table 3.14 gives comparable data about social expenditure for 'disability'. However, note that the OECD and Eurostat definitions are different, so that OECD estimated that the mean EUR15 social security transfer for 1994 was 19.7% of GDP, while Eurostat estimated that mean EUR12 social protection expenditure for the same year was 28.6% of GDP at market prices. The corresponding estimates for the UK were 15.4% and 28.1%.

Attempts are frequently made to relate sickness and disability rates to the wage-replacement rates of social security benefits in different countries, although these are frequently superficial and based on selected and unrepresentative data. As already noted, in almost every country the method of calculating the various possible elements of benefits paid (particularly for long-term incapacity benefits or disability pensions) is so complex that it is not possible to provide any typical estimate of the amount of benefit paid, what wage replacement level this represents or any ceiling. Table 3.15 is one attempt at such a comparison which shows little or no obvious correlation.

TABLE 3.14   Social benefits for 'disability' as % GDP, 1980–1998

	1980	1985	1990	1995	1996	1997	1998
UK	—	—	2.0	3.2	3.2	3.1	3.0
Ireland	0.6	0.8	0.8	0.9	0.9	0.8	0.7
Sweden	—	—	—	4.2	3.9	3.8	3.8
Norway	—	—	3.8	4.0	3.9	3.9	4.2
Finland	3.2	3.4	3.8	4.6	4.5	4.2	3.8
Denmark	2.5	2.4	2.8	3.3	3.3	3.2	3.4
The Netherlands	5.2	4.9	5.1	3.7[1]	3.5	3.3	3.2
Belgium	2.1	2.4	1.9	2.4	2.4	2.3	2.3
France	1.5	1.6	1.6	1.4	1.4	1.4	1.4
Germany	1.6	1.6	1.5	1.9	2.1	2.2	2.2
Mean EU12	1.8	1.9	1.9	1.9	2.0	2.0	2.0

[1]Marked fall 1994–1995.
From Eurostat (2000).

TABLE 3.15   Relationship between benefit levels and short- and long-term incapacity in different countries

Country	Wage replacement for sickness		Male sickness and disability as % of labour force (1995)		
	% wage replacement	Ceiling (ECU/week)	Temporary	Long-term	Total
Denmark	100	357	5.1	4.1	9.1
Germany	90	—	4.6	3.1	7.6
UK	80–90[1]	500	3.1	4.8	7.9
Sweden	80	500	3.3	3.7	7.0
The Netherlands	70	725	4.4	7.6	12.0
Belgium	60	357	3.0	4.1	7.1

[1]Estimated.
Based on data from Tables 2.4 and 3.4.

Conclusion

There is some variation between these different sources of data, as might be expected, but there do not appear to be any major inconsistencies. The UK appears to have broadly comparable levels of disability to other EU countries, and even if self-reported symptoms are slightly lower this probably only reflects cultural variation in reporting [see also Raspe (1993); P Croft, personal communication, 2002 (Raspe H, Matthis C, Croft P, O'Neill. Pain in the United Kingdom and Germany—are the British tougher? Unpublished report)]. It is not possible to draw any conclusions about relative rates of short-term sickness absence because so much is now paid by employers and omitted from the social security statistics in many of these countries. The UK has one of the lowest rates of industrial injury benefits. Eurostat's and Aarts' data suggest that the UK has the lowest rates of long-term incapacity benefits in the the EU countries they compared, although AS/tri suggest it is simply closer to the lower end of the EU range. This may be more true of women than men, and reflect the lower entitlement of women in the UK. The UK showed by far the largest relative rise in the total number on long-term invalidity benefits between 1980 and 1995, but this must be seen against longer-term trends and was probably largely a question of 'catching up'. UK expenditure on long-term invalidity benefits has risen faster than any of the other EU countries compared between 1980 and 1995, but is still (with Ireland) the lowest in Europe. Although musculoskeletal disorders are one of the most common causes of incapacity in all these countries, the UK seems to be unique in its dramatic increase in the *proportion* of long-term incapacity benefits accounted for by back pain. All these analyses show consistently that since the 1970s the Netherlands has had the highest rates of incapacity in any country studied, for both men and women, although some of the data suggest this is mainly for long-term incapacity and may be mainly for older workers. Contrary to popular myth, although Germany has had more stable levels of incapacity than the other EU countries compared and has even managed to reduce them slightly since the mid 1980s, all of these analyses suggest that the total level of incapacity in Germany is about the EU average, and the total figure hides a much higher level of long-term incapacity in older men and women.

4 Social security in individual countries

There is wide variation in the amount of information on individual countries in this review, depending on the availability of information, difficulty finding and accessing sources, and whether it is available in English.

The United Kingdom

Hill (1990) provides an introduction to *Social Security Policy in Britain*. Bolderson (1991), DSS (1993), Lonsdale (1993), Lonsdale & Aylward (1993, 1996) and Rowlingson & Berthoud (1996) provide earlier reviews of social security developments and trends in the UK.

The UK is the second largest EU country with a population of just over 58 million. At least until recently, the UK has had one of the highest marriage rates and the highest divorce rate in the EU with about 30% of births outside marriage and 19% of families with children headed by a lone parent.

In July 2001, the Department of Social Security (DSS) was combined with the Department for Education and Employment (DfEE) to form the DWP. References to the DSS and DWP are more or less interchangeable, depending on date.

The original Beveridge proposals introduced in 1948 were for NI based on contributions from employers, employees and the self-employed. Entitlement to benefits is still largely based on NI contributions although the majority of the funding now comes from general taxation. The original plan was that contributions should be actuarially based to reflect an individual's own prospective benefits, as in private insurance, but this was never implemented. Today, contributions are more a form of general taxation set according to overall revenue needs. Nevertheless, entitlement to NI benefits still depends on having earnings over a certain threshold, and having paid sufficient contributions over a sufficient period of time; being a resident or an employee is not sufficient in itself.

Bolderson (1991) provided a brief overview of UK developments since the Beveridge reforms in 1946–1948. From the mid 1960s, reflecting the changes in social attitudes to disability described above, there was increased government awareness of disability particularly in what was then the combined Department of Health and Social Security, and increasing academic interest and research. This was reinforced by an early government survey of disabled people. There was political pressure for an increasingly social administration approach and to elaborate on the Beveridge plan, and this led to an expansion of benefits. A whole range of additional statutory benefits was introduced in the 1970s, including IVB, Attendance Allowance (AA), Mobility Allowance and non-contributory benefits. These provided better support for long-term incapacity and support for disabled people who had not paid NI contributions. They applied the same Beveridge principles of providing for loss of faculty and function, incapacity for work and loss of the power to enjoy a normal life, but also extended social security for the disabled in that they were non-means tested, non-contributory and unrelated to the cause of disability.

Because of the way it has evolved, the present system of disability benefits is complex, involving a number of different benefits for different people in different circumstances and based on different principles (Lonsdale & Aylward 1993, 1996):

- NI benefits to cover specific risks, mainly for working people
- A system of non-contributory but means-tested benefits which act as a 'safety net' to provide a minimum income
- A number of 'category benefits' which are neither NI based nor means tested but depend on specific entitlement, e.g. maternity, single parents, severely handicapped.

Benefits for sickness and disability fall into all three types. Broadly, benefits provide income support for people who are incapable of work, help meet the extra costs of disability, compensate people for injuries and diseases incurred in the course of their employment, and top up earnings in work.

The original sickness benefits introduced by Beveridge were designed to cover short terms of sickness and assumed that most recipients would soon be fit to return to work, particularly once better health care was freely available to all under the new National Health Service. Unfortunately that dream was not realised. McKewon (1976), a Scottish doctor and epidemiologist, recognised that there is more to health than medical care: in a modern society, health depends more on healthy behaviour and the social and physical environment than it does on public health or professional health services. Glouberman (2001) listed at least 12 'determinants of health': income and social status, social support networks, education, employment and working conditions, socio-economic environments, physical environments, personal health practices, healthy child development, biology and genetic endowment, health services, gender and culture. McKewon (1976) concluded that health policy has to go beyond standard medical services to improve the health of the population, and must address social policy and poverty. The logical conclusion is that social security is as important to health as actual health services.

There were growing numbers of long-term sickness claimants towards the end of the 1960s, so Invalidity Benefit (IVB) was introduced for them in 1971. IVBs were generally slightly higher than sickness benefits, on the assumption that the long-term sick and disabled had greater needs. IVB also gave entitlement to additional benefits which eventually included an Invalidity Allowance for the younger disabled because it was assumed they would have greater loss of earning capacity, and an additional, earnings-related, disability pension for older claimants who had built up sufficient contributions. Provision for those who required care and attention (AA) was introduced in 1971 and for those who had difficulty walking (Mobility Allowance) in 1976.

Severe Disablement Allowance (SDA) was introduced in 1984 to replace two previous benefits for severely handicapped persons of working age who had never worked or who had not paid sufficient NI contributions. The initial plan was that claimants had to be aged less than 20 when disability began and incapable of all work due to at least 80% disablement.

Up until 1995, UK arrangements for social security sickness and invalidity benefits were similar to most EU countries, though from 1983 progressively more short-term sickness benefits were provided by the employer as SSP. Since 1995, the previous social security sickness and invalidity benefits have been replaced by Incapacity Benefit (IB). SSP is now provided by the employer for up to 28 weeks, while various levels of IB provide short-term cover for sickness for those who are not eligible for SSP and longer term cover for incapacity after SSP finishes.

Table 4.1 summarises the present UK social security benefits for sickness and incapacity.

In general, when someone returns to work their disability benefits stop. However, there are now a number of benefit rules which protect benefits on return to work, are designed to support return to work, or facilitate return to benefits if return to work is unsuccessful:

- Disability Living Allowance (DLA) is not affected by return to work (although return to work could raise questions about continuing need, e.g. for mobility component)
- Industrial Injury Disablement Benefit (IIDB) is not affected by return to work.
- 'Therapeutic work' on medical advice, <16 hours and <£60 per week
- Disabled person's tax credit and Working families' tax credit can supplement low earnings for disabled people coming off benefit
- Income Support (IS) and housing benefits may continue under certain circumstances to supplement low earnings.
- 'Back to work bonus', Child maintenance bonus and job grant—one-off payments of up to £1000 in certain circumstances, when coming off certain benefits and moving to full time work
- Housing benefits, council tax benefits and mortgage support may continue for 4 weeks
- Welfare to work benefit protection—if re-claim IB within 52 weeks, return to previous rate of benefit (+ various other 'linking' rules).

Table 4.2 shows the relative number of people on different disability and incapacity benefits and Table 4.3 the distribution of expenditure. Unless stated otherwise, all DWP statistics presented in this review refer to the number of 'recipients' of each benefit which for most benefits is the same as those 'beneficiaries' who actually receive cash payments. However, for IB, a significant number of people who fulfil the incapacity criteria do not have full NI entitlement

TABLE 4.1 Alternative UK social security benefits available to cover sickness and incapacity for those aged <65 years

Claimant	Benefits	Duration (weeks)	Amount per week (from April 2001)
Most employees	Statutory Sick Pay from employer	First 28	Basic £62.20 + employment agreements
	Short-term higher rate Incapacity Benefit	29–52	£62.20 + dependent allowances[1]
	Long-term Incapacity Benefit	53–retirement age	£69.75 + dependent allowances
			+ age <35 £14.65; age 35–44 £7.35
Self-employed, unemployed >3 months	Short-term lower rate Incapacity Benefit	First 28	£52.60 + dependent adult allowance
	Short-term higher rate Incapacity Benefit	29–52	£62.20 + dependent allowances
	Long-term Incapacity Benefit	53–retirement age	£69.75 + dependent allowances
			+ age <35 £14.65; age 35–44 £7.35
			+ £20 if on Incapacity Benefit from pre-1995
Not in regular employment, insufficient National Insurance contributions	Severe Disablement Allowance (>80% disablement)	Age 16–retirement age	£42.15–£56.80 + dependent allowances
	Or		
	Income Support (means tested)		£53.05 + dependent allowances
	+		+
	Disability Premium (ISdp)	Age 16–retirement age	£22.60
	or Severe Disability Premium		£41.55
In addition to the above:			
Injury at work or prescribed disease contracted in a specific occupation	Industrial Injury Disablement Benefit (>14% disablement)	29 weeks–death	20% £22.58 – 100% £112.90
Those whose disability puts them at a *disadvantage in getting a job*	Disabled Person's Tax Credit (means tested)	Age 16–retirement age	Supplement to low earnings:
			£56.05 + various enhancements + dependent allowances
Those who need help with personal care or mobility	Disability Living Allowance Care and Mobility components	Start age 16–65, continue to death	Care: £14.65–£55.30
			Mobility: £14.65–£38.65

Statutory Sick Pay is based on incapacity for the claimant's own occupation; Incapacity Benefit is based on incapacity for all work. Most of the other disability and disablement benefits are based on need and assessed by loss of faculty or disablement. Disability Working Allowance is based on disability and income.

[1]Adult dependent £31.15 for short-term Incapacity Benefit, £39.95 for long-term Incapacity Benefit; each child dependent short-term lower rate Incapacity Benefit nil, all others £11.35.

Most DWP statistics of 'incapacity' include the various types of Incapacity Benefit and Severe Disablement Allowance.

TABLE 4.2   Relative number of recipients of various disability and incapacity benefits (February 1998) (thousands)

Benefit	Total (all ages)	Working age[1]
Statutory Sick Pay	300	300
Incapacity Benefit – short-term, lower rate	109	109
– short-term, higher rate	103	103
– long-term	1459	1337
Severe Disablement Allowance	369	330
Attendance Allowance	1200	—
Disability Living Allowance (care and/or mobility)	1980	1228
Income Support + disability premium	858	858
Income Support + severe disability premium	370	370
Industrial Injuries Disablement Benefit	262	176
War Disablement Pension	270	76
Invalid Care Allowance	370	?

[1]Men 16–64; women 16–59.

TABLE 4.3   Relative spending on sickness and disability

Incapacity Benefit	44%
Disability Living Allowance	24%
Attendance Allowance	13%
Severe Disablement Allowance	5%
Other[1]	14%

[1]Statutory Sick Pay, Industrial Injuries Disablement Benefit, War Pensions, Invalid Care Allowance, Disability Working Allowance, etc.

to the benefit so do not receive the basic cash payment of IB but receive 'credits only'. These 'credits' provide access to a wide range of other financial benefits including NI contributions, other social security benefits and supplements including in particular disability premium if they fulfil the low income and means-tested criteria for IS, and relief of various charges; 53% of 'recipients' of IB now receive 'credits only'. All the other disability benefits considered here do not have any NI contribution requirements, so there are no 'credits only' and virtually all recipients are receiving the cash benefits, apart from very small numbers whose payments are suspended, e.g. when they are in hospital long-term.

The levels of benefits need to be assessed in context. Average UK male earnings are now £436 gross per week (Labour Force Survey Quarterly Supplement Winter 2000/01), which after tax and direct work-related costs such as travel, is equivalent to a net income of something between £300 and £350 per week. This is also approximately the same as the average total household income in the UK (DSS 2000b). So at first sight, flat-rate sickness and disability benefits in the UK [about £70 per week (Table 4.1)] provide very low wage replacement ratios, apparently much lower than in any other country in Europe apart from Ireland. However, all of the above figures refer to the basic rate of each benefit and give a false impression of what a sick or disabled person actually receives, because most recipients receive a range of additional benefits and supplements, while many also have other sources of family income.

DSS Social Security Statistics (2000) provided data on the overlap between the different disability and incapacity benefits (see also Swales & Davies 1998).

Only 40% of sick and disabled claimants of working age receive a single benefit and over 59% receive two or more benefits:

- The two main combinations are IB and DLA or DLA and IS
- 79% of IB beneficiaries (and 28% of those receiving IB credits only) also receive DLA
- 40% of IB beneficiaries (and 97% of those receiving IB credits only) also receive IS
- 89% of recipients of SDA receive DLA and 75% receive IS.

(This implies that for recipients of working age, approximately 80% of DLA functions as a supplement to IB and SDA.)

- 50% of people of working age who are in receipt of IIDB also receive IB (Leigh 2001) and 30% receive DLA (DSS Analytical Services Division estimate 1997).

IS disability premium is only paid (without further assessment) to claimants who already receive or are credited with another disability benefit. In addition:

- Nearly 700,000 people on IB since before 1995 still have 'transitional protection' of earlier entitlements and so receive an average of an additional £20 per week (DWP Analytical Services Division data July 2001)
- 13% of IB recipients receive additional payments for dependent(s).

The above analysis is limited to social security benefits. Certain benefits may also lead to entitlement to various 'top-up' housing, mortgage assistance, and other allowances or relief which can add up to significant amounts. Nor does this allow for Local Authority spending and benefits in kind.

It has been estimated (UK Government Green Papers 1998a,b) that as many as 90% of UK employees now have some form of occupational sick pay and about 75% are covered by occupational invalidity and pension arrangements (86% of men and 77% of women in full-time work, and 35% of women in part-time work) and in general these produce benefits comparable to other EU countries. In 1995, the last year when most employers received reimbursement for SSP, this amounted to £770 million per annum. (This is the best available estimate of SSP, though it was actually of DSS/Inland Revenue 80% reimbursement which was not the full SSP paid by employers. After 1995, reimbursement was severely curtailed and no estimate of SSP is available.) By 1995, 11 million employees were in a company pension scheme and 8 million people had a private pension (although there may be an unknown degree of overlap). The TUC (2000) estimated that employers also pay about £750 million per annum in civil litigation costs for industrial injuries. Many occupational and private pension schemes pay for early retirement due to illness or disability. Private pensions pay out a total of £30 billion a year, compared with DWP retirement pensions of £47 billion (the state also provides another £20 billion tax relief for pension contributions), though this is largely for people over retirement age and it is not possible to estimate how much is early retirement related to disability. However, DWP statistics show that 18% of long-term IB recipients are now receiving an occupational or private pension with an average value of £85 per week and 5% receive >£150 per week.

Moreover, this is still largely focused on individual earnings and does not allow for other sources of household income: 70% of IB recipients are married or cohabiting; 18% have a partner who is earning; there are no data on how many have a partner with an occupational pension; 6–9% have a partner who is also on IB (DWP Analytical Services Division data 2001). The end result is that recipients of IB are now spread fairly evenly across the income distribution and a quarter of recipients are now in the top 40% of income. This is also consistent with the 1996/97 Disability Follow-up to the Family Resources Study (Grundy et al 1999) which found that average gross weekly household income ranged from £146 for a disabled adult living alone (29% of the disabled) to £395 for a disabled adult living with a partner and children (32% of the disabled).

Thus the actual income of someone with long-term disability in the UK is much higher than appears from the basic flat-rate level of IB, at least *provided* they are male, have full NI entitlement and have a partner. Moreover, many IB recipients are unskilled and have limited earning capacity, far short of the average wage, and wage replacement ratios should be calculated on a more realistic estimate of the wages they would be likely to obtain and the hours they would be likely to work if they managed to obtain employment. On this basis, a recent analysis on the Policy Simulation Model showed that compared with 40 hours per week at the minimum national wage of £4.10 per hour, current IB recipients have a median wage replacement ratio of 70–90%.

Dorsett et al (1998) followed up 1947 people leaving IB between June and November 1996 and found that their net weekly income at the end of their IB claim was £171 and at interview 5–10 months later was £177. However, there were two sharply divergent courses of leaving IB. One-third left IB voluntarily, 68% of them returned to some form of work and their income at follow-up rose to £234. The other two-thirds were disallowed IB following the *All Work Test* (see below), only 19% of them returned to work and their income at follow-up ranged from £130 to £152.

Finally, about a quarter of disabled people, particularly if they are younger, female or single, and have limited NI entitlement to benefits (quite apart from the question of their disability), actually receive very limited financial benefits from the social security system above the very low level of basic IS for poverty. This is again consistent with the contrast between the average gross weekly household income of a disabled adult living with a partner and children (£395) and that of a disabled adult living alone (£146) (Grundy et al 1999).

To put it in a different context, Table 4.4 compares the relative value of alternative social security benefits, and shows that in almost every situation there is a financial advantage to being disabled or incapacitated rather than unemployed or in poverty.

Table 4.5 shows the age distribution of recipients of incapacity and disability benefits.

Most recipients of disability and incapacity benefits remain on benefit long-term with very slow turnover, but there is also a high turnover of short-term claims (Swales & Craig 1998). The Association of British Insurers estimate that the average duration of an SSP claim is about 3 weeks, which is similar to DWP estimates (Table 4.6). There is no data on SSP

TABLE 4.4 Basic weekly rates of different benefits for a single person aged 25–35 with no dependents

April 2001	Amount	Conditions	Duration
Jobseekers Allowance (Unemployment)	£53.05	Means tested Conditional on seeking work	6 months
Income Support (with no premiums)	£53.05	Means tested	Retirement age
Income Support + disability premium	£75.65–£94.60	Means tested	Retirement age
Long-term Incapacity Benefit	£84.40 (+£20 if from pre-1995)	Not means tested	Retirement age
Industrial Injury Disablement Benefit	£22.58–£112.90	Not means tested Independent of earnings	Life

TABLE 4.5 Age distribution of beneficiaries of Incapacity Benefit (IB) and Severe Disablement Allowance (SDA) (February 2001)

Age (years)	IB (%)	SDA (%)
<24	5	14
25–34	13	18
35–49	32	30
50–59	36	23
60–64	15	7
65+	—	7

From DWP Incapacity Benefit and Severe Disablement Allowance. Quarterly Summary of Statistics, Feb 2001.

TABLE 4.6 Duration of Statutory Sick Pay (SSP)

Duration of SSP (weeks)	% returned to work	% still off work
1	35	65
2	55	45
8	90	10
28	99	1

Based on Association of British Insurers statistics, personal communication, 2001.

for back pain separately, although from other international data it is likely to be longer than average.

DWP administrative data show that the average duration of spells of IB is: short-term, lower-rate 13 weeks; short-term, higher-rate 18 weeks; and long-term 2.26 years. However, because of the very skewed distribution, current recipients of long-term IB have been on benefit for an average of 5–6 years. Nearly half those currently receiving long-term IB were in receipt of Invalidity Benefit (IVB) before it was replaced by IB in April 1995, and are still on benefits.

There is very little turnover of those on SDA; the average duration of those currently on SDA is 16–17 years, and once on SDA few come off it except when they reach retirement age or die.

Disability

Estimates of the disabled population and their needs in society vary greatly with the source of the data, the way the information is obtained, the definitions used and the exact wording of the questions (Table 4.7):

- The Census and General Household Surveys asked whether people have a long-standing illness which limits their activities
- The OPCS Disability Surveys and the Disability follow-up to the Family Resources Survey used severity of disability scales
- The Labour Force Survey defined the disabled as those having a (self-reported) work-limiting, long-term, health problem or disability.

TABLE 4.7   Prevalence of disability (% of those aged over 16 living in private households)

Source	Date	Millions	%
Census	1991	6.4	14.9
General Household Survey	1993–1994	8.6	24.2
Labour Force Survey Summer	2000	5.4	15.0
OPCS Disability survey	1985	5.8	13.5
Disability follow-up to the Family Resources Survey	1996–1997	8.6	19.7

In addition, there are 0.52 million disabled people in communal establishments, although 80% of them are aged over 65 years (Census 1991).

The Labour Force Survey (Summer 2000) found that:

- There are >6.6 million people in the UK with some form of self-reported, long-term disability—nearly one-fifth of the working-age population
- The prevalence of disability increases with age: 9% of those aged 16–17 years, 34% of those aged 50 to state pension age
- 3.1 million disabled people (48%) are in employment (12% of all people in employment). However, disabled people are only half as likely as non-disabled people to be in employment
- Back and neck conditions account for 18% of self-reported disabilities
- Employment rates vary greatly with the type of disability: back and neck conditions are about average (46%); employment rates are lowest for people with mental illness (17%)
- Unemployment rates are nearly twice as high for people with long-term disabilities compared with non-disabled people (9.4% cf 5%)
- Disabled people are nearly seven times as likely as non-disabled people to be out of work and claiming social security benefits (40% cf 6%).

Table 4.8 shows that 43% of disabled people on social security benefits say they would like to work. However, when the question is made more stringent, only 7% of those on

TABLE 4.8 Disabled people's availability for work

	All social security benefits (%)	Incapacity Benefit (%)
Would like work	43	37
Available for work	15	7

Based on data from the Labour Force Survey, Summer 2000.

sickness or disability benefits say they would actually be available for work (Labour Force Survey, Summer 2000).

The prevalence of limiting long-term illness and disability reported in the General Household Surveys increased very slightly from about 15% to 17% between 1975 and 1995, although it fluctuated and there was no clear trend. This must be interpreted against a more dramatic rise from 21% to 35% for all self-reported illness over the same period, despite gradually improving objective health parameters. The 1996–1997 Disability Follow-up to the Family Resources Survey (Grundy et al 1999) suggested that the prevalence of disability reported in 1996–1997 was much higher than that reported in the 1985 survey and considered that this was not accounted for by any methodological differences. However, the authors emphasised this does not necessarily reflect a true increase in disability, but that responses to questions about disability may be more strongly influenced by the context in which they are asked and the general socio-economic and employment climate than is sometimes assumed.

Disability data from the Labour Force Surveys suggests that the number of people of working age reporting a long-term health problem or disability which affected their working life increased gradually from about 10% to about 14% of the population of working age between 1984 and 1997–1998, partly due to an increase in the number of older workers, though also due to changes in the definition and wording of the questions. However, a Technical Report (Labour Force Survey 1998) suggested this rise is probably due mainly to changing attitudes towards and increased awareness of disability rather than any 'real' change in the level of disability. The prevalence of most forms of pain and disability is slightly higher in women, although the difference is slight and this must be viewed against a general tendency for women to report bodily symptoms and concerns more readily. The prevalence rises markedly with age, from about one in seven of those aged 16–44, to about one in three of those aged 45–64 (Table 4.9). Again, these are all data from self-report questionnaires and must be interpreted accordingly.

TABLE 4.9 Prevalence of self-reported, limiting, long-standing illness

Age	Men (%)	Women (%)
0–15	7	7
16–44	14	16
45–64	31	32
65–74	42	40
75+	50	55

From General Household Survey (OPCS 1996).

The prevalence of self-reported disability varies with ethnic group (Table 4.10), although this is not reflected in DWP disability and incapacity benefits. (There are no published data on the ethnic distribution of benefits.)

TABLE 4.10   Ethnic variation in self-reported disability in various OPCS surveys

Ethnic group		% self-reported disability
White	– born in the UK	12.6
	– born in Ireland	17.0
Black	– Caribbean	11.0
	– African	7.0
Asian	– Pakistani	9.3
	– Indian	9.0
	– Bangaladeshi	9.0
Chinese		4.0

The 1996–1997 Disability Follow-up to the Family Resources Survey collected population data from >5000 disabled people about their disability, their extra needs and costs, their use of services and DSS benefits received (Craig 1996, Craig & Greensdale 1998). The measure of disability was based on the 1985–1988 OPCS Disability Surveys, and collected self-report data on difficulties in performing 13 everyday activities:

- Locomotion
- Reaching and stretching
- Dexterity
- Seeing
- Hearing
- Communication
- Personal care
- Continence
- Behaviour
- Intellectual functioning
- Consciousness
- Eating, drinking and digestion
- Disfigurement

A single disability index was produced by combining the individual's three most severe disabilities into a weighted sum. This bears some similarity to the assessment of need for DLA and the *All Work Test* for IB (see below). However, it can be seen from the items that they may, at least in principle, be more relevant to severe levels of disability and the elderly than to incapacity for work in those of working age. Craig (1996) pointed out this may produce a very different measure of disability than other measures.

The 1996–1997 Disability Follow-up to the Family Resources Survey (Grundy et al 1999) estimated that about 20% of the adult population of the UK had some self-reported disability according to the definition used. Many reported quite mild disability. About 4% of the adult population reported severe levels of disability with scores of 7 or more out of 10, but this was heavily skewed by age, with a prevalence of such severe disability rising from 1% of those aged 16–19 to 12% of those aged 80+ years.

From the disability surveys, back pain is the most common disabling condition in men and women (Table 4.11). It leads to one of the lowest levels of economic activity for any physical condition (Table 4.12). Perhaps surprisingly, then, the associated level of social security benefits for back pain is more or less in proportion to the prevalence (Table 4.13).

There are several detailed surveys of low back disability in Britain. Mason (1994) found that 11% of adults said that back pain had restricted their activities during the past 4 weeks. Almost all those aged 16–24 years only had restrictions for a few days. However, there was surprisingly little difference between those aged 25 to over 65 years. About one-third had restrictions for 1–5 days and about one-third had them for the whole 4 weeks. The effect on their life-style varied, and was mainly restriction of normal activities in the home, garden, sports or mobility.

TABLE 4.11   Prevalence of the main disabling conditions (as % of people with limiting health problems)

Disabling condition	Total	Men	Women
Back or neck	19	17	20
Chest or breathing	13	13	14
Heart, blood pressure, circulation	11	14	8
Legs or feet	11	12	10
Mental health problems	8	7	9
Arms or hands	6	6	7
Diabetes	4	5	3
Difficulty seeing or hearing	4	4	3
Skin	2	2	2

Based on data from Labour Force Survey (2000), Twomey (2001).

TABLE 4.12   Percentage economic activity by disabling condition

Skin	77
Diabetes	72
Chest or breathing	69
Difficulty seeing	55
Difficulty hearing	70
Heart etc	52
Back or neck	50
Legs or feet	48
Mental health	22
All long-term health problems	52

Based on data from the Labour Force Survey (2000), Twomey (2001).

TABLE 4.13   Comparison of relative proportion of various disabilities and main disabling conditions in recipients of various DSS benefits

Main disabling condition	Population report (prevalence) (%)	Incapacity Benefit (%)	Income Support + disability premium (%)	Severe Disablement Allowance (%)
Back or neck	19	22	18	14
Chest or breathing	13	15	15	6
Legs or feet	11	15	15	16
Mental health problems	8	14	14	6
Difficulty seeing or hearing	4	2	2	3
Diabetes	4	2	1	1
Skin	2	1	1	—

From Labour Force Survey (2000), DWP Statistics.
Approximately 50% of social security benefit recipients have more than one illness or disability, of which mental health problems are the most frequent secondary diagnosis.

Walsh et al (1992) reported the only population survey in the UK to use detailed clinical measures of low back disability. They assessed eight activities of daily living to give a total disability score from 0 to 16. Table 4.14 shows the 1-year and life-time prevalence of low back disability by age and sex.

Hillman et al (1996) carried out a community survey of 3174 adults aged 25–64 in Bradford in 1995. The point, 1-year and life-time prevalence of low back pain (LBP) was 19%, 39% and 59% with an annual incidence of 4.7%. Over a 1-year period, 50% of episodes were <2 weeks, 21% lasted 2–12 weeks and 26% were >3 months duration. In the previous

TABLE 4.14   One-year and life-time prevalence (%) of back pain, disability and time off work by gender

		Age				Total
		20–29	30–39	40–49	50–59	
Men						
Back pain	1-year	35.4	37.1	38.2	40.5	37.6
	Life-time	52.0	60.4	64.2	70.5	61.3
Disability score >8/16	1-year	4.1	5.8	6.6	5.3	5.4
	Life-time	8.2	12.6	20.8	23.1	15.9
Time off work	1-year	9.5	13.5	9.4	9.5	10.6
	Life-time	22.4	31.3	38.2	46.2	34.1
Women						
Back pain	1-year	27.0	33.6	43.7	35.7	34.8
	Life-time	45.2	53.8	62.3	63.7	55.8
Disability score >8/16	1-year	2.1	4.7	5.7	5.6	4.5
	Life-time	7.7	13.1	16.4	15.8	13.1
Time off work	1-year	6.1	5.1	9.8	6.5	6.8
	Life-time	16.9	18.4	29.8	29.8	23.3

From Walsh et al (1992).

12 months, 21.8% of employed people with LBP reported that they had taken time off work because of their back—a total annual prevalence of 6.4% for all adults aged 25–65. Sickness absence because of LBP declined with increasing age. The authors pointed out, however, that there could be considerable local variation and it is not possible to extrapolate these figures to the entire country.

The most recent Omnibus Survey conducted in March–June 1998 (ONS 1999) found that 40% of adults said they had suffered from back pain in the preceding 12 months. One-third of those with back pain said that it had restricted their activities in the previous 4 weeks; 5% of those aged 16–64 who were employed said they had taken time off work in the previous 4 weeks because of back pain, although only 2% had received a medical sick certificate; 13% of those aged 16–64 who were not employed gave back pain as one of the reasons.

All of these data are based on self-report which for various reasons is probably an over-estimate (Table 4.15).

TABLE 4.15 Varying estimates of the impact of back pain

Source of information	% adults of working age
Questionnaire—1 month prevalence of back pain	38
Questionnaire—restricted activities during last month or year (usually only for a few days)	10–15
Marked disability on a detailed disability questionnaire	6
Questionnaire—time off work in past year	5–10
Employment estimates of long-term work incapacity	Approximately 1
Social security benefits for long-term back incapacity	Approximately 0.3

Based on Waddell (1998).

There is conflicting data on any regional variation in the prevalence of LBP, disability, work loss or incapacity, and no convincing evidence of any significant UK regional variation in the underlying pathology or impairment (Waddell 1998).

Warton et al (1998) carried out a national survey in 1995–1996 of approximately 5000 DSS claimants who were not working, studying their characteristics and experiences and comparing those who reported a health problem that affected the kind of work they could do ('disabled' claimants) and those who did not ('others'). Disability was defined and measured by the claimant's response to a simple question: 'Do you have any health problems or disabilities which affect the kind of paid work which you can do?' However, there was no objective or external check on the accuracy of the responses and the analysis made no attempt to allow for possible selection bias. One-quarter of these claimants stated they were disabled: 32% of the disabilities were musculoskeletal; 85% expected their disability would last longer than a year. Disabled claimants were typically older, less qualified, less likely to have been employed before their current spell out of work, and more likely to live alone. Disabled and 'other' claimants were looking for the same kind of jobs and shared the same fears and concerns about returning to work, though 27% of disabled claimants had the additional concern that they would not be fit enough to work. Disabled claimants were more pessimistic about getting work, and the number of job applications declined more with age among disabled claimants than among the 'others'.

When they were re-interviewed 2 years later, 39% of all initially disabled claimants had recovered or failed to mention a health problem. For those over age 45 years, only 22% of disabled claimants recovered but 16% of the 'others' of that age developed a health problem during the follow-up period. During the 2-year period of the study, 56% of disabled claimants returned to work compared with 73% of the 'others', but more of the disabled only returned to part-time work and they were more likely to stop work again. The median period out of work for disabled claimants was 6 months or more, while for the 'others' it was 3 months or less. Disabled claimants who had been employed immediately before claiming benefits, who were still working part-time while on benefits, who had better qualifications and who had a driving licence were more likely to return to work.

This survey concluded that, effectively, disabled claimants are in double jeopardy. Not only do they have a disability which may affect their ability to work, disproportionate numbers also have limited qualifications and work experience which create further barriers to securing work.

Over the last 30–40 years, disability has had a progressively higher public profile and the 20th century was finally labelled 'The disabled century' (BBC2 10 June 1999). A report on institutionally disabled people in the early 1970s described them as 'the socially dead' and led to the concept of 'care in the community' though there was little actual shift in resources. However, there was gradually increasing social consciousness of disability, increasing demand for the rights of disabled people, and disabled people themselves developed a greater political voice and lobby. During the 1980s and 1990s, disabled people gained progressively greater civil rights enshrined in legislation, though the 1995 Disability Discrimination Act is still criticised by disabled people and their organisations because it does not include any power of enforcement. In the 1990s, disabled people have become more militant and the major rights focus has been on access: Direct Action Network (DAN) is now prepared to break the law to get public attention. Despite these political advances, disabled people still suffer major social disadvantage: 6 of 10 disabled people of working age are not in work; 3 of 4 disabled people live below the official poverty level. The latest emphasis is on 'Disabled Pride'.

The provisions of the Disability Discrimination Act to provide 'suitable and reasonable adjustments' to occupational duties or to offer alternative work can be applied to the dismissal or return to work of employees with a long-term disability of >12 months duration (as opposed to the recruitment of such individuals which is the primary focus of the Act). An example of one of the early cases was a health service worker who was sacked 16 weeks after sustaining a lifting injury to his back at work following which he continued to have chronic pain and whose orthopaedic surgeon could not predict when he would be fit to return to work. He claimed that he had been discriminated against as a person with a disability, but lost his employment tribunal claim at the employment appeal tribunal and in the Court of Appeal. However, by 2000, employment tribunals awarded compensation to 47 cases for discrimination on grounds of disability (Equal Opportunities Review www.eordirect.com).

Rehabilitation services

Beveridge (1942) did not make any detailed or specific proposals for rehabilitation services, but did stress throughout his report that they were a fundamental assumption of his social security plan. He put forward three general propositions:

- That rehabilitation must be continued from the medical through the post-medical stage until the maximum of earning capacity is restored and that a service for this purpose should be available for all disabled persons who can profit by it irrespective of the cause of their disability
- That cash allowances to persons receiving rehabilitation service should be the same as training benefit
- That rehabilitation services, like medical treatment, should be free and universally available.

The Tomlinson Report (Tomlinson 1943)—an *Inter-departmental committee on the rehabilitation and resettlement of disabled persons*—was produced about the same time. The opening words recognised that 'The successful rehabilitation of a person disabled by injury or sickness is not solely a medical problem' and that 'close co-operation between the Health and Industrial services is necessary throughout the whole process. Ordinary employment is the object and is practicable for the majority of the disabled—with the goodwill and co-operation of the representative organisations of employers and work people, in conjunction with the Health services and the responsible Government Departments'. The Tomlinson Report made recommendations on how this should be organised: about the responsibilities of various government departments, the establishment of a Joint Committee representing the departments concerned, and legislation for a register of disabled persons, employment quotas, resettlement and sheltered employment.

The Disabled Persons (Employment) Act 1944 was based on the Tomlinson proposals and introduced measures designed to assist disabled people (particularly ex-servicemen at the end of World War II) to re-enter the labour market. It was administered by the Department of Employment. There was an official register of disabled persons which enabled them to claim various kinds of assistance, but registration was voluntary. There was a distinction between disabled people who were considered to be capable of regular work and those considered unlikely to cope with ordinary competitive industry because of the nature or severity of their disability. Employers with 20 or more employees had to employ at least 3% of registered disabled people but this was impossible to enforce and was widely recognised to be ineffective. The sheltered employment programme was for the more severely disabled who were unable to compete on the open labour market: this scheme was very effective for individuals but the numbers were always limited and questions were raised about its cost-effectiveness. Employment Rehabilitation Centres (ERCs) provided for people who needed more help than simply job finding or employment counselling and assessment but only about 15,000 people completed ERC courses each year, and 88% of them were men. In the early 1990s the government also encouraged the growth of rehabilitation services in the voluntary and charitable sector but these probably only dealt with about 3000 people each year. After the 1995 Disability Discrimination Act, this entire system was dismantled and the disabled register, quotas and sheltered employment have now virtually disappeared.

Government and professional interest in rehabilitation flourished during and immediately after each World War to retrain disabled servicemen and establish remedial work, but in each case interest waned rapidly. After World War II, isolated employers like the RAF and the mining industry continued to provide rehabilitation. The Piercy Report (Piercy 1956) reviewed the general provision of rehabilitation, training and resettlement for all disabled people. Two decades later, the Department of Health and Social Security (England and Wales) published the Tunbridge Report (Tunbridge 1972) and the Scottish Home and Health Department published the Mair Report (Mair 1972), both of which considered the deficiencies and failures of current services and made recommendations on 'the future provision of rehabilitation services, their organisation and development'. Another two decades later, there was yet another consultative document from the Department of Employment (1990) but although this again laid out goals and principles it made no firm recommendations and little happened in practice. None of these reports had any real impact.

Despite the original recommendations of the Tomlinson Report and the implicit support of the Beveridge Report, the UK never developed a national rehabilitation service, unlike some EU countries such as Germany. The NHS and the social security system generally ignored rehabilitation issues which remained completely separate and unlinked to either health care or the receipt of benefits. Several experimental schemes during the 1960s and 70s to develop links between health care and employment came to nothing or were limited to individual efforts. At least up to 1992, there was also not much liaison between the Department of Social Security which provided benefits to replace earnings for disabled people and the Department of Employment which provided rehabilitation and other measures to foster re-employment among disabled people (Lonsdale & Aylward 1993, 1996). Consequently, there was very little link between sickness or invalidity benefits and rehabilitation. For many years, the policy for most sick and disabled people and their social support or re-employment was either/or. They were either assessed as incapable of work by a medical practitioner and therefore eligible for social security benefits, or they were assessed as capable of work and had to take their place in the job queues alongside everyone else. As already noted, prior to the introduction of the Disability Working Allowance (DWA) in April 1992, the UK system did not recognise 'partial incapacity'.

Rehabilitation services remained fragmented and unco-ordinated, but nevertheless by the late 1970s and early 80s there was a diverse range of hospital rehabilitation departments, RAF rehabilitation units, miners rehabilitation centres, medical and employment rehabilitation centres, special training centres, demonstration centres and various centres established by voluntary organisations. Given adequate government and professional support, these might have served as the basis to develop proper rehabilitation and vocational rehabilitation services. Unfortunately, that support was never forthcoming and recent years have seen the demise of many of these facilities and initiatives (Frank et al 2000).

Nocon & Baldwin (1998) reviewed rehabilitation in the UK and suggested that actual delivery has always fallen far short of the statutory provisions. In practice, most rehabilitation is provided by the NHS (and that largely by the hospital service) and takes the form of physiotherapy. Yet CSAG (1994a) found that in the early 1990s only 2% of NHS patients with back pain received physiotherapy within the first 3 months of sickness absence. Every report has stressed the key role of the general practitioner, but in practice most have little or nothing to do with occupational issues or the rehabilitation of their patients. Vocational rehabilitation facilities are much more limited and the potential of non-health-care settings is underdeveloped. Rehabilitation is a statutory element of some social services and implicit in others, but in practice social services do not recognise or implement this. In general, there is no clear definition and allocation of responsibility for rehabilitation. Nocon & Baldwin (1998) found considerable geographical variation, and some confirmation of the decline in the availability of rehabilitation over the past decade. In reality, only a small minority of sick workers in the UK receive any active or effective rehabilitation other than routine physiotherapy and this is often delayed.

The TUC (2000) produced a consultation document on rehabilitation in the UK—Getting Better at Betting Back. They pointed out that Britain's record on rehabilitation is unimpressive and that in general there still seemed to be a prevailing attitude that getting injured and ill people back to health was the sole responsibility of the NHS, and getting disabled people back to work was simply a matter of treating their medical condition. Unfortunately, this was often ineffective. They considered that occupational health services in the UK 'have withered over the past 20 years'. The TUC was concerned about the current lack of adequate provision and access to high-quality rehabilitation services in the UK, even while recognising that there were major obstacles to funding and development, and that remedying the situation might take considerable time. They pointed out that, traditionally, work-place injuries and rehabilitation have focused on serious physical trauma. These injuries were catastrophic and rare, and most people with such serious injuries did have access to rehabilitation. Their major concern now was for the 'less serious' but much more common and equally disabling 'work-place illnesses' such as back pain, musculoskeletal disorders and stress-related disorders. There was an implicit assumption throughout the consultation document that work is often the cause of these conditions, which from the remainder of the present review may be open to debate. Nevertheless, this consultation document raised a number of valid and important points.

The TUC estimated that British employers were paying about £750 million per annum in compensation to pay off people injured at work—rather than spending some of this money on rehabilitation to get them back to work.

The TUC proposed the fundamental principle that: 'People who are injured or made ill by their work should have a right to return to health and return to work so that they can maintain their earnings and continue their careers'.

- Employers should have a mechanism in place and an action plan to deal with work-related injury or illness. All too often, valuable time is lost either in arguments about what to do, trying to work out what to do, or simply ignoring the problem
- All employers should have a rehabilitation policy similar to the legislative requirement to have a health and safety policy
- Early intervention is the key to successful rehabilitation, so the rehabilitation process needs to be triggered almost immediately the injury or illness has been recognised
- Throughout, the active involvement of the injured worker and his or her representative(s) is vital
- It supports the Australian system of a non-medical 'case manager' whose primary duty is to the injured person and who should have sufficient control over resources to ensure that rehabilitation is effective
- The case manager and the injured person [and/or their representative(s)] should agree on a work plan which sets out the steps needed to restore health as far as possible and to return to work.

A British Society of Rehabilitation Medicine Working Party Report *Vocational Rehabilitation: the Way Forward* (Frank 2000), a College of Occupational Therapists conference (June 2001) and a *British Medical Journal* editorial (Disler & Pallant 2001) have all reiterated the same messages. Consistent criticisms throughout all of the reports and from disability pressure groups, academics and within government are the lack of provision, the lack of co-ordination and the division of responsibility between government departments and other agencies. However, despite repeated reports and recommendations, none of this has led to any real change in policy or provision of services. Frank (2000) concluded that 'looking back at the development of vocational rehabilitation (in the UK) from the time of the first world war….the development of services has been piecemeal, unco-ordinated, lacked adequate investment and been inadequate for society's needs. Moreover, looking at today's depleted services….they are woefully inadequate in the scope, content and standards which might reasonably be considered appropriate for the beginning of the twenty-first century'. Everyone, including disabled people, health professionals, policy makers and politicians clearly acknowledges the need for and the goals of vocational rehabilitation. Disabled people and the various professional groups involved are convinced of the value of rehabilitation but unfortunately there is a lack of hard scientific evidence on its effectiveness. Until that evidence is available, UK politicians and policy makers remain unconvinced and highly sceptical that expenditure on rehabilitation would be effective or cost-effective.

Current political reforms do aim to get people off benefit and into work, which should be beneficial for the individual, the Exchequer and society (UK Government 1998a,b). HM Treasury tends to focus on the labour market and (dis)incentives and job availability is a major issue, but other factors also help to determine the ability and willingness of individuals to compete in the labour market. Gardiner (1997) reviewed 42 early experimental schemes in the UK to get people 'from welfare to work':

- Training and education programmes
- Job search measures

- Incentives for employers
- Public job creation
- Out-of-work benefits
- In-work benefits
- Assistance with job-related costs
- Transitional assistance measures.

Gardiner (1997) also identified the major barriers individuals faced in returning to work:

- Personal characteristics such as work experience, health problems and caring responsibilities
- Disincentives for spouses to work created by the benefits system
- Problems due to loss of assistance with mortgage costs on moving into work
- Uncertainty about making the transition, particularly relating to the possible reclaim of benefits in the future
- Lack of information on the options available.

Overall, they considered that these schemes probably could have a significant impact, but there was insufficient data to draw any firm conclusions.

Chitty & Elam (1999) edited papers from a joint DSS/National Centre for Social Research seminar *Evaluating Welfare to Work*. In this seminar, Lewis & Walker (1999) also reviewed UK initiatives over the past decade and concluded that 'the evidence shows that relatively few people are long-term unemployed through choice and that, instead, those who find themselves out of work for long or recurrent periods are trapped by a combination of barriers'. They summarised the barriers as:

- The individual's own (lack of) skills and experience or 'human capital'
- The labour market
- Broader social and psychological circumstances
- The benefit system itself.

Lewis & Walker (1999) categorised the content of key return to work initiatives as:

- Out-of-work benefits
- Job search support
- Training and education
- Work experience
- Employer incentives
- Transitional arrangements
- In-work benefits and work incentives.

Finally, Lewis & Walker (1999) listed what they considered to be the successful features of welfare-to-work policies:

Content:

- Information about the financial viability of work
- Job search support and career guidance

- Investment in human capital
- Employer subsidies and incentives
- In-work benefits and transitional support
- Addressing multiple issues.

Delivery:

- Conditionality and active signing regimes
- Streamlining delivery
- Delivery through personal advisers
- Flexibility in delivery
- The role of compulsion
- Targeting delivery
- Role of contracted providers
- Delivery of welfare to work to employers.

The New Deal for Disabled People (1998) (UK Government Green Paper 1998a, www.newdeal.gov.uk) funded some 20 small Innovative Schemes to test new ways of helping disabled people into work. No complete report on these schemes has yet been published and anecdotally most of them failed to produce any good evidence of effectiveness. However, one scheme showed promising preliminary results. Watson *et al* (2001) studied 84 IB and Jobseekers Allowance recipients with chronic LBP who had not worked for a mean of 38 months (44% on IB; 65% actually stopped work because of LBP). The initial study was in Salford and the study was then replicated in Bristol. A partnership between employment, health and vocational training agencies provided an occupationally focused rehabilitation programme of physical rehabilitation, psychological support and vocational counselling, all based on pain management principles. Fifty-six per cent of those who were referred joined the programme; 97% who started completed the programme; and 39.5% of those who completed the programme were employed at 6-month follow-up (Salford 43%, Bristol 36%). A further 26% were in job training, education or voluntary work. These studies were small but the results are very impressive and show that at least some of these apparently intractable patients can be helped into employment provided suitable cross-agency support is provided. Further roll-out and a proper randomised controlled trial is being planned by the DWP.

Back pain is currently one of eight priority areas for the UK Health and Safety Executive (HSE). In May 1999, the Department of Health and HSE jointly launched 'Back in Work' pilot initiatives in England and Wales. The objectives were:

- To identify and develop innovative ideas to tackle back pain in the work place
- To develop and disseminate good practice
- To improve work-place health and raise its status.

Nineteen small pilot studies were commissioned and funded for up to £50,000 and each ran for 12 months from 2000 to early 2001: 13 of 18 addressed prevention, 12 of 18 the delivery of various forms of treatment, and 12 of 18 'rehabilitation'; 14 of 18 specifically dealt with manual handling; 11 of 18 to at least some extent considered general working practices and policies.

Because of the limited funding and time scale, most studies were barely able to set up and run for a few months and it was not possible to conduct proper outcome evaluation. The full report is presently being collated and written up, but preliminary results have been presented (DoH/HSE 2001). From these it appears that:

- The pilot studies generally consisted of various small groups of health professionals 'doing their thing'. There were some interesting and productive new collaborations, e.g. between employer, union, occupational health and manual handling, but no really innovative approaches
- The employees were generally satisfied with the services they received. Employers' reactions were more mixed: some were satisfied and supportive but others were more sceptical
- There is no evidence that any of the pilot schemes had any real impact on back pain, sickness absence or long-term incapacity (although no evidence does not necessarily mean no effect).

The DWP are conducting feasibility studies for much more extensive Job Retention and Rehabilitation Pilot (JRRP) schemes. About 4–6 JRRPs throughout the UK will run from September 2002 for 2 years, each funded for £2–3 million and covering the entire population of a selected area (e.g. Glasgow). People who have been on sickness absence for any reason (of which back pain, other musculoskeletal and mental health conditions are the most common) will be screened to identify those with >50% risk of going on to chronic incapacity. These patients will be randomly allocated to a health-care intervention, an occupationally focused intervention, the two combined or a control group of usual NHS care. Each JRRP involves an extensive multidisciplinary team and will test innovative packages of health care and occupational interventions based on the current evidence. The primary outcome will be the proportion going on to IB at 28 weeks.

Social security reforms in the 1980s

By the late 1970s, the political argument was between building upon and extending the Beveridge design versus rationalising and extending means testing of social security benefits (Hill 1990). During the 1980s, the UK social security system experienced increasing structural problems particularly within the public pension and health-care sectors (Ollson et al 1993). Social security accounted for nearly one-third of all public expenditure, was the fastest growing sector of public expenditure and was the largest employer of non-industrial civil servants (and still is). In contrast to the expansion of the 1970s, during the 1980s a changed political climate and concern about rising social security expenditure led to progressive cuts in state provision of benefits for the disabled.

The spiralling costs of welfare led to political reaction and welfare retrenchment. Grimshaw (1999) considered that the Thatcher government which came into power in 1979 'saw the welfare state as one of the prime causes of poor economic performance. Its funding required high taxation, it discouraged work and investment, and encouraged welfare dependency. The cushioning effects of social programmes led workers to sustain unrealistic wage demands that destroyed competitiveness'. The Thatcher ideology encouraged individuals to provide for themselves with minimal state provision for need and increased reliance on private charity and help. Anything more than minimum state provision led to welfare dependency and undermined the individual's commitment to self improvement ('moral hazard'). Conservative governments from 1979 to 1997 argued that reform of welfare was essential and had the clear intent of 'rolling back the state' and keeping the lid on public spending. This welfare retrenchment at a time of economic turmoil weakened the safety net just when more people were facing job and financial insecurity. Particular concerns (from the perspectives of costs and of social need) were and remain pension provision, long-term care for the elderly, mortgage protection and unemployment insurance.

During the 1980s, the Conservative government implemented a consistent and long-term policy to transfer a large part of the economy to the private sector. Best known were the privatisation of public companies, the compulsory tendering of major parts of the public service, and changes in the housing sector, but there were also major changes in the social security system. For example, the UK is now the only EU state in which private pension schemes, including both company pensions and individual arrangements, can substitute for part of the statutory state scheme rather than simply supplement it. The goal of Thatcherism was to reduce state involvement and expenditure, but in practice demographic changes, the increased number of pensioners and rising unemployment actually had the opposite effect. Paradoxically, also, the shift to more means testing increased social security administrative costs. Apart from that fundamental political shift, however, the reforms also addressed some very real social security problems. The previous system of sickness benefit had a major structural problem of effectiveness. There was duplication of work between employers and the Department of Social Security, with both paying benefits during most short spells of sickness, so many claimants received parts of their benefits from two sources. In the 1970s and 1980s there had been a tremendous growth in occupational sick pay which was used as a political justification to reduce the need for the state to cover these early periods. Incentives to work were also considered to be reduced by the combined effects of high benefits and tax exemptions.

In 1983, responsibility for short periods of sickness was largely transferred to employers in SSP. The duration was initially for 6 weeks in a tax year, but was progressively extended by 1986 to cover up to 28 weeks in any one period of sickness. These 28 weeks of incapacity do not have to be continuous, and spells of sickness that are separated by <8 weeks can be linked together. The statutory minimum level of SSP is still low compared with most European countries, although higher sickness benefits are generally considered a natural and important part of employment contracts. It is estimated that 91% of the work force now have some occupational sick pay (UK Government Green Papers 1998a,b), although there are considerable differences in wage replacement levels and the duration of sick pay between various groups of employees. White collar workers and public employees generally have 90–100% wage replacement. Blue collar workers, however, generally have much lower wage replacement, often closer to the statutory minimum SSP level. Initially, when the scheme started in 1983, employers were able to reclaim in taxation 100% of the SSP they paid. From 1985, they also received allowance for the NI contributions they paid on workers while they were receiving SSP. However, the continuing growth in occupational sick pay led to the government reducing these allowances and from 1991 employers could only recover 80% of SSP paid, although special arrangements were made for small employers in certain circumstances. Trade unions and employees criticised the decrease to 80% repayment of SSP, but the government argued that it had been balanced by other changes in the NI structure. After 1995, reimbursement was severely curtailed. Independent assessment from Scandinavia in the early 1990s (Olsson et al 1993) considered that the SSP system in the UK had been implemented efficiently and that government, employers and trade unions generally regarded the system as functioning well. One of the major aims of SSP and these progressive changes was to shift the incentives and responsibility for control of sick pay on to employers, although politicians claimed it also improved the partnership between government and employers. In theory, both employers and trade unions should be well aware that profitability and wages were directly influenced by the costs of sickness absence. In reality, a recent study of The Cost of Sickness Absence (UNUM 2001) found that UK employers, managers and human resources departments still do not have proper statistics or accounting of sickness absence, are unaware of the costs, and generally underestimate the real costs by at least a half.

Olsson et al (1993) also pointed out that by the late 1980s the rather high level of social exclusion in the UK was regarded as a persistent and very serious problem. Marginalisation through early retirement and invalidity benefits was increasing year by year, despite the fact that UK employers had to pay more of the costs. The reasons for this trend were not clear, although some observers suggested that institutional and individual incentives in the sickness and invalidity benefit systems might have an important and growing influence. One of the major possible disadvantages of the arrangements at that time might be to increase the financial incentive on employers to get rid of workers who were at increased risk of long-term sickness. Even if terminating employment involved short-term financial costs to the employer, these were measurable and often outweighed by the probable long-term savings on uncertain future sickness costs and production losses. Once employment was terminated, that worker was no longer the responsibility of, or of interest to, the unions. And once someone was on long-term invalidity benefit and/or employment-related pension, the costs no longer fell directly on the employer, but on the NI or Pension Funds. The fallacy, of course, was that ultimately society must bear these costs through taxation and pension contributions, of which employers shoulder a large share. For the individual case, however, the long-term gain to the employer of terminating employment was 100% relief of any direct costs, while the long-term costs were indirect, diluted and dependent on future levels of taxation and pension fund contributions.

The Social Security Act of 1986, implemented by 1988, was based on three main objectives:

- The social security system must be capable of meeting genuine need. Resources should be directed effectively to areas of greatest need

- The social security system must be consistent with the government's overall objectives for the economy. The tax burden on future generations should be reduced. Incentives for people to take up work should be improved. The system should encourage greater individual responsibility and choice
- The social security system must be simpler to understand and easier to administer.

In practice, the main effort at that time was to reduce and simplify the administration of social security benefits. The previous Supplementary Benefits were regarded as complex, too easily available, insufficiently targeted, difficult and costly to administer, and very costly, so they were replaced by IS which aimed to encourage individual responsibility and choice, be easier to administer and control, and less costly.

A small but significant reform in 1988 attempted to facilitate return to work. Benefits could be retained while people attended rehabilitation courses and the therapeutic earnings limit was greatly increased. Unfortunately, that had little impact in practice.

More generally, Marsh & Rhodes (1992) and Bradshaw (1992) questioned whether the Thatcher policies were effective in practice. They transferred some of the costs of sickness to employers, stopped full indexing of benefits and increased means testing, but social security expenditure and disability benefits continued to grow.

Invalidity Benefits up to 1992–1993

Hills (1997) provided data on UK welfare spending from 1921 to 1995 (Figure 4.1). There was a slight peak in the early 1930s at the time of the Great Depression, and a steady rise after World War II until the mid 1970s. From 1973 to 1996 it fluctuated with the economic cycle. Total welfare spending includes social security, health, education, pensions,

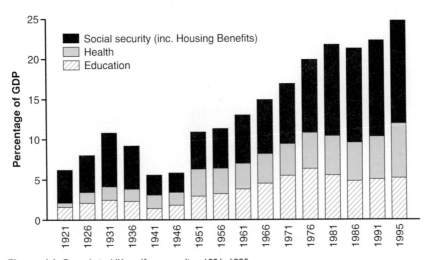

Figure 4.1 Growth in UK welfare spending 1921–1995

Reproduced from Hills (1997) with permission

housing and personal social services (Figure 4.2). From 1973, the share of health and social security gradually increased. Social security expenditure rose from 4.7% of GDP in 1949–1950 (the first full year of the post-Beveridge social security system) to 12.3% in 1992–1993 (the last year before the major reform). From 1978–1979 to 1992–1993, it grew an average of 3.7% per annum in real terms which was equivalent to an underlying rate of around 3% if benefits to the unemployed were excluded (DSS 1993).

During the 1970s and 80s the number of people on IVB grew by 215%. In contrast, there was a negligible rise in the number of people on Severe Disablement Benefit (SDA). The number of people on IS with disability premium (ISdp) only started to increase in the late 80s. Table 4.16 shows the growth in the number of people on IVB from 1971 when the benefit was first introduced until 1991, just before the 1992–1993 reforms.

The number of women on IVB was always less than the number of men for three main reasons: the smaller proportion of women in the labour market, the significant proportion of woman working part-time with earnings below the threshold for membership of the National Insurance (NI) scheme, and the married women's option (described below). However, although the number of women was always lower than men in absolute numbers, the rate of increase was greater for women. Between 1971 and 1991, there was a 192%

TABLE 4.16 Number of recipients of Invalidity Benefit from 1971–1991 by age and sex (thousands)

Age	1971		1980–1981		1990–1991	
	Men	Women	Men	Women	Men	Women
<40	31	14	60	37	84	77
40–49	46	18	72	25	126	75
50–59	106	46	162	51	291	140
60–64	139	2	176	5	273	37
65+	12	0	47	0	201	0
Total	334	81	517	116	976	330

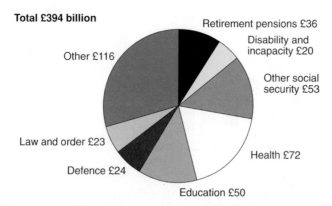

Total £394 billion

Retirement pensions £36
Disability and incapacity £20
Other £116
Other social security £53
Law and order £23
Defence £24
Health £72
Education £50

Figure 4.2 Distribution of UK government expenditure 2000 (billions)

increase in the number of men and a 307% increase in the number of women on IVB. Some of the increase among women could be explained by a change in the social security rules which enabled more married women to claim certain NI benefits from which they had previously been excluded. Up to that time married women could choose to pay a reduced rate of NI contributions which meant they were not entitled to most NI benefits including IVB. In 1976 this option was abolished although those already on the reduced option could choose to continue. Together with the increasing number of married women entering employment, this meant that more married women then fulfilled the contribution conditions of IVB and so the number of married women eligible for and receiving IVB rose faster than men or unmarried women. Although IVB no longer exists, this general trend is likely to continue as more women come into the NI system.

By far the greatest increase in receipt of IVB was among older men and women. By 1991 about 80% of men and about 50% of women receiving IVB were aged 50+ (Table 4.17). Unlike many other social security benefits, people on IVB who reached the state retirement age (60 for women, 65 for men), could choose to stay on IVB for a further 5 years rather than transferring to the state old-age pension. The immediate advantage was that IVB was not taxable in contrast to the state old-age pension which was counted as taxable income. Between 1971 and 1991, men over retirement age still on IVB showed a dramatic increase from 12,000 to 201,000 (from 4% to 21% of all male recipients). Women over retirement age showed a similar increase over the same period from 2000 to 37,000 (from 2% to 11% of all female recipients). From 1979, the proportion of IVB recipients with occupational pension schemes and the proportion of income from occupational pension schemes also increased (Central Statistical Office 1989).

All the above data are about the increasing number of people on IVB (the IVB *population*), but in contrast Table 4.18 shows little change in the number of *new* recipients starting IVB each year from 1980 to 1991.

This is shown graphically in Figure 4.3. In contrast to the size of the IVB population which more than doubled between 1980 and 1991, over that period there was actually a slight initial decline in the number of new awards to men while the number of new awards to

TABLE 4.17 Age distribution of Invalidity Benefit recipients (1991)

Age	IVB (%)		SDA (%)		Isdp (%)	
	Men	Women	Men	Women	Men	Women
<40	9	23	59	33	45	37
40–49	13	23	16	21	25	27
50–59	30	42	12	28	30	36
60–64	28	11	7	11	n/a	n/a
65+	20	0	6	7	n/a	n/a
Total (thousands)	976	330	116	178	192	182

TABLE 4.18   Annual number of new spells of Invalidity Benefit 1980–1991 for those under pension age (thousands)

Year ending	Total	Men	Married women	Other women
June 1981	357	277	58	22
June 1982	296	223	54	19
April 1983	299	220	55	24
April 1984	273	202	53	18
April 1985	264	193	53	18
April 1986	276	201	56	20
April 1987	278	197	63	18
April 1988	276	196	58	22
April 1989	280	198	58	24
April 1990	284	208	52	24
April 1991	288	204	57	27

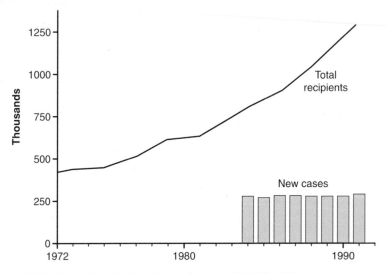

Figure 4.3 Numbers of Invalidity Benefit awards in the UK, 1972–1991

both married and other women remained about the same. At that time, the government actuary's department estimated that over the next 60 years, demographic trends alone would predict a relatively stable annual number of men starting IVB but an increasing number of all women starting IVB because of changing patterns of female participation in the labour market and changes in the NI rules.

The size of the benefits population depends on the number starting benefit, how long they stay on benefit, and the number coming off benefit. These statistics show that the large increase in the number of IVB recipients was not due to any increase in the number of people coming on to benefit, but rather due to more people staying on IVB longer and fewer coming off benefit (Figure 4.3). However, there were some differences between men and women. In 1981, 45% of men who started IVB were still on it by the end of the first year, but by 1989 that figure had risen to 79%. Those leaving IVB were most likely to do so during their first or second year on benefit, but very few left after the second year. The pattern was similar for both married women and other women, but although more women were getting IVB and they were tending to stay on benefit longer, they were still more likely than men to return to work within the first year.

Lonsdale & Aylward (1993, 1996) summarised the number of disabled people on various benefits at the end of 1991 (Table 4.19).

TABLE 4.19 Number of recipients of various disability and invalidity benefits (1991)

Invalidity Benefit (IVB)	1,306,000
Income Support with a Disability Premium (ISdp)	365,000
Severe Disablement Allowance (SDA)	294,000
Industrial Injury Disablement Benefit (IIDB)	192,000

All of those on ISdp would be receiving some other form of disability benefit. Some of those on IIDB might also be receiving other benefits.

To put this in perspective, DSS (1993) estimated the number of people (in thousands) on various social security benefits at any one time in 1992–1993 (in a total population of approximately 55 million and employed population of 27 million) (Table 4.20).

TABLE 4.20 Number of people receiving various social security benefits in 1992–1993 (thousands)

Sickness Benefit	135
Statutory Sick Pay	330
Invalidity Benefit	1490
Attendance Allowance	765
Disability Living Allowance	935
Severe Disablement Allowance	320
Industrial Injury Disablement Benefit	295
Total sickness and disability benefits	4270
Retirement Pension	9910
Unemployment Benefit	715
Income Support	5320
Housing Benefit	4315

Factors influencing the growth of the numbers on Invalidity Benefit

The National Audit Office (1989) prepared an independent report on the growth of recipients of IVB during the 1980s. This report found no major increase in the incidence of incapacitating disease but considered the evidence suggested the growth was due to non-medical factors. They identified three principal trends underlying the growth: each year more people came on to the benefit than came off and on average individuals were receiving benefit longer; the average age of recipients was increasing; and the proportion of married women receiving benefit was increasing. Although benefit conditions had been tightened, the numbers receiving IVB were expected to continue to grow.

Lonsdale & Aylward (1993, 1996) reviewed a number of DSS research projects during the 1980s which studied factors that might influence the receipt and duration of IVB. Most of these studies were econometric and ranged from an analysis of Census data for 1971 and 1981, to a programme of research into the 'wider costs of unemployment' using Family Expenditure Survey data, to an analysis of a sample of NI statistics.

Many of these studies considered the interaction between labour market processes and disability insurance. In the early part of the 1980s, rising unemployment coincided with an increase in the numbers of people in receipt of IVB, and it was thought that higher unemployment and worsening labour market conditions induced withdrawal from the labour market through a discouraged worker effect (Disney & Webb 1991), and an increase in the proportion of men settling for the status of being disabled (Piachaud 1986). Another argument for a causal association between the growth of unemployment and IVB was suggested by Disney & Webb (1990) to be more employer discrimination at times when there was a surplus of labour. 'When unemployment is rising, employers can choose from a greater pool of applicants and so will tend to pay greater attention to the past history of applicants such as medical records.'

Piachaud (1986) analysed census data from 1971 and 1981 on men aged 55–69 and found that both the levels and changes in the number of men defined as disabled were related to levels and changes in unemployment. Any increases were predominantly in the older age groups. He concluded that the impact of unemployment was to make older men accept disability status more readily when their job prospects were poor. He attributed about half the rise in disability to the worsening labour situation, and about half to other factors such as an increase in the value of IVB relative to unemployment benefit, and changing individual, medical certification or administrative standards of disability.

Holmes et al (1991) analysed a 1% sample of IVB recipients between the years 1975–1976 and 1983–1984 to examine the determinants of starting and remaining on IVB and the difference between men and women. Both men and women had an increasing likelihood of starting IVB with increasing age, if they had a history of sickness-related benefits, if they lived in areas of poor housing, poor employment structure and high unemployment, if they had been registered unemployed, if they were low paid, or if they were older and entitled to higher IVB rates. There were some differences between married and other women. The number of married women starting IVB was particularly related to labour market conditions such as the local rate of female unemployment and local job opportunities. Non-married women were more likely to start IVB the higher their rate of benefit entitlement.

Holmes et al (1991) found similar determinants of the time people remained on IVB. Both men and women were more likely to remain on IVB the older they were (especially in the age group 55–65), the lower their level of previous earnings and the higher the level of benefit received, if they had a history of sickness-related benefits, or if they lived in areas of poor housing and high unemployment. People aged 55–65 who were in an occupational pension scheme were likely to stay on IVB longer, although the opposite effect occurred in younger age groups. Among recipients who had been on IVB for more than a year, the longer an individual had been on IVB, the longer he or she was likely to remain on it: 'duration dependence'.

Holmes et al (1991) also found that over the period under study, there was an increase in the proportion of new claimants with characteristics associated with longer claim duration. There was an increase in the average age of new claimants, the proportion who were contributors to an occupational pension scheme, married women, and those with a history of unemployment.

Disney & Webb (1990) used Family Expenditure Survey data from 1979 to 1984 to show that the growth of IVB receipt was faster in geographical regions where unemployment grew more rapidly. On multivariate analysis, they found variations in IVB receipt across time and region to be positively and significantly associated with variations in the rate of unemployment, the proportion of the eligible population aged 55+ years, and the wage replacement rate of IVB. These findings were repeated using a number of different econometric methodologies and in every analysis Disney & Webb (1991) found the dominant variable to be unemployment: higher unemployment was associated with greater numbers on IVB.

The puzzle, as Disney & Webb (1991) found when they extended their analysis to the latter part of the 80s, was why IVB continued to increase even when unemployment rates began to fall. It is possible that to some extent this was an artefact: the fall in the official unemployment rate was based on those receiving unemployment benefit which might not be an accurate reflection of those available and looking for work (Beatty et al 1997). Nevertheless, this was unlikely to account fully for the continuing trend.

Several of the above research findings might help to explain the continued rise in IVB. First, Holmes et al (1991) found that the longer someone was on IVB the longer they were likely to remain on IVB (duration dependency) and an increasing proportion of new claimants also had characteristics associated with long duration claims. So an increasing proportion of IVB recipients would have a reduced chance of coming off benefits, producing a 'hysteresis effect'. Once on IVB for a few years, recipients were likely to have lost contact with, and knowledge about, the labour market. Their skills might have been superseded by others. Their drive and confidence in applying for and securing a job might have fallen. They were likely to be less attractive to employers when there was a surplus of labour, particularly if it was younger and cheaper. The older they were, the stronger these effects were likely to be.

Secondly, the number of recipients of both unemployment benefits and IVB, and the relationship between the two rates, might be influenced by changes in the social security benefit rules. Improved employment opportunities could have been offset by the rising financial attractiveness of IVB which was also more generous than unemployment benefit. The basic rate of IVB plus the higher-rate Invalidity Allowance (IVA) was worth over 50%

more than the basic rate of unemployment benefit. In addition, while the basic rate of IVB and IVA increased in line with inflation, the Additional Pension component had increased much more, and an increased proportion of recipients received Additional Pension among all age groups. As already noted, tightened eligibility for unemployment benefit could also have increased the incentive to claim an alternative benefit like IVB. All the studies summarised above found that not only unemployment but also benefit levels affected the likelihood of receiving IVB. If falling unemployment was to reduce the number on IVB, the effects would need to occur among the older men who formed the bulk of IVB recipients. The incentive for them to return to work was rather weak because of the attractiveness of IVB through its non-taxable status and relatively higher value.

In all of these studies, the three common factors associated with the increasing numbers on IVB were unemployment, age and benefit levels. It seemed clear that higher rates of unemployment generally or locally, being in an older age group, and entitlement to higher rate of IVB were all factors which increased the likelihood of receiving and remaining on IVB during the 1980s. Disney & Webb (1991) suggested that there might then be a hard core of IVB recipients, particularly those who were older, who had been on IVB longer, or who were receiving higher financial levels of benefit, who would be likely to remain on IVB regardless of the level of unemployment. Once a person is assigned incapacity status, this may become almost irreversible in the current economic climate and especially if the person was approaching retirement age anyway.

Dorsett et al (1998) commented retrospectively on the underlying assumptions about the rise in the number of people claiming disability benefits at the time of introducing IB. One view saw the rise in the number on IB recipients in terms of two factors:

- The characteristics of people claiming benefit, particularly that a significant proportion were people capable of (at least some) work who should therefore not be receiving benefits
- The excessive ease with which some people appeared to be able to claim and receive IVB. Methods of assessing incapacity were inadequate and administered by family doctors who were (over)sympathetic to their patients' self-report of incapacity for work rather than based on the true severity of their medical condition.

Since many recipients were men in their 50s and early 60s, it was assumed that IVB was simply providing an alternative financial and socially acceptable route into early retirement.

Dorsett et al (1998) again stressed that very little of the increase in the numbers of IVB was explained by increased claims but rather by people remaining on IVB longer, and argued this was due mainly to demographic changes and technical issues. Demographic factors included the changing age structure and the increasing number of women in the work force. There were changes in the labour market which made it harder for IVB recipients to move off benefit and into work. The most important technical issue was that IVB could continue tax-free beyond retirement age.

Berthoud (1998) suggested that what had happened was that the 'employment threshold' had gradually moved down the severity scale, so that a large number of people claimed benefits on the grounds of incapacity in the 1990s who would not have been doing so in the 1970s. Some observers concluded that these were people who were capable of work despite their health problem, but they had made a conscious choice to depend on social security rather than work. Berthoud contested that these incapacity trends must be seen in the context of much wider and systematic shifts in employment patterns. He suggested the growth was more likely to be due to two simultaneous and interacting social changes:

- As the supply of labour had expanded faster than demand, employers had become more selective in their choice of staff. Marginal workers, such as disabled people, had been disadvantaged and excluded
- Social attitudes about work and who should work had changed. It had become accepted that if people had health problems and if these made it difficult for them to work, they need not work and social security benefits were an entitlement with less stigma than previously. Disabled people now demanded the same recognition and status as pensioners.

Medical assessment

A report by the National Audit Office (1989) on the growth of IVB focused particularly on the roles of general practitioners (GPs) and the Regional Medical Service (RMS) in the control process. This was followed by an internal review within the Benefits Agency Medical Services.

Up to 1992, all disability and invalidity benefits relied heavily on medical assessment and certification. Medical certification by the caring physician (usually the patient's own family doctor or GP) was the core administrative mechanism in the initial claim for sickness benefit, SSP and IVB. In 1988, GPs signed approximately 14 million certificates, of which some 4 million were for people who had been sick for at least 6 months. The RMS provided independent medical assessments for the DSS which occupied a pivotal role in the administrative mechanism which controlled access to, and exit from longer-term benefits. In 1988, approximately 750,000 claimants were referred to the RMS, and in about 80% of cases the RMS medical adviser agreed with the GP that the claimant was unfit for work (National Audit Office 1989). Medical assessments for SDA, IIDB, AA, War Pensions and Supplementary Benefit were carried out by medical advisers employed directly by the DSS.

For IVB, claimants had to be 'incapable of work by reason of some specific disease or bodily or mental disablement'. For benefit purposes, work meant employment or self-employment and could be on a full- or part-time basis. The medical certificate provided by the caring physician rested (and still rests) on the doctor's opinion that:

- The patient is unable to work because of their physical or mental disorder (limitation) *or*
- Although physically and mentally capable of work, it would be prejudicial to their health to undertake it (restriction).

When the patient had been incapable of work in their normal occupation for 6 months or more and was likely to remain incapable of that work, the certifying doctor was expected to consider the patient's fitness for alternative work.

Most medical certificates are based primarily on physical or mental incapacity for work and DWP assessments for IVB (and IB) focus almost entirely on that question. However, with a condition like back pain, many caring physicians also appear to have some lingering concern about work possibly being 'prejudicial to their health' based on an outmoded model of injury and avoidance of activities that might provoke or aggravate symptoms. This approach is increasingly difficult to justify in the face of increasing scientific evidence and current clinical guidelines that the best management for back pain is to keep active. The DSS has always taken a more stringent view about possible 'harm' and in practice have limited this to conditions where work may result in 'a substantial risk to the mental or physical health' of the patient or others.

The National Audit Office (1989) surveyed GPs and found that 38% had received no routine training or advice on medical certification, and only 19% had consulted the DSS guidance handbook which was issued to all GPs. Only 47% recognised their responsibility to assess their patient's fitness for alternative work, and in practice few considered that option (Ritchie et al 1993).

In practice, although medical factors alone were supposed to be used to measure incapacity to work for benefit purposes, other factors such as sex, age and experience could not be ignored. 'In practice, capacity to find and keep a job, even for people with identical impairments, will be affected by the interaction of their impairment with factors such as their age, sex, qualifications and experience, accessibility and employer discrimination' (Rowlingson & Berthoud 1996). It is therefore not surprising that a DSS study by Ritchie et al (1993) found that many complex factors influenced family doctor's judgements of their patient's capacity for work when issuing sick certificates. The patient's medical condition and its impact on employment potential was always high on the list. However, it was almost immediately linked to a whole range of non-medical factors, including the patient's prospects of finding work, their age, their motivation to find work, the financial and psychological consequences of returning to unemployment or job search, and the potential for rehabilitation or training. NHS doctors whose primary professional responsibility was to care for their patients often found it impossible to separate the medical condition from these social issues when assessing capacity or incapacity for work. This was likely to be even more difficult with certain conditions like psychological or psychosomatic symptoms, subjective complaints or chronic conditions with a fluctuating course. The National Audit Office (1989) survey also found that GPs were influenced by very practical considerations about the impact of loss of benefit if a medical certificate was refused (43%), particularly allowing for the patient's family and social circumstances, and Job Centre requests to claimants to obtain a sick certificate (28%).

Up to the 1980s, the major cross-check on GP certification and further medical information for longer-term benefits were provided by independent medical assessments carried out by medical advisers from the RMS or employed directly by the DSS. The RMS was previously part of the Department of Health (DoH), these doctors were employed by the DoH (many of them being GPs employed on a part-time basis), and their primary responsibility was to health care. Medical assessments for the DSS were a secondary part of their work, carried out on a quota basis. Some had little interest and most had little training in disability assessment, and this led to a lack of clear evidence and a lack of objective, robust decisions. There was no quality control. Mental health problems were particularly difficult to assess and it became almost impossible to exclude claimants from benefit. Pain and subjective conditions such as fatigue, ME and back pain with 'psychological overlay' were equally difficult. The 'easy' decision was to pass many claimants as 'fit within limits' without giving any clear assessment of fitness or unfitness for their regular work or for alternative work.

The RMS had provided a reasonable service to the DSS in earlier times when only small numbers of benefit claimants needed to be assessed, but they were unable to maintain this service as the numbers of claimants increased greatly from the 1960s onward. By the late 1980s, both the DSS Benefits Agency and the National Audit Office were dissatisfied with the RMS. The National Audit Office Report (1989) found that many of the part-time staff in the RMS had inadequate training and were uncertain about their role in the DSS benefits system. There was concern about the poor quality of some medical reports, the number of cases requiring a second opinion or an independent consultant's reports, and ensuing delays. There was lack of training, guidance and monitoring. The National Audit Office Report was particularly critical of significant weaknesses, administrative delays and lack of control of the whole process of awarding benefits by local DSS offices. Anecdotally, from the early 1980s, the political and administrative 'climate' of IVB was considered to be one of increasing leniency and lack of monitoring and control by the DSS. In contrast, claimants for the various other disability benefits were assessed by medical advisers employed directly by the DSS, who were mostly full-time, had more training in disability assessment, and had a primary responsibility to the DSS. Eligibility and assessment for these benefits were always more tightly controlled and enforced.

Lonsdale (1993) pointed out that in practice the social security definition of incapacity had also been widened by an extensive body of appeal case law that developed over time and made it more difficult for adjudicators to disqualify recipients from IVB. During the 1980s, an increasing number of adjudications were made without a medical examination. Of those who were independently medically examined for the DSS, the proportion assessed as capable of some form of work fell from 27% in 1981 to 18% in 1991 (Lonsdale & Aylward 1993, 1996).

As a result of these criticisms, the medical assessment service previously provided by the RMS was taken over by the DSS itself in England from April 1991, in Scotland from 1992 and in Wales from 1993. From that time, between about 1992 and 1994, doctors employed directly by the Benefits Agency Medical Service progressively took over assessment work for all disability and incapacity benefits. These doctors were mainly full-time, more experienced and better trained in disability assessment, and this had a particular impact on problems like back pain. During the same period the Benefits Agency introduced a rudimentary form of functional assessment (at the time when the All Work Test was being developed—see below). The medical assessment form used a matrix which linked assessment to decisions, and back pain was used as the first example because of its frequency and importance. There was also much tighter quality control and administrative control of medical assessments and awards of benefits.

These structural changes were paralleled by and reflected cultural developments in the whole Benefits Agency medical assessment system, from about 1991 to date. There was increasing recognition of the need for training, leading to the emerging speciality of Disability Assessment Medicine, which has had a separate professional qualification since April 2000 and has been accredited with the General Medical Council as a separate speciality from June 2001. All Benefits Agency Medical Services doctors must now be 'approved' which involves specific training, successful completion of several stages of the approval process, and the continuing demonstration of satisfactory work standards.

There was also progressive focus on and scrutiny of social security problem areas, including back pain, with efforts to improve assessment of these particular conditions. Accumulating scientific evidence and changed clinical thinking about back pain, and the Clinical Standards Advisory Group Report on back pain (CSAG 1994a) were acknowledged by the Benefits Agency Medical Service to have had significant impact on social security thinking. These changes progressively affected all benefits, first IVB, then DLA and finally IB with the introduction of the *All Work Test* from April 1995. That process has continued since.

Welfare reforms from 1992–1993

By the early 1990s, the 'soaring cost' of social security and claims that it was 'out of control' got a great deal of political and media publicity in the UK. The Secretary of State for Social Security set out the aim 'to improve the system to make it better focused to protect the vulnerable, to ensure we all have the means to cope with the needs and contingencies of modern life and to make sure the system does not outstrip the nation's ability to pay'. It is perhaps telling that most of the government publications (DSS 1993; Lilley 1993; Social Security Advisory Committee 1993) were all about expenditure. Even if it was against a background of increasing political consciousness of the rights of disabled people, there was little fundamental debate about social needs, or utilisation of resources, or the choices society faced in addressing these needs and demands.

In the Mais Lecture, the Secretary of State (Lilley 1993) set out some propositions for reform:

- There are no easy solutions
- The reform of something as vast as the social security system is best carried out sector by sector rather than by the 'big bang' approach
- Any effective structural reform must involve either better targeting or more self-provision, or both
- Means testing is not the only way of targeting benefit more closely on need
- The existing array of benefits—contributory, universal and income-related—are rather more targeted than some comment suggests
- No one has the right to opt out of contributing to help those who cannot provide for their own needs but there is no reason in principle why people should not (in addition to contributing to others) opt to make provision for themselves privately rather than through the State system

- Contracting out inevitably involves a switch from pay-as-you-go to fully funded provision
- Disincentives are inherent in statutory benefits
- The more the provision for needs and risks is monopolised by the State the less the incentive to work and save to provide for them.

The Ninth Report of the Social Security Advisory Committee (1993) made additional comment on several of these propositions.

Disability Living Allowance

AA was previously available for severely disabled people of any age, under quite strict criteria of disablement. AA was replaced in April 1992 by DLA for those under age 65, and continued as AA under different rules for those over age 65. In general, the new eligibility criteria were less stringent. As a result of the OPCS reports on disability (see above), DLA was deliberately set at several levels to extend lower levels of benefit to people under age 65 with lesser degrees of disability who still required help.

DLA (Table 4.21) is a non-means-tested and tax-free benefit for severely disabled people under age 65, consisting of two components:

- A *care* component, for those who need help with personal care to attend to bodily functions or a need for supervision/watching over to prevent substantial danger, or help to prepare a cooked main meal

TABLE 4.21   Benefits Agency DLA leaflet 1991

DLA		
is a new benefit for disabled people		
Customer service	Cost effective	High quality process
Customer choice	Single adjudication for Care and Mobility	Review process is seen to be meaningful
Customer dignity respected		
Medical involvement is the exception, not the rule	Make best use of scarce resources	Disabled people are involved in the process
Streamlined processes for the rapid clearance of claims, reviews and appeals	Essential evidence only	Independent appeals process
	Maximum use made of existing information	Independent, non-medical adjudicators
Effective enquiries	Streamlined processes for rapid clearance of claims, reviews and appeals	Special rules cases dealt with quickly and sympathetically
Targeted publicity providing clear positive messages		
Reliance on information provided by the customer	High quality and effective communication	
SELF ASSESSMENT			
Medical involvement the exception, not the rule	Emphasis on effect rather than medical condition	Essential evidence only	Reliance on information provided by customer

- A *mobility* component (higher rate), for disabled people who are either virtually unable to walk or in whom the exertion required to walk would lead to a serious deterioration in their health, or (lower rate) who are able to walk but need guidance or supervision out of doors from another person.

AA continued for all those over age 65 who needed help with personal care or needed supervision, but it did not include any mobility component.

The introduction of DLA, AA and DWA was accompanied by a fundamental change in the assessment system, which moved away from medical examination to self-assessment as the main source of information about the impact of disability (Lonsdale & Aylward 1993, 1996). This decision owed more to intense campaigns by the disability lobby and political pragmatism than to any independent evidence. The DSS received few complaints and considered that many claimants, at least for AA, were 'pleased by the standard of medical examinations and the services they received'. However, disabled people and organisations representing them expressed concerns that such examinations did not always offer the best method of determining a person's care and mobility needs. Some claimants found the examinations intrusive and distressing. A medical examination, even lasting an average of 1.5 hours, might only assess the disabled person's clinical condition and resulting disability at one point in time, which might not be representative of the global and continuing needs which disability imposed. Objective disability evaluation as used in the US might be most scientifically valid, but is complex, time-consuming, costly, and might be considered intrusive and insensitive by disabled people. So it was decided that assessment should focus more on what disabled people themselves and those who cared for them, either professionally or personally, had to say about the practical everyday effects of disability. Self-assessments were judged to be the most obvious way of achieving this. There was widespread consultation which gave a resounding endorsement for this approach from disabled people and organisations representing them. The design and format of the new claims packs adopted a clear layout, large print and easy to understand language. Indeed, one of these claims packs won an award for the clarity of its language. However, it was also recognised that not all disabled people would find it easy to complete the self-assessment sections, so a number of supporting arrangements were made to provide flexibility. The questions focused on disability rather than impairment because surveys had shown that disabled people generally found them easier to answer and more relevant, e.g. it may be easier to say that one can not walk (the disability) than to explain the medical reason why one can not walk (the impairment).

The major weakness of the DLA assessment is that it is heavily dependent on the claimant's own report of their functional capacity, and *self-report* has different connotations from *self-assessment*. From the clinical literature on back pain, such self-report of disability depends not only on the underlying medical condition but may also be strongly influenced by psychosocial factors (see Figure 1.3). It is also open to conscious exaggeration.

The possible advantages of the self-report form as a control mechanism on claims are that it does impose a more stringent demand on the claimant to provide detailed information, and the psychometric properties could permit some checking on the validity of the pattern of responses. In practice, claimants quickly adapted to the new claims system, with assistance from advisers and support agencies. At that time, it was not politically acceptable to introduce any form of psychometric checking on validity.

In practice, one of the main controls on claims is to compare the claimant's self-assessment of disability and needs with what is regarded as 'normal' for their particular condition. The *Disability Handbook* (Aylward et al 1998) provides such guidance to assist DLA/AA adjudicators and tribunals. If the lay adjudicator still cannot decide the claim on the basis of the claimant's self-assessment form together with any accompanying information from relatives, carers or professionals, they refer the claimant to the Benefits Agency Medical Service for independent medical examination which attempts to judge the effect(s) of the claimant's medical condition on each functional area. So although routine and unnecessary medical examination is avoided, doctors still have a key role.

Sainsbury et al (1995) evaluated DLA and AA awards. By that time the number of DLA awards was 50% higher than originally forecast. The new lower rate criteria did successfully distinguish between people with differing levels of need, but the distinction was blurred. Lower rate recipients were only slightly less severely disabled, but tended to have particular disability in personal care, dexterity, seeing and communication. The majority of claimants had no or few difficulties with the application form although a substantial minority, particularly those with mental illness, had a lot of problems, despite the mechanisms to assist these people. Satisfaction with the benefit was closely correlated with whether the application was successful.

Disability Working Allowance

At the same time, in April 1992, concern about the possible financial disincentives facing a disabled person wishing to return to work led to the introduction of the Disability Working Allowance (DWA). The immediate aim of DWA was to eliminate the benefits trap in which a disabled person returning to part-time, relatively low-paid work might be worse off than being on benefits. DWA was a completely new type of benefit which provided a graduated 'top up' to earnings to maintain a positive incentive to work. It differed from previous disability income replacement benefits in that it was targeted at disabled people who wished to do some work yet still needed some support. So it was designed to provide long-term help for people who had a significant disability, and short-term rehabilitative help for people recovering from an illness. This was really the first UK attempt to address the problem of partial incapacity.

Before it was introduced, the DSS estimated that 50,000 people might receive DWA. About 20,000 claims for DWA were received in the first 6 months but only 2100 were allowed. Many claims were made by people who were not entitled to the allowance, usually because they were not already receiving one of the qualifying benefits to which DWA applied, or they were not in paid work. Research indicated that some people made claims without reading the information provided. Others did read and understand the information but nevertheless made a claim so that the DSS could check whether or not they were really ineligible. This particular problem gradually improved and by 1996 the allowance rate had risen to about 80%.

In practice, only 3371 people received DWA in the first year and after 4 years by March 1995 there were still only a total of 10,595 recipients (Arthur & Zarb 1997). Rowlingson & Berthoud (1996) studied why there was this low take-up in a cross-sectional study of 1113 potential and 324 actual DWA recipients and a cohort study of 2192 peoples starting DWA. They found that two-thirds of the potential claimants for DWA had not heard of the new benefit while knowledge and understanding of the rules about DWA was also low. Most of the recipients of DWA had only heard about the benefit once they were already in work. Only 5% of those who were aware of DWA had ever applied for it. In general, only about 5% of DWA recipients had actually been encouraged into work by the availability of the DWA benefit. Those disabled people who were on DWA were likely to be more severely impaired, working shorter hours or self-employed. Rowlingson & Berthoud (1996) concluded that DWA did function as a medium-term subsidy to disabled people in low-paid work but that it had a very minor impact on the number of disabled people who moved into work.

In their survey, Rowlingson & Berthoud (1996) found that the average net individual weekly income of those who were on the various incapacity benefits but not working was £117, those who were working and receiving DWA was £131 and those who had returned to work and were not receiving DWA was £199. DWA was achieving its aim of removing the benefits trap but provided a very modest supplement over not working. Many recipients of the non-means-tested incapacity benefits would be no better off working with DWA.

Rowlingson & Berthoud (1996) summed up the reasons why DWA had not been successful at getting disabled people into work. Many disabled people felt unable to work and had very low expectations of working again. Those who could or wished to work wanted to move into full-time 'proper' jobs but there were major barriers to obtaining work including the overall lack of jobs, employers' attitudes and impairments. The available jobs were unattractive because of low pay which provided a financial disincentive but they were also part-time and low status and pay was only part of the problem. Awareness of DWA was low and even those who were aware of DWA did not take it into account because they wanted to be independent of the state when they moved into work.

In April 1995 there were a number of structural changes, extension to longer working hours and certain training situations, and a modest increase in the value of DWA, the main aim of which was to improve uptake and provide greater incentives for people to leave sickness or incapacity benefits and start work while at the same time maintaining the original safeguards in case claimants had to give up work again due to their illness or re-injury. Arthur & Zarb (1997) reviewed the impact of these changes in a survey carried out in July 1996 in a sample of 2800 people who had received DWA between April 1995 and April 1996. They found that the annual number of applicants for DWA had nearly doubled and the total number of recipients rose to 17,000 by March 1996. There was increased awareness of DWA and it influenced the decision to start work in about half *of those who were receiving it*. Overall, however, the impact was still modest.

The aims of DWA were laudable but that particular benefit scheme is perhaps best summed up as 'a noble failure'. This is why there is continuing political effort in the UK to develop alternative arrangements to support partially incapacitated people who are able and wish to do some work. Since 1993–1994, IVB allowed for claimants who were 'fit within limits' to have limited earnings. Reduced Earnings Allowance was introduced as a supplement for those with limited earnings potential. From April 2000, DWA was replaced by a new Disabled Person's Tax Credit which aims to provide more generous help and make more support available to more disabled people.

Incapacity Benefit

IB was introduced in April 1995 as the main NI benefit for people who are unable to work because of illness or disability, and replaced previous NI sickness and invalidity benefits. Most short-term sickness is covered by SSP and the main focus of IB is on longer-term incapacity once SSP finishes (although short-term, lower rate IB does provide cover for shorter-term sickness for those who are not covered by SSP).

The original policy objectives of IB (Social Security Incapacity for Work Act 1994) were:

- To focus incapacity provision across the social security system on those people whose medical condition is such that it would be unreasonable to expect them to seek or be available for work
- To improve help with the transition back to work
- To achieve a system that is simple for staff to understand and operate
- To maximise customer satisfaction through simple and fair arrangements
- To ensure no cash losers at the point of change
- To reduce areas of duplication between state and private provision
- To improve targeting of benefits by re-structuring the rates of benefit.

The three main elements of the reforms were:

- A new, functionally based incapacity test (the *All Work Test*)
- A new benefit structure (IB)
- Bringing this benefit into the taxation system.

Claimants have to be 'incapable of work by reason of some specific disease or bodily or mental disablement' (Social Security Contributions and Benefits Act 1992). IBs are designed to help people who are incapable of work because of the effect(s) of their medical condition, and it is these effect(s) which distinguish long-term incapacity from long-term unemployment. 'Work' in this context is taken to mean 'work that the person can reasonably be expected to do'—'focusing only on the effects of their medical condition'—and not making any allowance for non-medical factors such as age, skill, or the availability or likelihood of obtaining work. During the first 28 weeks of incapacity 'reasonable expectations' are based on the person's incapacity for their usual occupation, but after 28 weeks 'reasonable expectations' are based on their incapacity for any form of work ('all work') and not only their previous occupation. Recipient of IB can receive various other DSS benefits, but not unemployment benefit (subsequently Jobseekers' allowance) and IB now ceases at the state retirement age when recipients are automatically transferred to retirement benefit. IB is counted as taxable income.

For SSP and the first 28 weeks of incapacity the test is whether the person is incapable 'by reason of some specific disease or bodily or mental disablement of doing work which they could reasonably be expected to do in the course of the occupation in which they are engaged' (Social Security Contributions and Benefits Act 1992). This is usually assessed by the treating physician who issues a medical certificate using the criteria discussed above, although a DSS Bulletin from the Chief Medical Adviser (1988) has advised doctors to reconsider these criteria, using the RCGP (1996) clinical guidelines for acute back pain as an example that the best management and advice for many patients may be to stay active and at work.

After 28 weeks, incapacity must be for 'all work'. Many serious medical conditions qualify automatically or if they are certified by a DWP doctor, e.g. blindness, severe or progressive neurological, neuromuscular, cardiorespiratory or immune deficiency disease, active and progressive inflammatory polyarthritis, severe mental illness, severe learning disability, or terminal illness. Previously undiagnosed potentially life-threatening conditions that require investigation, severe uncontrolled or uncontrollable disease, patients who will have major surgery or other major therapeutic procedure within 6 months, and conditions where work would lead to substantial risk to the patient or others are also accepted automatically. About 16% of recipients have such severe conditions and are exempt, while another 2% are exempt on the grounds that they receive the highest rate care component of DLA. All other claimants (just over 80%) must satisfy the *All Work Test*.

The structural changes introduced with IB included new benefit rates and additions, making the benefit taxable, the abolition of the previous earnings-related additional pension for new claimants, and stopping IB at the state retirement age. A number of other changes were designed to help IB claimants back to work, including improvements to Disability Working Allowance, a 2-year training linking rule, and extra help from the Employment Service for ex-IB recipients. It was forecast that over the first few years these changes (and particularly the introduction of the *All Work Test*) would find 240,000 ex-IVB claimants and 160,000 new IB claimants capable of work, who would be disallowed benefits with major savings.

The All Work Test

Eligibility and assessment for IB differs fundamentally from assessment for DLA/AA. The first and most fundamental difference is that claimants can only apply for DLA/AA after disability has been present for 3–6 months, and payment of benefits does not begin until the claim is approved; IB claimants start to receive benefits automatically as soon as they become eligible when they reach the end of SSP and only then is their claim assessed retrospectively and benefits stopped (but not reclaimed) if their claim is disallowed. Self-assessment of disability in activities of daily living and personal care may be most relevant to DLA/AA but is only weakly correlated to capacity for work (see Figure 1.4). The continuing increase in the numbers on IVB and experience with DLA following the introduction of the self-assessment system suggested the need for stricter cross-checking of the claimant's own report. In line with general European trends back to a biomedical concept of disability, there was seen to be a need to move away from 'self-assessment' and to 're-medicalise' the assessment procedure.

The introduction of IB was therefore accompanied by a new *All Work Test*. To define and assess disability reliably required:

- A clear and simple definition of incapacity which focuses only on the effects of the medical condition
- A process perceived as fair, readily understood by claimants and by those applying it
- A reduced role for GPs in controlling access to long-term IB
- Arrangements for expert consideration of the information provided about the claimant's medical condition.

The basic approach remained that all DSS assessments should be based primarily on the claimant's own assessment of the effects of disabilities, rather than quantifying impairment and/or assigning a medical diagnosis. 'This is intended to allow you to give information about the effect of your medical condition and the resulting physical or sensory disabilities upon your capacity for all types of work' (Disability Rights Handbook 1996). 'Self assessment with confirmation where necessary has been made simple and straightforward' (Lonsdale & Aylward 1993, 1996). Routine decisions are made by lay adjudicators, but social security doctors have a critical role in the determination of eligibility for IB. All claims are initially scrutinised by a social security doctor and no claimant can be disallowed IB without a medical assessment by the *All Work Test* which provides 'confirmation where necessary'.

It may help to follow the progress of a claimant for IB through the system:

1. For the first 7 days of sickness, a worker may self-certificate and receives SSP from their employer
2. For up to 28 weeks, the caring NHS physician issues routine medical certificates (Med 3) and most workers receive SSP from their employer. Doctors are required by law to issue medical certificates to their patients free of charge and to provide related factual information to the DWP on request. These workers on SSP are not notified to the DWP and do not appear in DWP statistics. Alternatively, if no SSP is available to them and they fulfil the NI conditions of entitlement, they submit a claim for IB and start on short-term, lower-rate IB from the DWP
3. 2 weeks before the end of SSP, the employer gives the worker a form to submit to the DWP and claim IB. Provided only that the worker fulfils the NI contribution criteria, he or she then starts to receive IB and appears in DWP statistics as receiving benefit while their claim is being considered
4. Once the claimant starts on IB, the DWP requests the caring NHS physician to issue a

Med 4 certificate giving slightly more medical and diagnostic detail. The NHS caring physician generally then has no further involvement in the DWP process, unless their patient develops a new condition, deteriorates or appeals against a DWP decision. This certificate is scrutinised by a DWP doctor. Serious or exempt conditions as listed above are automatically accepted and the patient continues on IB without any further assessment. (These serious and exempt conditions now account for just under 20% of applications for IB)

5. The remaining 80% stay on IB meantime, and are sent a self-assessment questionnaire which collects similar information to the *All Work Test* (see below). (About 5% do not return the questionnaire and their IB is then stopped)

6. A DWP doctor reviews the returned questionnaire, together with all previous Med 3 and Med 4 medical certificates, any factual reports and previous claims. That doctor makes a balance of probabilities decision on whether or not the claimed level of disability is consistent with and supported by the medical evidence (with quality assurance of this decision process)

7. a. The doctor decides if the claimed level of disability is consistent with and supported by the medical evidence, and an appropriate period of 3, 6, 12 or 24 months (rarely now permanently). The claimant's questionnaire is then passed to a social security lay adjudicator who calculates if the score is >15, in which case the claim is accepted. IB is paid for the period decided by the social security doctor, and is then reviewed. (This accounts for about 25% of cases.) If the score is <15, the claimant is referred to the Department's Medical Services for independent medical assessment by the *All Work Test*, and in the meantime continues to receive IB

   b. If the DWP doctor's decision is that the claimed level of disability is not consistent with and is not supported by the medical evidence, the claimant is referred to the Department's Medical Services for independent medical assessment by the *All Work Test*, and in the meantime continues to receive IB. [Unless the sick person goes back to work or fails to return their questionnaire, no claimant can have IB disallowed without a medical examination. In total, about half the applications for IB (excluding serious and exempt cases) are now sent for examination by the *All Work Test* although in the early days of IB it was as high as 65%]

8. The medical adviser's report is returned to the DWP Adjudication Officer who re-scores the doctor's descriptors on the *All Work Test*, and compares them with the claimant's questionnaire to see if the medical evidence supports the claimant's self-assessment. The lay Adjudication Officer then assesses all the evidence and makes the final decision whether or not to award IB. (Internal DWP statistics suggest that Adjudication Officers over-rule the medical advisor's recommendation by 'bumping up' the scores of claimants without good reason in 15% of cases.) Although this is listed as the 'award' of IB it is actually a decision to either continue or disallow the IB that is already being paid

9. Claimants who are disallowed benefit at any stage have various rights of appeal. (About 6–7% of disallowed claimants appeal and about 40% of these appeals are successful)

10. Overall about 79% of claims for IB are allowed and 21% are ultimately found to be ineligible and their IB is then stopped.

It should be emphasised that the *All Work Test* is not simply the self-assessment questionnaire or the medical assessment but the entire process of scrutiny, examination and adjudication. The claimant's initial questionnaire, the medical adviser's report and the DWP Adjudication Officer's judgement all focus on the same key functional areas and descriptors. The *All Work Test* applied by a trained and approved doctor provides a more substantial bulwark against the weakness of a self-reporting system, while retaining full allowance for the claimant's own account of his or her functional limitations and restrictions. The final decision on award of benefit is not by the examining doctor, but by the lay adjudicator who must consider not only the medical evidence but all of the other evidence.

The *All Work Test* was developed from extensive consultations and pilot studies. Several alternative approaches were considered. Simply tightening up existing assessment procedures was not considered to be robust enough to ensure that benefits would be targeted on those who were incapable of work because of the effect(s) of their medical condition. A new test of impairment, although used in some other countries such as the US and Australia, was considered to be too cumbersome, difficult and costly to administer, and impairment of different bodily parts was poorly related to capacity for work (see Figure 1.4). Existing DSS assessment of disablement, as used for IIDB and Disability Working Allowance (DWA), was again considered to be too cumbersome, difficult and costly to administer, and inappropriate to assess incapacity for work. Indeed, many recipients of IIDB and DWA were working. Functional Capacity Evaluation—performing a standardised set of movements and tasks with objective measurement and assessment by a specially trained physiotherapist or occupational therapist—was widely used in the US and fulfilled many of the goals in principle, but was likely to be very time-consuming, cumbersome and costly, and might be regarded as too demanding and intrusive by some claimants. There was insufficient scientific evidence to justify the use of 'iso-machines' which were also very expensive, very time-consuming and impractical for the large numbers requiring assessment. After rejection of these various alternatives, the chosen test was based on medical incapacity and focused on the claimant's ability to perform a range of activities related to work.

The *All Work Test* was developed from well established clinical measures of disability and standard psychometric principles, and focused on a range of activities of daily living relevant to capacity for work. The final test took the form of an independent medical assessment of:

- Functional areas, e.g. walking, sitting, lifting, etc. (Table 4.22)
- Descriptors—clearly worded statements of disability ranked according to their incapacitating effect in each functional area (Table 4.23)
- Thresholds for benefit—the level in each functional area at which the incapacitating effect is such that the person cannot reasonably be expected to work
- Lower thresholds—the level in each functional area at which the incapacitating effect begins to impair capacity for work, even if the person may still reasonably be expected to work.
- Scores for each lower incapacitating effect so that their combined effect may be added together (Table 4.23).

TABLE 4.22   The 14 functional areas of the *All Work Test*

1. Walking on level ground with a walking stick or other aid if such aid is normally used
2. Walking up and down stairs
3. Sitting in an upright chair with a back, but no arms
4. Standing without support of another person or the use of an aid other than a walking stick
5. Rising from sitting in an upright chair with a back but no arms without the help of another person
6. Bending and kneeling
7. Manual dexterity
8. Lifting and carrying
9. Reaching
10. Speech
11. Hearing with a hearing aid or other aid if normally worn
12. Vision in normal daylight or bright electric light with glasses or other aid to vision if such aid is normally worn
13. Continence
14. Remaining conscious other than for normal periods of sleep

TABLE 4.23   Descriptors and scoring for the functional area of walking in the *All Work Test*

Descriptor	Points
● Cannot walk at all	15
● Cannot walk more than a few steps without stopping or severe discomfort	15
● Cannot walk more than 50 metres without stopping or severe discomfort	15
● Cannot walk more than 200 metres without stopping or severe discomfort	7
● Cannot walk more than 400 metres without stopping or severe discomfort	3
● Cannot walk more than 800 metres without stopping or severe discomfort	0
● No walking problem	0

Each functional area is graded by the medical adviser on 4–7 descriptors which are each scored from 0 to 15 points (Table 4.23). There are four additional descriptors of mental disabilities, although these are each only scored 1–2 points.

Table 4.24 shows the pattern of functional limitations in pilot studies in which 58% of claimants had musculoskeletal incapacities.

TABLE 4.24   Pattern of functional limitations in the *All Work Test*

Bending and lifting	25%
Walking	21%
Standing	18%
Psychiatric morbidity	10%
Rising	8%
Reaching and stretching	7%
Manual dexterity	4%
Sensory impairments	4%
20% had associated pain	

From DSS In-House Evaluation Study III.

To 'pass' the test (i.e. to be accepted as incapacitated for work) requires a total of 15 points. What is important is whether the ability to perform work-related activities is substantially reduced, not the point at which work becomes impossible. Certain key activities may be sufficient individually, e.g. 'cannot walk more than 50 metres without stopping or severe discomfort' or 'cannot sit comfortably for more than 10 minutes without having to move from the chair'. Alternatively, the cumulative effect of several lower thresholds may add up to a score of >15 points. With a condition like back pain it is clearly very easy to reach the 15-point threshold with a combination of sitting, standing, walking, bending and lifting all being limited to some extent by pain.

The role of the independent medical adviser is to reach an accurate assessment of disability, bringing together information gained from observation, questionnaire, medical evidence and examination, and with due awareness of all the biopsychosocial issues involved. The doctor must systematically assess each of the functional areas and descriptors, record the supportive evidence, and form a judgement based on all of this evidence over time. The medical adviser must justify his or her selection of descriptors and ratings by robust evidence gained from the interview, clinical examination and available medical evidence. The principal source of guidance is the *Incapacity Benefit Doctor's Handbook* (BAMS 1999) which provides detailed background, instruction and guidance on the entire process. There is strict quality control and medical assessments are screened for inconsistencies between the claimant's self-report, the medical evidence and the doctor's professional judgement. The medical adviser applying the *All Work Test* is trained to be aware of the relationship between the medical condition, physical impairment, disability and capacity for work, and the potential impact of psychological factors or possible exaggeration, to point them out to the lay adjudicator and to justify his or her professional findings and opinions. Recognition of these issues, and the need for training and 'approved' status for examining doctors, was part of the genesis of the emerging speciality of Disability Assessment Medicine.

Swales & Craig (1997) evaluated the *All Work Test* in a survey of nearly 1200 cases in November 1995, 6 months after it was introduced; 49% of the sample had back pain. The main purpose was to assess reliability by comparing the DSS examining doctor's assessment with an independent study doctor's assessment (Table 4.25).

Claimants were much less likely than the examining doctor to chose descriptors with very low scores and much more likely to chose those with very high scores. On the *All Work Test*, the DSS doctor and independent study doctor agreed that 25% of claimants were incapable of work and 52% capable, with overall agreement on 77%. In 15% the DSS doctor considered them capable and the study doctor incapable, and in 8% the DSS doctor considered them incapable of work but the study doctor capable. In a subgroup of 88 claimants with back pain and a secondary mental diagnosis, 24% were assessed as unfit for work largely on physical grounds and a further 38% on combined physical and mental grounds

Swales (1998b) collected data on *All Work Test* scores for a further group who were disallowed between June and November 1996. Of those disallowed, 18% had back

TABLE 4.25 Reliability of the *All Work Test*

	Total physical assessment Score 15+ (%)
Claimant	70
DSS doctor	33
Independent study doctor	27

Claimed functional limitation	No significant problems Assessed by DSS doctor (%)
Walking	65
Rising from sitting	62
Sitting	55
Bending/kneeling	52
Standing	44

	Incapable of work (%)
DSS doctor	52
Independent study doctor	46
Claim allowed (final DSS decision)	60

From Swales & Craig (1997).

conditions, 25% had other musculoskeletal conditions and 14% had mental health conditions, which is a higher proportion of back and musculoskeletal conditions than among those awarded IB. Men and those aged under 40 were more likely to have back conditions. In just over two-fifths of cases, both the independent medical examiner and the Adjudication Officer gave a score of 0, as did a quarter of claimants! In cases who had both a physical and mental health assessment, 70% were given a physical score of 0.

Pilot evaluations of 536 subjects also compared the *All Work Test* with previous assessments (Table 4.26).

TABLE 4.26 Comparison of the *All Work Test* with other forms of assessment

	Incapable of work (%)
All Work Test	46
Previous IVB assessment	60
Comprehensive clinical assessment	46

From DSS In-House Evaluation Study II.

The major strength of the *All Work Test* is that it focuses on the effects of the claimant's medical condition on key functional areas that are directly relevant to capacity for work. It is concerned solely with whether the claimant is fit for some form of work, and medical assessment for IB does not require any quantitative assessment of partial incapacity or remaining earning capacity. The *All Work Test* has high clinical validity and good psychometric properties. It is relatively simple, quick and cheap to administer, and has high face validity.

Porter (1997) surveyed early claimant reactions to the delivery of IB. Not unexpectedly, successful claimants were broadly satisfied with the new benefit and the *All Work Test* while unsuccessful claimants were more critical. Unsuccessful claimants saw the new system as being designed to discourage claims irrespective of merits. They felt the *All Work Test* undermined and under-valued their work skills, and underestimated the disadvantages that disabled people faced in the labour market. They felt that DSS medical assessments were intended to 'trick' claimants into giving answers that might disqualify their claims and that assessments were deliberately harsh.

Berthoud (1998) also suggested that 'The main criticism of the new test has been the exclusive focus on medical criteria', illustrating this by 'the primacy of doctors in the design and evaluation of the points system' while 'experts in disabled people's position in the labour market (disability organisations, specialists in occupational health, disablement employment advisers and employers themselves) were hardly represented'. 'More generally, the procedure excluded from consideration the vital interaction between impairments and their social context (such as age and previous experience) which determines the real outcome.'

The appeals service

Although few claimants probably realise it, the Appeals Service is completely independent of the DWP and is answerable directly to the Secretary of State for Social Security, although by the nature of its task it must work closely with the DWP. It is an independent, professional service whose function is to provide independent, impartial and authoritative decisions. The Social Security Act 1998 made major changes to the Appeals Service and the appeals process with the aim of improving efficiency and providing speedier, more accurate and fairer decisions in a more uniform, understandable, adjudication system. Nevertheless, it retains a legal structure and rules, which are inevitably highly complex and difficult for the layman to understand.

In 1999, the Appeals Service handled 330,000 appeals for all social security benefits, an increase from 230,000 per annum within the previous 4 years. Despite the increased caseload, the average waiting time reduced from 42 weeks to 20 weeks in the year to September 1999. The President of the Appeals Service is a Judge, and it employs 67 full-time and 650 part-time lawyers, 750 part-time doctors (who are completely separate from the DWP Medical Service), 450 lay disabled members or carers, and 1000 civil servants. All part-time members must work at least 20 days per annum to have sufficient experience, and over the past 2 years there has been increasing emphasis on training and quality control. The Appeals Service now has an annual budget of £55 million.

The basic remit of the appeals process is to review whether DWP decisions on individual cases (which by the nature of the system always consist of the DWP disallowing a claim for benefits and the claimant's appeal against that decision) are correct according to the social security legislation and rules. The appeals tribunal reviews the existing evidence and the claimant may chose to attend for interview. Most appeals tribunals for the main disability benefits consist of a legal and medical member, and for DLA a third lay member. The legal member is chairman of the tribunal, and in certain circumstances the chairman may hold the appeal alone. The members of the appeals tribunal generally do not carry out any physical examination, although if the tribunal considers the available evidence is insufficient to reach a decision, it can then instruct a further 'expert' examination of the claimant on questions of medical fact.

In training, the guiding principles are that appeals hearings should be courteous and dignified and attempt to bring out the best in the claimant, give the claimant the opportunity to say what he or she needs and wants to say, and leave the claimant with the feeling that the hearing was fair. In reviewing the original DWP decision and the claimant's appeal against that decision, this often involves the members of the appeals tribunal deciding whether the claimant's, the medical and any other evidence about disability are consistent and believable, even if this is strictly constrained by the time available (an hour or less) and may be largely an intuitive process. It is not a question of moral judgements for or against the claimant or deciding if he or she is 'worthy' or 'unworthy'. Whatever the theory or practice from the perspective of the Appeals Service, claimants' satisfaction with the process depends above all else on the outcome of the hearing and whether their appeals were successful.

After the appeals tribunals, the final stage of appeal is to the Appeals Commissioners who provide a judicial review on questions of law, akin to the higher appeal Courts.

By the legal nature of the system, appeals tribunals and particularly Commissioner's decisions form the case-law which provides the background to future DWP practice. Decisions which over-turn DWP decisions inevitably have greater impact on DWP adjudicators. This probably tends, however erratically and gradually, to liberalise the decision-making process from the initial DWP interpretation and application of the original legislation and legislative intent.

Trends since 1992–1993

Table 4.27 shows the annual number of new awards of the various incapacity and disability benefits over the past decade. There is no information on how many claimants are awarded more than one benefit each year but it is probably few, so total new awards is the arithmetical sum of all four benefits. This gives a conservative estimate, and if there is greater overlap the trends since 1994–1995 would probably be even more marked.

Table 4.28 estimates the total number of recipients currently on the main incapacity and disability benefits. As noted earlier, approximately 60% of recipients get more than one of the incapacity and disability benefits, which must be allowed for in calculating the total number of people on these benefits (DSS Social Security Statistics 2000). The primary and most important benefits are IB and SDA, and these are mutually exclusive. Eighty per cent of working-age recipients of DLA receive other incapacity and disability benefits and should not be counted twice; 50% of those on IIDB also receive IB and should again not be counted twice. The disability premium for IS is only paid to recipients of one of the other incapacity and disability benefits, so these people are already included in the other statistics.

TABLE 4.27   Number of new awards of incapacity and disability benefits for all conditions (thousands)

	Invalidity Benefit/ Incapacity Benefit[1]	Severe Disablement Allowance	Industrial Injury Disablement Benefit	Disability Living Allowance	Total awards of all incapacity and disability benefits[2]
1990–1991	850	19	—	—	
1991–1992	926	21	12	—	
1992–1993	918	19	13	308	1258
1993–1994	904	21	14	257	1196
1994–1995	978	28	19	280	1305
1995–1996	866	33	18	298	1215
1996–1997	905	34	21	299	1259
1997–1998	869	25	16	260	1170
1998–1999	740	13	15	213	981
1999–2000	706	12	13	215	946

[1] Including credits only.
[2] This is a simple total of the number of awards of benefit, not of recipients, as there is no information on how many claimants are awarded more than one benefit in each year.

TABLE 4.28   Total number of recipients of the main incapacity and disability benefits for all conditions current at one point in time each year (thousands)

	Invalidity Benefit/ Incapacity Benefit[1]	Severe Disablement Allowance	Industrial Injury Disablement Benefit	Disability Living Allowance	Total[2]
1990	1518	285	—	—	—
1991	1678	293	—	—	—
1992	1897	302	166	1000	2482
1993	2114	316	171	1145	2745
1994	2249	330	180	1308	2931
1995	2406	348	193	1491	3149
1996	2524	384	199	1688	3346
1997	2420	385	212	1853	3282
1998	2404	395	217	1980	3304
1999	2344	391	212	2042	3249
2000	2281	386	219	2110	3199

[1] Including credits only.
[2] Allowing for the overlap due to many recipients being entitled to more than one disability benefit, total benefits for incapacity and disability = IB + SDA + (IIDB × 0.5) + (DLA × 0.20).

The total number of recipients was therefore calculated as IB + SDA + (IIDB × 0.5) + (DLA × 0.20). This gives an approximate total for recipients of all ages (including some on IIDB and on DLA and up to 2000 a diminishing number on IB who were over working age) of all incapacity and disability benefits (although not including AA which is purely for those over retirement age and largely goes to the elderly). There are however several assumptions to this calculation:

- The overlap between the different benefits is the same for those of working age as for recipients of all ages
- The overlap between the different benefits has remained constant between 1990 and 2000.

The above estimate of total recipients (Table 4.28) compares with summary data published by the DWP (Table 4.29). The total in Table 4.29 is not directly comparable to Table 4.28 as it only includes recipients of working age and does not include IIDB, although it does include IS with disability premium.

TABLE 4.29   Total recipients of working age of incapacity and disability benefits (thousands)

	Incapacity benefits only[1]	Incapacity and disability benefits	Disability benefits only[2]	Total incapacity and disability benefit recipients
May 1997	1634	982	193	2809
May 1998	1608	1025	207	2841
May 1999	1609	1043	213	2865
May 2000	1621	1058	223	2902

[1]Incapacity Benefits including credits only, Severe Disablement Allowance and Income Support with disability premium.
[2]Disability Living Allowance (some of these recipients may be working).

The 1995 reforms were mainly directed to controlling entry to benefits and the statistics show they clearly had the intended impact (Table 4.27). The rising trend in the number of new awards of IVB and IB was reversed more or less immediately. The impact on all of the other incapacity and disability benefits was delayed, peaking slightly later in 1996–1997. Altogether, the total number of new awards fell 27% between 1994–1995 and 1999–2000.

The impact of this reduced inflow on the pool of current recipients is diluted by the large proportion who have been on benefits long term and are unlikely to come off. The number of recipients of IB peaked in 1996–1997 and since then has fallen by 9% (Table 4.28) with a 22% fall in the number of long-term beneficiaries (Table 4.30). The numbers of recipients of SDA and IIDB have more or less plateaued since about 1997, which is consistent with the very small outflow from these benefits (Table 4.28). These reductions are counter-balanced by the large and continuing increase in the numbers on DLA (Table 4.28). This is to some extent inevitable in the early years of any new benefit but there is clearly a major problem with this benefit (see below). However, from the statistics on overlap between these various benefits (DSS Social Security Statistics 2000), DLA appears to be functioning very largely as a supplement to one of the other disability benefits rather than going to different people (see page 118). Overall the progressive increase in the total number of recipients of incapacity and disability benefits up to about 1996 has now halted and since then the number appears to have more or less plateaued (Tables 4.27 and 4.28).

Incapacity benefit

Table 4.30 shows the steady rise in the number of recipients of long-term incapacity benefits, which increased four-fold in the 20 years up to about 1994, despite no evidence of any

TABLE 4.30 Number of beneficiaries of long-term Invalidity Benefit or Incapacity Benefit (short-term higher and long-term rate but excluding short-term lower rate) for all incapacities at the end of each statistical year (benefits paid, excluding credit only)

	Men	Women	Total
1972	334	81	415
1973	355	81	436
1974	366	78	444
1975	373	79	452
1976	400	79	479
1977	422	84	506
1978	462	97	559
1979	505	107	612
1980	506	109	615
1981	517	116	633
1982	553	130	683
1983	593	144	737
1984	638	159	797
1985	673	177	850
1986	706	193	899
1987	754	214	968
1988	808	240	1048
1989	860	266	1126
1990	917	293	1210
1991	976	330	1306
1992	1063	376	1439
1993	1156	424	1580
1994	1217	464	1681
1995	1262	505	1767
1996	1217	485	1702
1997	1151	488	1639
1998	1080	485	1565
1999	994	471	1466
2000	929	487	1416

commensurate rise in disability. The UK Government Green Papers (1998a,b) suggested that over this period, IVB and IB had proved a simple but costly method of governments keeping down the unemployment numbers. In some cases, IVB and IB had become a more generous form of unemployment benefit or a supplement to income in early retirement, which was never the intention.

In February 2001, just over 6% of the working-age population of Britain was claiming social security benefits on the basis of sickness or disability (DWP Quarterly Summary of Statistics 2001). Since the April 1995 reforms, the number of men on IB has fallen by about one-fifth and the number of women has plateaued (Table 4.30). There has been a general fall in the numbers receiving all categories of IB, not only long-term benefits, and a much greater fall in the number over pension age as a result of progressively abolishing the right to stay on IB after reaching the state retirement age (Table 4.31). Table 4.32 shows the number of new spells of IB commencing since 1995. Overall, there has been a fall of about 15%. The greatest fall is in the number starting short-term lower-rate IB, which in view of the nature of that benefit may reflect changing entitlement to SSP. There is no epidemiological evidence of significant change in levels of sickness, and this is reflected in the lack of change in the numbers coming off SSP and on to short-term higher-rate IB. There has been a fall of about one-third in the numbers commencing long-term IB, which is where most of the efforts at tighter control have been targeted. There is little change in the numbers commencing credits only, although in view of the fall in total numbers, they represent a gradually increasing proportion of new recipients.

Table 4.33 shows that the fall in the number of new awards of IB since its introduction in 1995 has been due mainly to a 15% fall in the number of claims. There is no clear pattern in the total award rate, although there has been a slight increase in the number of new awards which consist of credits only.

TABLE 4.31 Quarterly statistics for number of recipients of all rates of Incapacity Benefit (including credits only) since introduction in April 1995 (thousands)

		Short-term lower rate	Short-term higher rate	Long term	Credit only	Number over pension age[1]
1995	May	128	—	1699	557	287
	Aug	122	94	1656	573	279
	Nov	124	104	1622	579	262
1996	Feb	124	100	1602	580	246
	May	121	106	1580	590	231
	Aug	121	105	1565	598	217
	Nov	126	106	1545	608	201
1997	Feb	120	106	1533	614	188
	May	118	105	1520	628	172
	Aug	119	107	1498	646	154
	Nov	116	108	1482	662	139
1998	Feb	111	103	1461	665	122
	May	104	100	1445	668	106
	Aug	98	97	1428	679	89
	Nov	98	91	1415	696	76
1999	Feb	98	88	1377	710	52
	May	92	87	1379	719	44
	Aug	92	88	1361	733	29
	Nov	93	91	1336	746	11
2000	Feb	94	89	1327	750	—
	May	93	90	1320	759	—
	Aug	93	91	1323	779	—
	Nov	94	92	1327	796	—
2001	Feb	96	92	1330	805	—

[1] Over age 65 for men, 60 for women.

The first three columns are mutually exclusive. Some of those receiving credit only and those over pension age may also appear in the first three columns.

From DWP Incapacity Benefit and Severe Disablement Allowance: Quarterly Summary of Statistics. February 2001.

TABLE 4.32 New spells of Incapacity Benefit commencing in each quarter

		Short-term lower rate	Short-term higher rate	Long term	Credit only	Total
1995	Aug	89	27	8.0	81	205
	Nov	98	26	8.8	85	218
1996	Feb	99	24	9.8	75	208
	May	94	26	10.3	76	205
	Aug	88	22	7.9	88	206
	Nov	96	24	8.1	97	225
1997	Feb	90	22	8.0	81	201
	May	82	23	7.4	81	193
	Aug	87	23	6.6	95	211
	Nov	86	24	6.5	94	210
1998	Feb	82	23	6.7	80	191
	May	75	23	6.4	76	180
	Aug	73	21	6.2	82	182
	Nov	75	22	6.1	87	190
1999	Feb	75	23	5.4	85	188
	May	66	21	5.8	78	171
	Aug	64	21	5.5	75	166
	Nov	69	24	6.2	83	181
2000	Feb	69	22	5.9	72	169
	May	68	24	6.4	78	177
	Aug	66	22	6.5	82	177
	Nov	68	24	6.2	77	175
2001	Feb	69	23	6.0	65	162

From DWP Incapacity Benefit and Severe Disablement Allowance: Quarterly Summary of Statistics. February 2001.

TABLE 4.33 Claims/award rates of Incapacity Benefit since introduction in 1995

	New claims	Awards of Incapacity Benefit	Awards as % of claims	Credit only awards	Credit only as % of all awards	Total awards	Total awards as % of claims
1995–1996	1,072,456	453,680	42	338,740	43	792,420	74
1996–1997	1,067,919	495,560	47	340,800	41	836,360	78
1997–1998	1,012,827	455,380	45	348,880	43	804,260	79
1998–1999	926,229	409,980	44	330,360	45	740,340	80
1999–2000	911,807	379,960	42	308,340	45	688,300	75

DWP Incapacity Benefit Key Fact sheet July 2001.

From July 1997 to April 1998 there were 26,778 appeals to the Independent Tribunal Service: 26% were paper hearings of which 2% were successful; 74% were oral hearings of which 37% were successful (all as % of total appeals). Claimants who attended or were represented at the hearing were more likely to be successful (Parliamentary Written Answers 31 July 1998).

Swales (1998b) studied DSS administrative data on those who left IB between April 1995 and February 1997 and tracked them for 1 year. About half claimed a new benefit within 6 months, the majority within 1 month. The most common benefits claimed soon after leaving were Unemployment Benefit (Jobseekers Allowance) and IS, although in the longer term and more gradually, a significant minority returned to IB and then tended to remain on it for at least 12 months.

Dorsett et al (1998) followed a 'flow sample' of 2263 people who left IB between June–November 1996, interviewing them between 5–10 months later with additional postal follow-up to the end of 1997. They were mainly long-term recipients with a mean duration on IB of 25 months (voluntary leavers who had been on IB <23 weeks were excluded); 62% of leavers had musculoskeletal conditions, including 39% who had problems with their back or neck (although 57% also had multiple conditions). Leavers were spread fairly evenly from age 25 to 55, but unlike those staying on IB there were relatively fewer leavers over age 55 years. Two-thirds of those surveyed had left IB after being disallowed by the All Work Test while one-third left voluntarily. Almost 90% reported some continuing health problems at the time of leaving benefits and at follow-up (even those leaving voluntarily) and the majority experienced some continuing disadvantage in the labour market. Among those who were disallowed benefit by the All Work Test and who remained out of work, 70% still regarded themselves as sick or incapacitated rather than unemployed. Overall, 76% of leavers reported continuing difficulty with heavy work and 63% had further time off because of sickness or for treatment.

At the time of follow-up, more than one-third were in full-time work. However, there was sharp divergence: 66% of voluntary leavers were in full-time work but only 21% of those who were disallowed were in full-time work. Half the voluntary leavers returned to their previous job and half to new work. The majority even of those disallowed had been 'economically active' in some way at some time since coming off benefit, but even those who were in full-time work had low earnings which were little different from their previous benefits. More than a quarter had returned to IB, 13% of voluntary leavers and 35% of those disallowed. More than one-fifth continued to rely on other social security benefits, 11% of voluntary leavers and 27% of those disallowed. Those who were aged <55 years, better qualified, previously employed or had an employed spouse or partner were more likely to return to work. Those who appealed the disallowance of their benefits were least likely to return to work. Scores on the All Work Test did not correlate well with subjects' own judgement of their disability, and leavers' own subjective estimates of their health were a better predictor than the All Work Test of return to work. Nevertheless, the main barriers to return to work were reported to be associated with age, qualifications and local job availability rather than disability.

Dorsett et al (1998) concluded there were two sharply divergent exits from IB (Table 4.34). Those for whom IB covered a period of temporary disability and who retained a strong attachment to work tended to recover their health at least enough to regain their place in the labour market even if with some remaining disadvantage. Those with a strikingly lower attachment to work tended to have persisting lower levels of economic activity after leaving IB. Those who appealed against disallowance of IB had particularly poor outcomes:

TABLE 4.34   Destination of Incapacity Benefit leavers a year later

	Voluntary leavers (%)	Disallowed leavers (%)
In full-time work	66	21
Returned to Incapacity Benefit	13	35
Not working, on other social security benefits	11	27

From Dorsett et al (1998).

most did not return to any form of paid work, they remained sick and disabled, and they suffered the greatest loss of earnings. Although the right to appeal is essential, the process of appeal appeared to act as a brake on recovery and any form of job search or economic activity. In many ways these appellants remained 'in limbo' for considerable periods of time. Dorsett et al (1998) concluded that simply disallowing people from IB and then leaving them to find their own way into employment did not work.

More recent DSS administrative data (May 1999) again showed that 28% of new claimants of IB and 70% of new claimants of DLA were on some form of benefit 3 months earlier; 56% of new claimants of IB had some form of benefit history over the preceding 4 years.

Despite the halt in the upward trend in IB, the UK Government Green Papers (1998a,b) considered that the *All Work Test* was still a key part of the problem. It is an all or nothing test which focuses on what disabled people cannot do rather than what they can do, and writes off some people as unfit who might be able to do some, possibly new or assisted, form of work. It gives the wrong messages to disabled people who are trying to make the most of their potential. Once people 'pass' the test they are often consigned to permanent disability with limited prospect of returning to work.

Severe Disablement Allowance

SDA was originally designed for people who were disabled from childhood due to severe congenital or developmental conditions, who were never able to work or pay NI contributions and so had not gained entitlement for IB. It has always and still includes a large proportion of severely handicapped people who are the classic example and public image of 'disabled people'. There were originally high standards of disablement which were enforced rigorously. The numbers of recipients and social security expenditures on SDA have always been small compared with other disability benefits (Table 4.28).

Previously, claimants for SDA over age 20 had to pass the *All Work Test* and then also be assessed at >80% disablement. From 1996, they no longer had to take the *All Work Test* but had a one-stage assessment of disablement.

The number of people receiving SDA was rising very gradually in the early 1990s, but rose more rapidly between 1993 and 1996 (Table 4.28) and since this time has more or less plateaued (Table 4.35). As previously noted, by the nature of their disability, most recipients of SDA stay on this benefit for many years. Taking existing cases at April 1995, Table 4.35 shows that there has been a very gradual fall in their numbers with time, generally due to

TABLE 4.35 Quarterly statistics for numbers receiving Severe Disablement Allowance since May 1995 (thousands)

		Total beneficiaries	Pre 13.4.95 cases	Post 13.4.95 cases
1995	May	325	319	5
	Aug	330	317	12
	Nov	338	314	24
1996	Feb	344	310	34
	May	350	306	44
	Aug	355	302	53
	Nov	361	298	64
1997	Feb	364	291	72
	May	367	283	84
	Aug	369	277	92
	Nov	369	272	98
1998	Feb	369	268	102
	May	370	264	105
	Aug	370	261	109
	Nov	370	258	113
1999	Feb	369	253	116
	May	370	252	119
	Aug	370	248	121
	Nov	369	244	125
2000	Feb	367	241	127
	May	366	237	129
	Aug	365	234	131
	Nov	366	232	134
2001	Feb	367	229	138

From DWP Incapacity Benefit and Severe Disablement Allowance: Quarterly Summary of Statistics. February 2001.

reaching retirement age or death. Between mid 1995 and late 1997 there was a marked increase in the number of new cases. Since late 1997 the number of new cases has fallen and the number coming on more or less balances the number leaving so that the number on SDA has remained more or less constant. This corresponds roughly to the introduction of IB and the changed rules of entitlement for SDA itself which both came into effect in about 1995–1996. About this time, there was also a simple change in computer programming which prompted Benefits Agency staff to consider benefit claimants' eligibility for SDA. By 1998 just over two-thirds of new recipients of SDA were aged over 20. Yet in contrast there was little change in the number of disabled recipients below that age, which is what would be expected from the more or less constant prevalence of severe congenital or developmental disabilities. Because of the lower rate at which benefit was paid, 70% of claimants for SDA got no real help from the benefit and had to rely on means-tested IS.

Disability Living Allowance and Attendance Allowance

The number of recipients on DLA has risen faster than for any other incapacity or disability benefits (Table 4.28), at about 19% per annum since it was introduced in 1992–1993.

Swales (1998a) surveyed 1200 people awarded DLA since April 1994. About half those receiving any form of DLA were aged >50 years and half those receiving the care component were aged >80 years. Most had more than one disabling condition with an average of nine specific care needs, and the majority of recipients got both mobility and care awards. The middle rate was the most common care award and the higher rate the most common mobility award. Musculoskeletal and mental or nervous system conditions were most common. Swales (1998a) considered there were some imbalances and overlaps in the current system of entitlement and also cast doubt on the quality of DSS decisions about the award of DLA and the adequacy of the evidence on which these decisions were based.

The Disability Living Allowance Advisory Board (Grahame 1998) discussed the future of DLA and AA, and expressed serious misgivings about the way these benefits had been structured and administered over the previous 5 years. It commented that the number of people receiving DLA and AA was much higher than predicted, due to:

- Higher take-up (due to effective publicity)
- Many disabled people receiving help with applications from welfare rights personnel and disability organisations
- A noticeable degree of over-statement of need and a significant degree of incorrect payments
- Adjudication officer practices:
  - insufficient understanding of the disabling condition
  - inadequate corroboration of the disabling condition by the claimant's own doctor
  - failure to request adequate medical evidence
  - failure to select the most appropriate source of medical evidence
  - misinterpretation of the available medical evidence
  - managerial pressure to increase throughput and reduce administrative costs
  - tendency to give awards for life, ignoring the possibility of improvement
- A high reversal rate of disallowed claims at Benefits Agency review or Disability Appeals Tribunal
- A series of legal judgements by Commissioners, Court of Appeal and the House of Lords had progressively broadened entitlement beyond the original policy intention
- A significant degree of avoidable physical and psychological disablement resulting from lack of investment in local clinical and rehabilitation services leading to delayed or ineffectual management of treatable diseases.

It considered that there was statistical evidence for many of these facts and that DLA and AA awards were 'in conflict with the facts' in 63% of cases. Moreover, two-thirds of awards were made for life, but one-third of these were to people whose condition might be expected to improve.

Conversely, however, population surveys have suggested that the take-up rates for these benefits among disabled people who would be eligible for them are low, even among those who are severely disabled (Table 4.36). This probably applies most to elderly disabled people.

Berthoud (1998) argued that the crucial question is whether the large increase in DLA benefits is going to disabled people who need them or to a wider group of claimants who do not.

TABLE 4.36 Take-up rates for benefits among disabled people who would be entitled to them

DLA Care Allowance	30–50%
DLA Mobility Allowance	50–70%
Attendance Allowance	40–60%

From Craig & Greendale (1998).

He reviewed the evidence that some DLA benefits are being paid to people with lesser degrees of disability who do not incur extra costs, that the DLA criteria and their application do not target the benefit well enough, and that some people exaggerate, but all to a limited extent. He concluded that about one-tenth of DLA benefits may be going to the wrong people, but this is greatly outweighed by the large number of people with more severe disabilities who are not receiving the benefit to which they would be entitled. Regarding the method of assessment, Berthoud pointed out that one of the main policy intents when DLA was introduced in 1992 was to make the benefit easier to claim, in contrast to IB where the policy intent was to make it harder to claim. It is then illogical to criticise DLA for its success.

However, all of this ignores recent DWP statistics which suggest that most DLA benefits to people of working age are now being paid to people on IB or other disability benefits (see page 118), which raises questions about whether it really is meeting additional costs of disability or simply serving as a financial supplement to other benefits.

Trends of benefits for back incapacities

Because of the major changes which have occurred in disability and incapacity benefits since the early 1990s, it is simpler to look separately at trends up to 1991–1992 and those during the 1990s, which permits use of more comparable statistics in each comparison.

Incapacity and disability benefits up to 1991–1992

CSAG (1994b) collated spells and days of Sickness and Invalidity Benefit statistics from 1953–1954 to 1991–1992 to demonstrate the societal impact of back incapacities (Table 4.37). Between the early 1950s and the late 1970s, the number of spells of sickness and invalidity benefits for back incapacity rose three-fold, although up until the mid 1970s the rate for women remained about half that for men relative to the numbers at risk. Over the entire period from 1953 to 1992, the number of days of benefit paid rose exponentially: eight-fold for men and 24-fold for women. This was partly explained by the increasing number of women eligible for these benefits, but more recently also by some tendency towards gender equality, although total spells, days and rates of back incapacities for women all remained lower than for men. These data underestimate the increase since the mid 1980s, because a progressively greater proportion of short-term sickness was covered by SSP and excluded from these DSS figures.

Table 4.38 shows the relatively greater increase for back incapacities compared with all other incapacities.

TABLE 4.37 Total Sickness and Invalidity Benefits for back incapacities from 1953–1954 to 1991–1992 (including people receiving credits only)

	Spells (thousands)		Days (thousands)			Rate (days/thousand population)	
	Men	Women	Men	Women	Total	Men	Women
1953–1954	274	37	6477	1200	7677	453	219
1954–1955	277	39	6496	1344	7840	452	249
1955–1956	300	42	7127	1439	8566	491	269
1956–1957	320	44	7508	1393	8901	514	264
1957–1958	323	44	7663	1440	9103	519	276
1958–1959	354	47	8420	1569	9989	567	309
1959–1960	384	51	9183	1696	10,879	614	340
1960–1961	382	51	9053	1639	10,692	600	331
1961–1962	403	54	9744	1756	11,500	639	354
1962–1963	422	57	10,193	1765	11,958	665	359
1963–1964	463	60	11,079	2132	13,211	720	437
1964–1965	504	65	11,865	2093	13,958	769	431
1965–1966	522	61	12,410	1974	14,384	803	411
1966–1967	545	65	13,176	2127	15,304	855	451
1967–1968	575	68	14,008	2125	16,134	916	461
1968–1969	662	86	15,692	2464	18,156	1029	542
1969–1970	683	86	16,385	2396	18,781	1081	537
1970–1971	653	88	16,204	2438	18,642	1074	558
1971–1972	616	90	15,461	2433	17,894	1030	564
1972–1973	678	94	16,410	2594	19,004	1099	604
1973–1974	701	102	16,665	2675	19,340	1127	633
1974–1975	709	104	17,012	2713	19,725	1107	—
1975–1976	—	—	—	—	—	—	—
1976–1977	759	130	18,803	3376	22,179	1209	—
1977–1978	833	155	21,589	4434	26,023	1391	—
1978–1979	843	191	21,575	4805	26,380	1390	—
1979–1980	830	212	25,452	6323	31,775	1640	—
1980–1981	—	—	26,090	7011	33,101	1671	—
1981–1982	—	—	26,526	7978	34,504	1698	—
1982–1983	—	—	26,148	8867	35,015	1682	—
1983–1984	—	—	21,491	7449	28,940	1397	729
1984–1985	—	—	24,947	8647	33,594	1600	811
1985–1986	—	—	27,324	10,645	37,968	1734	973
1986–1987	—	—	28,193	11,652	39,845	1800	1049
1987–1988	—	—	32,191	14,303	46,494	2059	1262
1988–1989	—	—	35,755	16,840	52,595	2285	1458
1989–1990	—	—	39,776	19,816	59,592	2548	1680
1990–1991	—	—	44,358	22,903	67,261	2847	1927
1991–1992	—	—	52,821	28,549	81,371	3409	2428

Notes:

1. Data for spells are not given after 1979–1980 as an increasing proportion of shorter spells were omitted from DSS statistics.

2. Benefits paid are not equivalent to work loss because approximately half of all sickness absence for back pain is now covered by Statutory Sick Pay (CSAG 1994b) while 46% of those on incapacity and disability benefits were previously unemployed (DWP data 2001).

3. Data for female rates from 1974–1975 to 1982–1983 are not given due to lack of accurate population-at-risk figures for this period.

TABLE 4.38   The relatively greater increase in sickness and invalidity benefits for back incapacities (including credits only)

	1978–1979	1991–1992	% increase 1978–1979
	Days (% of total)	Days (% of total)	to 1991–1992
All incapacities	371,041,500 (100)	573,522,900 (100)	54.6
Musculoskeletal diseases	60,103,600 (16.2)	161,107,500 (28.1)	—
Back incapacities	26,380,000 (7.1)	81,370,700 (14.2)	208.5
All other musculoskeletal incapacities	33,723,600 (9.1)	79,736,800 (13.9)	136.4
All circulatory diseases	56,655,100 (15.3)	108,570,500 (18.9)	91.6
All mental disorders	57,586,200 (15.5)	105,849,300 (18.5)	84.5
All respiratory diseases	53,746,100 (14.5)	40,399,800 (7)	−24.8

Incapacity and disability benefits 1990–2000

Tables 4.39 and 4.40 show the same trends of total annual spells and days of all incapacities and back incapacities during the 1990s, comparable to the earlier IVB data in Table 4.36.

TABLE 4.39   Total annual spells of Sickness and/or Invalidity Benefits April 1990–April 1995 and Incapacity Benefits April 1995–March 2000 (including credits only) (thousands) by gender

	Spells of certified incapacity		Back incapacities
	All incapacities	Back incapacities	as % of total
Men			
1990–1991	1651	227	13.7
1991–1992	1815	259	14.3
1992–1993	1926	289	15.0
1993–1994	2038	313	15.4
1994–1995	2153	332	15.4
1995–1996	2238	286	12.8
1996–1997	2187	292	13.4
1997–1998	2133	278	13.0
1998–1999	1988	261	13.1
1999–2000	1899	254	13.4
Women			
1990–1991	730	107	14.7
1991–1992	807	130	16.1
1992–1993	882	144	16.3
1993–1994	958	160	16.7
1994–1995	1037	168	16.2
1995–1996	1136	156	13.7
1996–1997	1125	160	14.2
1997–1998	1158	157	13.5
1998–1999	1131	152	13.5
1999–2000	1125	148	13.2

TABLE 4.40 Total annual days of Sickness and/or Invalidity Benefits April 1990–April 1995 and Incapacity Benefit April 1995–March 2000 (including credits only) (thousands) by gender

	Days of certified incapacity		Back incapacities as % of total
	All incapacities	Back incapacities	
Men			
1990–1991	355,994	44,358	12.5
1991–1992	402,729	52,822	13.1
1992–1993	436,513	60,769	13.9
1993–1994	468,835	69,382	14.8
1994–1995	507,892	75,462	14.9
1995–1996	599,524	74,908	12.5
1996–1997	588,773	75,901	12.9
1997–1998	578,718	74,988	13.0
1998–1999	546,674	72,022	13.2
1999–2000	526,747	70,554	13.4
Women			
1990–1991	146,974	22,903	15.6
1991–1992	170,794	28,549	16.7
1992–1993	190,730	32,400	17.0
1993–1994	211,412	36,438	17.2
1994–1995	237,494	40,509	17.1
1995–1996	297,662	42,652	14.3
1996–1997	298,284	43,973	14.7
1997–1998	309,736	43,982	14.2
1998–1999	309,408	43,984	14.2
1999–2000	314,960	43,566	13.8

(Note that all of these IB statistics are based on a 1% sample and include people who receive credits only.)

From 1990 to about 1994, there was a gradual rise in the number of spells and days of IB for all incapacities for men and women. Back incapacities reflected the general trend, although spells and days of back incapacities rose slightly faster than other incapacities, so that back incapacities accounted for a gradually increasing percentage of all incapacities, especially for men.

From about 1995–1996, after the introduction of the new IB and the *All Work Test* in April 1995, these trends were reversed and spells and days of all incapacities fell slightly in men and plateaued in women. Spells of back incapacities fell more markedly in 1995–1996 so that the proportion of spells and days of all incapacities accounted for by backs fell from about 15–17% to about 12–14% in every set of data. Since 1995–1996, spells and days of IB for back incapacities have simply mirrored all incapacities in both men and women so the percentages have remained steady.

Tables 4.39 and 4.40 give the total number of spells and days of these benefits paid each year which provides the most complete measure of the societal impact of back pain and are the most comparable to the earlier data in Table 4.37. This is presented visually in Figure 4.4.

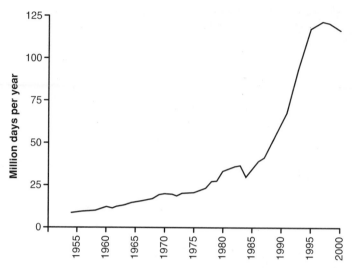

Figure 4.4 UK trends of Incapacity Benefits for back pain, 1990–2000

However, this may obscure changes because many of these people have been on benefits long-term and are unlikely to come off them. It is also difficult to relate this total figure to the number of people because one individual may have more than one spell on benefit in the year. Therefore, changes may be more obvious in analyses of the number of new awards each year (Table 4.41) and of the number of recipients currently on benefit at one point in time each year (Table 4.42).

TABLE 4.41 Spells of Incapacity Benefits commencing each year (including credits only)

	All incapacities	Back incapacities	Backs as % of all incapacities
1989–1990	838,900	120,200	14.3
1990–1991	849,700	131,700	15.5
1991–1992	926,200	156,800	16.9
1992–1993	917,900	159,500	17.4
1993–1994	903,500	154,000	17.0
1994–1995	977,900	161,600	16.5
1995–1996	866,200	116,900	13.5
1996–1997	905,300	128,900	14.2
1997–1998	869,200	110,300	12.7
1998–1999	740,500	93,600	12.6
1999–2000	706,000	89,000	12.6

Table 4.41 shows that new awards of IB for all incapacities rose steadily to a peak in 1994–1995 and then from 1995–1996 declined so that by 1998–1999 they were lower than in 1989–1990. New awards of IB for back incapacities showed the same rising and falling trend, but were even more marked, so that from 1989–1990 to 1993–1994 the percentage of all awards accounted for by backs increased from 14.3 to 17% and then from 1994–1995

TABLE 4.42   Number of people on Incapacity Benefit at the end of March/beginning of April each year (including credits only)

	All incapacities	Back incapacities	Backs as % of all incapacities
1990	1,518,100	202,500	13.3
1991	1,678,300	231,500	13.8
1992	1,897,300	279,600	14.8
1993	2,114,100	320,800	15.2
1994	2,249,100	357,300	15.9
1995	2,406,500	381,400	15.8
1996	2,524,000	334,700	13.3
1997	2,420,300	324,900	13.4
1998	2,404,200	321,500	13.4
1999	2,343,700	319,000	13.6
2000	2,281,000	308,000	13.5

has progressively fallen again to 12.6%. The number of people receiving IB at March–April each year (Table 4.42) shows the same pattern, although all of the changes are less marked because of dilution in the large numbers of people who remain on IB long-term.

Severe Disablement Allowance 1989–2000

Back conditions account for a much smaller proportion of SDA than of IB. In contrast to IB, there are more women (60%) than men (40%) on SDA, and more women are on SDA for back conditions. Back conditions now account for about 4% of SDA in women and about 2.5% in men. The proportion of SDA accounted for by back conditions has remained more or less constant throughout this period for women, but has risen from about 1% to about 2.5% for men.

The number of new awards (Table 4.43) and the total number of people in receipt of SDA for all disabilities (Table 4.44) rose progressively faster up to 1996–1997. The number

TABLE 4.43   Annual number of new awards of Severe Disablement Allowance

	All disabilities	Back disabilities	%
1989–1990	19,800	800[1]	4.0[1]
1990–1991	19,000	500[1]	2.6[1]
1991–1992	21,300	1100	5.2
1992–1993	18,600	1500	8.1
1993–1994	21,400	1500	7.0
1994–1995	27,900	1800	6.5
1995–1996	32,600	2500	7.7
1996–1997	34,100	2300	6.7
1997–1998	24,500	<1000[1]	—[1]
1998–1999	13,300	<1000[1]	—[1]
1999–2000	12,000	<1000[1]	—[1]

[1]These numbers are too small to be statistically reliable on the sample used.

TABLE 4.44 Number of people in receipt of Severe Disablement Allowance

	All disabilities	Back disabilities	Back pain as % of all disabilities
March 1990	284,600	8600	3.0
March 1991	293,300	8000	2.7
April 1992	302,100	8800	2.9
April 1993	315,700	9700	3.1
April 1994	329,500	11,400	3.5
April 1995	348,300	12,700	3.6
March 1996	384,800	13,000	3.4
March 1997	385,500	14,100	3.7
March 1998	395,000	13,400	3.4
March 1999	391,200	12,600	3.2
March 2000	386,000	12,000	3.1

of new awards and the total number of people in receipt of SDA for back disabilities showed a similar pattern, with a particular increase in the proportion of new awards for back disabilities between 1989–1990 and 1992–1993 (although these statistics are based on small samples and are less reliable). There was a dramatic reversal in these trends in 1998, with a fall of one-third in the number of new awards for all disabilities, and a fall of two-thirds in the number of new awards for back disabilities. Most recipients of SDA remain on benefit for many years so diluting any change, yet these trends in new awards have been sufficiently strong to reduce within 2 years the number of people on SDA for all disabilities and for back disabilities and the proportion accounted for by back disabilities.

Disability Living Allowance 1992–2000

Tables 4.45 and 4.46 show the number of new awards and the number of people currently in receipt of DLA from 1992–1993. DLA only started in April 1992, and no comparable diagnostic statistics are available for the previous Mobility Allowance and AA prior to that time.

TABLE 4.45 Annual number of new awards of Disability Living Allowance

	All conditions	Back pain	Back pain as % of all conditions
1992–1993	308,200	19,800	6.4
1993–1994	256,900	21,300	8.3
1994–1995	279,900	24,300	8.7
1995–1996	298,100	28,800	9.7
1996–1997	299,400	31,000	10.3
1997–1998	259,600	23,300	9.0
1998–1999	213,700	16,800	7.9
1999–2000	215,400	17,800	8.3
2000–2001	243,900	18,800	7.7

5% sample, % based on unrounded figures.

TABLE 4.46   Number of people in receipt of Disability Living Allowance

	All conditions	Back pain	Back pain as % of all conditions[1]
Feb 1993	1,144,700	81,800	7.1
Feb 1994	1,308,000	97,100	7.4
Feb 1995	1,491,300	115,000	7.7
Feb 1996	1,687,600	137,400	8.1
Feb 1997	1,853,100	159,800	8.6
Feb 1998	1,980,200	172,600	8.7
Feb 1999	2,042,300	177,000	8.7
Feb 2000	2,110,200	184,400	8.7
Feb 2001	2,210,600	192,600	8.7

5% sample.
[1] % based on unrounded figures.

Table 4.45 shows that there was a slight initial peak of new awards when DLA was introduced in 1992 and then a gradually increasing number of new awards each year, with a progressive build up in the number of people in receipt of DLA for all conditions up to 1996–1997. Over that period, the number of new awards of DLA for back pain rose more rapidly, accounting for an increasing proportion of all awards of DLA although the proportion always remained much lower than for IB. Between 1997 and 1999, there was a marked fall in the number of new awards of DLA for all conditions, with back pain falling even more rapidly to below the 1992 level and forming a smaller proportion of new awards. This fall appears to be due to a falling number of new claims rather than a falling success rate of awards. Because few people come off DLA except on death or entering long-term care, the number in receipt of DLA has continued to rise gradually since 1997 with the number in receipt of DLA for back pain reflecting the general trend and accounting for a constant proportion of all DLA (Table 4.46).

Industrial Injuries Disablement Benefit 1992–2000

Diagnostic statistics for IIDB are only available from 1992 (Tables 4.47 and 4.48). In the IIDB statistics it is difficult to determine exactly which ICD codes represent back injuries. DWP statistics for 'back injuries' in Tables 4.47 and 4.48 include ICD 10th revision codes M45–M51, M53, M54, S33 and also S34 (previously ICD 952, which is defined as 'Spinal cord lesion without evidence of spinal bone injury', but which the DWP Analytical Services Division use to code 'spinal injuries, otherwise unspecified'). Code A11 includes 'injuries to back, trunk and others' of which an unknown proportion are back injuries (although unrelated Australian workers' compensation statistics suggest that >80% of 'trunk injuries' are upper or lower back injuries). This coding problem appears to be unique to IIDB and does not apply to any of the other benefits discussed here.

Between 1991–1992 and 1994–1995 there was a 50% increase in the annual number of new awards of IIDB for all industrial injuries and since then the number has more or less

TABLE 4.47 Annual number of new awards of Industrial Injuries Disablement Benefits

	All injuries	Back injuries	ICD code 959.1 (All)[2]	Back and trunk injuries as % of all injuries[2]
1991–1992	12,030	1795	1743	29
1992–1993	12,575	1948	2003	31
1993–1994	14,270	2142	2123	30
1994–1995	18,905	1544	4964	34
1995–1996	17,580	1032	5238	36
1996–1997	20,880	1001	5793	33
1997–1998	15,600	1300	4100	34
1998–1999[1]	15,400	1100	3700	31
1999–2000	12,500	500	3400	31

[1] Provisional figures.
[2] There are no definite data on the relative proportions of back and trunk injuries.

TABLE 4.48 Number of Industrial Injuries Disablement Benefits currently being paid (with a threshold of at least 14% disablement)[1]

	All injuries	Back injuries	ICD code 959.1 (All)[2]	Back and trunk injuries as % of all injuries
April 1992	166,073	15,736	17,288	20
April 1993	171,184	17,114	18,505	21
April 1994	180,036	19,025	21,157	22
April 1995	192,664	18,952	27,970	24
April 1996	198,901	19,217	31,884	26
April 1997	212,071	19,716	37,105	27
April 1998	216,802	20,253	38,956	27
April 1999	211,600	19,900	38,300	27
April 2000	219,200	19,900	41,600	28

[1] A few recipients may be receiving benefits for more than one award for more than one injury, but that is probably <5% and is unlikely to have a significant effect on the total statistics.
[2] There are no definite data on the relative proportions of back and trunk injuries.

plateaued (Table 4.47). In the earlier period the number of new awards for back and trunk incapacities rose more rapidly, so that the proportion of all new awards of IIDB accounted for by back incapacities rose from 29% in 1991–1992 to 36% in 1995–1996. Since 1995–1996 the number of new awards for back and trunk incapacities has gradually fallen so that the proportion of all new awards of IIDB accounted for by back incapacities has fallen to 31%. Between 1992 and 1997 the number of recipients of IIDB for all industrial injuries increased by 21% and since that time has plateaued (Table 4.48). The number of recipients of IIDB for back and trunk incapacities has shown a similar but more marked pattern, so that the proportion of all IIDB accounted for by back and trunk incapacities rose from 20% in 1992 to 27% in 1997 and since that time has plateaued.

From 1994 to 1995 there was a dramatic fall in the number of new awards for back injuries and an equally dramatic rise in the number of new awards coded All, which more or less balanced each other, so that total back plus trunk injuries remained a fairly steady proportion of all injuries. The most likely explanation seems to be that (for whatever reason and mechanism) there was a change in coding practice at that time, and it is not possible to interpret this as meaning any real change in the number of back injuries. These statistics have therefore been accepted as 'back + trunk injuries'.

Income Support with disability premium

There are no diagnostic-specific statistics for ISdp.

Total social security benefits for back incapacities 1990–2000

Tables 4.49 and 4.50 summarise total numbers of new awards and of current recipients of all incapacity and disability benefits for back conditions.

As already noted, approximately 60% of recipients get more than one of the incapacity and disability benefits, and this overlap must be allowed for in estimating the total number of people on these benefits. The primary focus of this analysis was taken to be incapacity for work in those of working age. Only about 60% of those on DLA are now aged 18–65 years so the number receiving DLA was adjusted by × 0.60 to estimate those of working age only. The total number of working-age recipients was then calculated as IB + SDA + (IIDB × 0.5) + (DLA × 0.20). There are again several assumptions in this calculation:

- The age distribution and overlap between the different benefits is the same for back pain as for all conditions
- The overlap between the different benefits is the same for those of working age as for recipients of all ages
- The overlap between the different benefits has remained constant between 1990 and 2000.

TABLE 4.49   Total number of new awards for back incapacities and disability each year (thousands)

	Invalidity Benefit/ Incapacity Benefit[1]	Severe Disablement Allowance	Industrial Injury Disablement Benefit[2]	Disability Living Allowance	Total back incapacities[3]	Backs as % of all incapacities
1991–1992	157	1.1	3.5	—	—	—
1992–1993	160	1.5	4.0	20	185	14.7
1993–1994	154	1.5	4.3	21	181	14.4
1994–1995	162	1.8	6.5	24	194	14.9
1995–1996	117	2.5	6.3	29	155	12.7
1996–1997	129	2.3	6.8	31	169	13.4
1997–1998	110	<1[4]	5.4	23	140	12.0
1998–1999	94	<1[4]	4.7	17	118	12.0
1999–2000	89	<1[4]	3.9	18	112	11.8

[1] Including credit only.

[2] Back and trunk.

[3] Arithmetical sum: note that strictly this is the number of awards which may not exactly correspond to the number of individuals as a few may receive more than one award in a year.

[4] Based on very small samples.

TABLE 4.50 Total number of recipients of benefits for back incapacities and disability at one point in time each year (thousands)

	Invalidity Benefit/ Incapacity Benefit[1]	Severe Disablement Allowance	Industrial Injury Disablement Benefit[2]	Disability Living Allowance[3]	Total back incapacities[4]
1990	203	8.6	No data	—	—
1991	232	8.0	No data	—	—
1992	280	8.8	33	Start DLA	—
1993	321	9.7	36	49	359
1994	357	11.4	40	58	400
1995	381	12.7	47	69	431
1996	335	13.0	51	82	390
1997	325	14.1	57	96	387
1998	322	13.4	59	104	386
1999	319	12.6	60	106	383
2000	308	12.0	61	110	373

[1] Including credits only.
[2] Back and trunk.
[3] Of working age.
[4] Allowing for the overlap due to many recipients being entitled to more than one disability benefit. Total benefits for incapacity for work due to back conditions = IB + SDA + (IIDB × 0.50) + (DLA × 0.20).

There is again no information on how many claimants are awarded more than one benefit each year for back pain but it is probably few, so the total new awards was calculated as the arithmetical sum of all four benefits. This gives a conservative estimate, and if there is some more overlap the trends since 1994–1995 would probably be even more marked.

These trends are presented visually in Figure 4.5.

In the early 1990s, there was a progressive increase in the number of new awards of IVB and IB for back conditions and backs accounted for a gradually rising proportion of new awards (Table 4.41). Altogether, however, the total numbers of new awards of all disability and incapacity benefits for back conditions and for all conditions remained relatively steady (Tables 4.27 and 4.49). Since 1994–1995 there has been a dramatic fall in new awards of all disability and incapacity benefits for back conditions (Table 4.49, Figure 4.5). Most of the fall is accounted for by IB, which fell 27% in 1995–1996 and more gradually since. There has been a comparable fall in new awards of SDA since 1995–1996 and in new awards of IIDB and DLA since 1996–1997. Overall, new awards of all incapacity and disability benefits for back conditions have fallen 42% since 1994–1995, while awards for all other conditions have fallen 25% (Tables 4.27 and 4.49). In 1995–1996, the proportion of all awards accounted for by back incapacities fell from almost 15% to about 12–13% and since this time has fluctuated about that level (Table 4.49). Data on IB shows this has mainly been a matter of fewer claims which have fallen 42% for back incapacities compared with 21% for all other incapacities (Table 4.33).

Once recipients are off work and on benefits for 12 months or more, most remain on benefits for years, often to retirement age, so changes in the number of new awards have

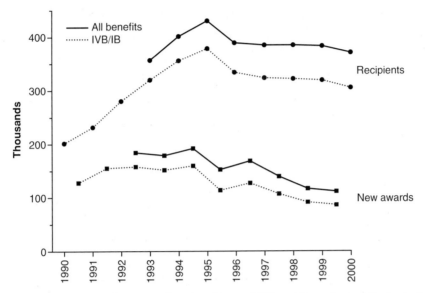

Figure 4.5 Numbers of new awards and recipients of UK social security benefits for back incapacities, 1990–2000

a slower impact on the stock of existing recipients (Table 4.50). As expected from the rising number of new awards for back pain up to 1995, the total number of recipients on incapacity and disability benefits for back conditions also increased rapidly up to that time (Figure 4.5). The number on benefits for back incapacities rose faster than those on benefits for other incapacities, so that backs accounted for a gradually increasing proportion of all recipients of these benefits. Since 1995, the rising trend of recipients has been halted. The number of people on IB for back conditions has fallen 19% since its peak in 1995 (Table 4.50) and the days of IB paid annually for back conditions has also passed its peak (Table 4.40). SDA-paid-for back conditions peaked slightly later in about 1997. IIDB- and DLA-paid-for back conditions appear to have plateaued in the last few years. Overall, the number of people of working age receiving incapacity and disability benefits for back pain rose approximately 60% between 1990 and 1995 and since then has fallen by 13% (Table 4.50, Figure 4.4). This recent fall appears to be specific to back conditions, while the total number of people receiving incapacity and disability benefits for all conditions has remained more or less constant (Tables 4.27 and 4.28).

These trends need to be interpreted against changes in health care for back pain and social security changes in the 1990s.

The increasing number of people receiving social security benefits for back conditions for several decades up to 1994–1995 to some extent reflected trends for all conditions. This was probably related to the changing social, economic and employment situation and probably also changing individual and social attitudes to work, sickness, incapacity and benefits (Croft 2000). Over most of that earlier period, however, the number of new awards and particularly the number of people on benefit for back incapacities increased more than for other incapacities, so that backs accounted for an increasing proportion of all incapacity and disability benefits. This might reflect individual and social attitudes and behaviour about back pain, and medical attitudes and practice, both in clinical management and sick certification. To some extent, back pain may also have formed a proxy for more general health, psychosocial or social problems.

Since 1995, the trend has reversed. There is no *a priori* reason to expect any biological explanation, and the epidemiological evidence reviewed earlier showed no change in the prevalence of back pain over the past decade.

Just over half the fall in new awards of benefits for back conditions mirrored changes in all conditions. Health and Safety legislation in the early 1990s obliged employers to reduce hazards at work and the Disability Discrimination Act 1995 obliged them to make reasonable adjustments to keep people with disabilities at work, although there is little evidence these had much impact. The main fall in IB followed immediately on from the change from IVB and the introduction of the *All Work Test* in April 1995. Increasing difficulty getting IB in 1995–1996 and more liberal availability of DLA and SDA might explain the temporary increase in awards of the latter benefits. The general fall was counter-balanced by an increase in DLA, although in practice this acts mainly as a supplement to IB. All of these statistics to some extent reflect the timing of changes in the assessment system. Thus, just over half the fall in awards for back conditions is probably explained by changes in the control mechanisms of the social security system.

Rather less than half the fall in awards was unique to back conditions. It is possible these social security or legislative changes could have had a differential effect on a subjective complaint like back pain, although there is no direct evidence of this. Probably more important, these trends coincided with more active medical management of back pain. There is little evidence this has had much direct impact, but it is possible changed medical thinking about back pain could have a more indirect effect. Health care and social support occur within a broad framework of social attitudes and practices about back pain, and about associated, sick certification, and social security benefits, and there is now emerging evidence these are changing (Waddell 2002b).

Some may argue these improvements are cosmetic and simply reflect greater difficulty getting social security benefits rather than any 'real' change in back pain, although a similar comment could apply equally to the rising trend up to 1995. It is also possible there could have been a shift in certification practice, e.g. there was a 15% increase in new awards of IB for mental and behavioural disorders from 1996 to 2000. However, this was the only condition to rise, there is no direct evidence of transfer between these diagnoses, and this rise was insufficient to accommodate the fall in back conditions.

It is unlikely that any single factor explains the changing trends, but rather the cumulative interaction of many influences. The real explanation, both of the earlier rise and the recent fall, may be enigmatic but fundamental cultural change (Waddell 2002a,b). To put it another way, perhaps sick certification and social security benefits for back pain are becoming less fashionable. Irrespective, these statistics show a very real, major and rapid shift in social behaviour related to back pain in the UK since the mid 1990s, and this differs from other conditions.

These findings are also consistent with a number of more general hypotheses about back pain in the context of social security:

- Back pain is largely a 'proxy'
- Psychosocial factors predominate
- Incapacity is related to illness behaviour and the sick role
- Certification legitimises disability and incapacity
- These trends are unresponsive to optimum clinical management
- There is a need for health-care professionals to have a broader perspective and role
- Society plays a critical role.

Moreover, the corollary is that:

- Better physical 'treatment' is unlikely to make much difference, although better 'management' may have some impact
- 'Proxy' may simply shift to another 'acceptable' label
- Psychosocial factors will still predominate
- There will be a minimal net effect on social security expenditure
- Social engineering is important
- Cultural change is paramount.

From this perspective, the rise and fall in social security benefits for back pain in the last few decades of the 20th century may best be interpreted as a social or 'cultural' phenomenon rather than a biological phenomenon. To put it another way, perhaps back pain simply became more and then recently less fashionable as a diagnosis for sick certification and social security benefits.

The major improvement has been in the number of people developing chronic back pain and incapacity who claim and start benefits. The challenge now is to find a better health-care or rehabilitation answer for the large number of people with chronic back pain who presently often remain on benefits long-term.

Welfare reforms since 1998–1999

New Labour came to power in 1997 and Grimshaw (1999) summarised Tony Blair's version of social democracy, the 'Third Way': 'For Tony Blair, the First Way is Individualism or Thatcherism whose weakness lies in its neglect of social solidarity and national cohesion. The Second Way is old-fashioned socialism with its commitment to nationalisation, redistribution of wealth and comprehensive welfare provision. The Third Way remains committed to ideals of social solidarity, social inclusion and opportunities for poor people to better themselves, but is pragmatic about how to achieve these goals. In the new mixed economy which it advocates, there will be a synergy between the public and private sectors, utilising the dynamism of the markets but with the public interest in mind. The government's role is to ensure that business is confident, successful and profitable by fostering innovation, promoting competitive skills and investing in education and training to equip citizens with the skills that employers need. Citizens in the new dispensation have a responsibility to work if they are able and to equip themselves through lifelong learning with skills that will attract a range of employers. ... Third Way government is strongly committed to public spending restraint. ... Welfare provision will be far from universal, and as far as they can, citizens will be encouraged to provide for themselves.' This political ideology has been reflected faithfully in public policy since 1997, with the primary emphasis on promoting work and welfare reform being directed mainly to controlling costs. Symbolically, the Department of Social Security and the Department for Education and Employment were amalgamated in summer 2001 into the DWP (with no mention of social security or welfare).

The UK Government Green Paper (1998b) *A New Contract for Welfare: Support for Disabled People* concluded that although the UK social security spending on benefits for those with long-term illness or disability had risen progressively to £24 billion per annum, it was failing to meet both key principles of encouraging work for those who can and providing security for those who cannot work. In particular, the social security system had drifted away from its original purpose: benefits were now going to some people for whom they were not intended while other disabled people for whom these benefits were intended were missing out. The system did not adequately meet the needs of those disabled early in life nor the most severely disabled people on the lowest incomes.

The Disability Living Allowance Advisory Board (Grahame *et al* 1998) was specifically considering DLA, but many of their comments may be equally relevant to all disability and incapacity benefits. They posed the fundamental questions:

- What is the benefit for?
- Who is the benefit for?
- How should claimants' needs be assessed (by subjective or objective tests)?
- How can the benefit be targeted to the right people?
- How should the benefit be administered?
- What are the benefit's links to community (or health) care?

and reiterated that any proposals should meet the following principles:

- Any changes must be seen to be fair and equitable to people with disabilities
- A convincing case must be made for any suggested removal or extension of entitlements
- Limited resources should be targeted to those in greatest need. At the same time the genuine needs of people with lesser disabilities should not be neglected.

Their principal recommendations were that benefits (particularly DLA) should be targeted at the most severely disabled, with the express aim of helping with the extra costs incurred due to *severe* disability. After 5 years' experience of these benefits, they concluded that self-report of disability was unreliable and produced both under- and over-statement of disability. As the sole source of information or in conjunction with inadequate medical information it produced poor adjudication decisions. They recommended that assessment should in future be based on a combination of self-report using a simpler form and mandatory professional confirmation from a multi-disciplinary assessment which covered all aspects of disability and rehabilitation. Most awards should be time-limited and not for life.

The underlying philosophy and principles of disability and incapacity benefits are discussed further in *The welfare state debate* section of the present review (see p000). Current UK reforms (UK Government Green Papers 1998a,b) are designed to make sure that where the state is providing help, most resources should go to those with the greatest needs.

In practice:

- Work is the best form of welfare for people of working age
- Break down barriers to work for disabled people
- Commitment to raising standards in education and training
- Tackling poverty and deprivation/attacking social exclusion.

The specific objectives of structural and process changes were to:

- Facilitate optimal early management
- Encourage work retention rather than incapacity
- Emphasise abilities rather than functional limitations
- Contribute to cultural change among health professionals
- Support re-education, re-skilling, rehabilitation back to work
- Review gateways to benefits.

The UK Government Green Paper (1998b) made a number of specific proposals to implement these principles, which were incorporated into the Welfare Reform Bill 1999:

- The Single Gateway, Personal Adviser and ONE service
- Change the *All Work Test* to a *Personal Capability Assessment*
- Restore the link of IB to work and NI contributions
- Changes to IB aimed to reduce obstacles and disincentives to return to work
- Disabled Person's Tax Credit
- Disability Income Guarantee. Incorporate SDA into IB
- A fairer balance between public and private pension provision.

The New Deal for Disabled People (NDDP) initiative was introduced in February 1999 and the New Deal for 50 Plus in April 2000, along with a number of New Deals for young unemployed, long-term unemployed and lone parents (www.newdeal.gov.uk). These were to varying degrees case-management programmes with a Personal Adviser to guide the individual through the system and drawing in a number of employment-related services to improve employability and place them in employment. The NDDP is under the joint responsibility of the Department for Education and Employment (DfEE) and the Department of Social Security (now combined in the DWP), although led by DfEE. Its aim is to help disabled people to move into work or remain in work:

- Improvement in the various benefit rules which protect benefits on return to work, are designed to support return to work, or facilitate return to benefits if return to work is unsuccessful (see earlier)

- The Personal Adviser service and the ONE service
- Funding of about 20 small 'Innovative Schemes' to test new ways of helping disabled people into work
- Larger scale Job Retention and Rehabilitation Pilots in several areas of the country which are due to start in 2002.

New Deal for 50 Plus (www.newdeal.gov.uk) aimed to meet the needs of older people who are on social security benefits and looking for practical help to find work. Help was provided with jobsearch skills, costs of travelling to interview, work-based learning or training, work trials and training grants. New Deal for 50 Plus paid an extra £60 tax-free per week on starting full-time work and guaranteed a take-home wage of at least £180.

The major structural proposal of NNDP was that there should be a single gateway to social security, so that all people with long-term sickness or incapacity could be assessed and helped without delay, while they still had the potential to rehabilitate and return to work. Each claimant would have a personal adviser who would help them access information about work, benefits and other government services available. Attendance for interview with the personal adviser to discuss the options for work and other paths to independence would become a condition of receiving benefits as well as ensuring that claimants received the benefits they were entitled to. Two models of service delivery were tested: first, the DfEE Employment Service itself received separate funding to deliver the Personal Adviser Service; secondly, independent sector organisations took the lead in partnership with other private sector organisations, public authorities and the Employment Service.

Arthur et al (1999) reported on the first year of pilot studies of the Personal Adviser Service in six areas of the country. Overall, there was general lack of knowledge of the service and uptake was low. It was most likely to be used by those who were younger, better qualified and still more closely attached to the labour market. Most clients who used the service felt it was helpful although they did not have a strong sense of being involved in a planning process. Employers were more critical of the service, although they were generally positive about its potential. There was insufficient data from these pilots to draw any conclusions about the effectiveness of the service at returning clients to work.

The next stage in the development of the 'single gateway' for people of working age was the introduction of the ONE service. This brought together the Employment Service, Benefits Agency and Local Authorities at a single point of contact to provide an integrated common service tailored to meet the needs of individuals. The objectives were (Green et al 2000):

- To put more benefit recipients in touch with the labour market through the intervention of their Personal Adviser
- To increase the level of sustainable employment by getting more benefit recipients into work
- To ensure that more clients experience effective, efficient service that is tailored to their personal need
- To change the culture of the benefit system and the general public towards independence and work rather than payments and financial dependence.

Several pilot versions of ONE were introduced in 12 areas around the UK between June and November 1999. Initially, participation was voluntary, but from April 2000 lone parents, unemployed, sick and disabled claimants were required to attend the first meeting with the Personal Adviser as a condition of receiving benefits. Green et al (2000) surveyed claimants during the first, voluntary phase. About two-thirds of benefit claimants had heard of ONE, although less that a half of lone parents and only a third of sick or disabled claimants were actually offered an interview. Overall, 30% of lone parent and 21% of sick or disabled respondents to the survey actually attended an interview. The main reasons sick and disabled claimants gave for attending were that they thought they had to or it might affect their claim (41%), it would help them with their claim for benefits (41%), to see what it had to offer (41%) or because they wanted a job (22%). The main reasons sick and disabled claimants gave for refusing an interview were health problems which prevented them looking for work (50%), they were not ready to talk about work (26%) or they already had a job and were expecting to return to work (20%). Sick and disabled claimants who attended interview were more likely to be under age 25 and to have no qualifications, and less likely to belong to an ethnic minority, live with a partner and dependent children, or to have a mental or behavioural disorder. Sick and disabled claimants who did attend interview were more likely to have discussed benefit-related issues (79%) (one-seventh of which included in-work benefits), training and finding work (51%) and special help or services available (26%). Overall, 85% of those who attended a ONE interview felt the advice they received was 'quite or very helpful'. From qualitative interviews, the success of ONE depended very much on the individual claimant's circumstances and needs and on the individual adviser's skills. However, one of the practical limitations is that ONE does not actually provide any return to work services but simply advises or refers the client to where these services are available. The sample was too small and the assessment too early to assess whether ONE had any impact on claimants returning to work.

Subsequent analysis suggested that the NDDP Personal Adviser Service pilots engaged 7% of the target population in an initial interview and 69% of those interviewed were taken on to the case-load. By November 2000, 64% of those taken on had left the case-load and 59% of them had found paid work. Overall, 11% of participants in the Personal Adviser Service moved off IB compared with 7% of non-participants, but because of the low engagement rate the Personal Adviser Service only achieved this for 1.8% of the original target population.

The UK Government Green Paper (1998b) also proposed that the emphasis of the All Work Test should shift from a negative focus on incapacity to a more positive focus on remaining capacity. In a Parliamentary written answer (28.10.98), the Secretary for State pointed out that the All Work Test 'does not mean that people who satisfy the test are unable to do any work at all: it simply establishes that their incapacity is such that it would be unreasonable to expect them to seek work as a condition for getting benefit. In practice, many people who satisfy the All Work Test may be capable of doing some work given the right help and support'.

The All Work Test was renamed the Personal Capability Assessment in April 2000. In principle, it now focuses more on what people can do rather than on what they cannot do (which are not necessarily reciprocal), and collects 'information or evidence capable of being used for assisting the person in question to obtain work or improve his prospects of obtaining it'. Together with a wider assessment of claimants' capacities and employability, this information can then be used to help them plan for a return to work and to provide the help and support they need to do so and increase their independence. The initial idea was that the *Personal Capability Assessment* would also be administered as early as possible before people lose contact with the labour market and there would be legislative powers to administer it within the first 28 weeks of incapacity, i.e. even before entitlement to IB. In practice, the timing and initial stages of the new *Personal Capability Assessment* are identical to the *All Work Test*, administered after people have started benefit and with the same self-report form followed if necessary by thorough medical examination and assessment. After medical examination (which is commonly at least 3–4 months after starting IB, i.e. 9–12 months after stopping work) the medical examiner prepares a standard medical report on incapacity (exactly as previously in the *All Work Test*) but also now prepares a separate 'capability report' about what work-related activities the person might still be able to do and what sort of help they might need to do them. Legislation has freed the DWP to pass this confidential medical information to other agencies involved in rehabilitation and re-employment. In practice, there are doubts if the *Personal Capability Assessment* has yet made any difference. The *All Work Test* and the medical report on incapacity are used by medical examiners and adjudicators to decide eligibility for benefits, exactly as before. Legislation does not allow the adjudicator to see the 'capability report' so it cannot influence the decision on eligibility for benefits. In practice, for purely logistical reasons, the 'capability report' is not available to the Personal Adviser either at the stage of first interview, so it does not inform or assist the ONE service, at least until a later stage in the process when it may be too late to be of much assistance.

The reforms also restored the link between IB and work and NI contributions. Entitlement to IB now depends on employment, earnings above a certain level and NI contributions in one of the last three complete tax years. So the long-term unemployed are no longer eligible and IB will cease to be a form of more generous support for long-term unemployment.

A number of changes to IB aimed to reduce obstacles and disincentives to return to work. Recipients may earn up to £15 per week, undertake unlimited voluntary work, and work for a trial period while still on benefits. There are grants to assist those starting work. People who come off IB to start work and then have to come back on to benefit within a year return immediately to their previous level of benefit.

From October 1999, Disability Working Allowance was replaced by Disabled Person's Tax Credit.

As part of the goal to direct disability benefits to those in greatest need, the level of benefit to those severely disabled has also been increased substantially. The most severely disabled people with the greatest care needs and the lowest incomes, and families with severely disabled children who depend on IS will get a Disability Income Guarantee. From April 2001, SDA was incorporated into IB.

It was also proposed to introduce a fairer balance between public and private pension provision. When IB was introduced fewer people had any occupational or private pension and very few retired early. Now a majority of people have some occupational or private pension and early retirement is common. IB is now sometimes paid on top of a reasonable pension, in effect topping up early retirement. Under the new rules, an occupational pension of up to £85 per week does not affect IB. From April 2001, for any occupational or private pension >£85 per week, IB is reduced by 50 pence for each additional £1 per week of occupational or private pension. In effect, claimants who are retired and have an occupational and/or private pension greater than about £9,000 per annum do not receive any IB.

It was again proposed that the claims system and adjudication of claims for DLA and AA should be reviewed. DLA and AA should no longer be 'life awards' but should be subject to regular review. To date, this has not been implemented.

A number of related welfare projects are designed to help and encourage people with a long-term illness or disability to retain or regain their links with the labour market:

- The 1995 Disability Discrimination Act, the Disability Rights Task Force and the Disability Rights Commission
- The New Deal for Disabled People, Department for Education and Employment investment in specialist disability services, and the Access to Work Programme
- Action to make work pay, including the national minimum wage, the new Disabled Person's Tax Credit and benefit changes to remove disincentives to work.

It will be several years before it is possible to assess what impact these recent reforms will have on social security trends in incapacity and disability benefits and for back conditions in particular.

Ireland

The Republic of Ireland is the smallest country in the EU with a population of 3.6 million. A higher proportion of the population are aged 15–64 than in any other EU country, with only 11.5% over age 65. The population is growing slower than in most EU countries. Until recently, there was a high rate of negative migration but that has now reversed and there is now slight positive immigration. The causes of Ireland's unemployment were essentially structural ones which prevailed up to the early–mid 1990s. Within the last few years, the unemployment rate has been significantly reduced to 4.5% which is one of the lowest in the EU.

Evolution of Irish Welfare System

The Irish Social Welfare System originated in its 19th-century union with the UK and developed in a piecemeal manner over many decades. Some of the early schemes, such as old-age pensions and NI, were directly applied from Britain while the influence of the Poor Law continued until the mid 1970s. Even since independence in 1921, the Irish social security system has continued to take account of developments in Britain and there are still close links between the social security departments. So it is not surprising that Ireland still has a similar pattern to the UK of social insurance, universal benefits and social assistance.

Prevailing economic conditions inevitably set the scene for social welfare developments. For example, there was a marked contrast between the depressed economic conditions of the 1950s when few social welfare developments took place, and the 1960s and early 70s when economic growth permitted a number of social welfare developments. Changing attitudes to the desirability and extent of state intervention were important, e.g. the anti-interventionist philosophy of the Catholic Church was said to have had a profound influence up to the 1960s. Political pressure groups were also important, e.g. the Trade Union movement has campaigned for better social welfare provisions throughout, while the growth of the women's movement from the early 1970s campaigned for the interests of women. Ireland's entry into the EEC in 1973 had both direct legislative and broader comparative influences on social welfare developments.

The Report of the Commission on Social Welfare (Curry 1986) distinguished several phases in the development of the Irish Welfare System. The first phase, from 1838 to 1920, was largely dominated by the Poor Law but also saw the beginning of British welfare systems prior to independence. The second phase, from 1921 to 1952, saw post-independence developments culminating in the establishment of the Department of Social Welfare in 1947. In the third phase, from 1953 to 1986, the rate of development of the Social Welfare System varied greatly with the economic situation, with little more than consolidation in the 1950s, expansion in the 1960s and early 70s, which was arrested from the mid 1970s– early 80s. The final phase dates from the publication of the major Report of the Commission on Social Welfare in 1986 and economic prosperity as a member of the EU.

The English Poor Law had been in operation from the 16th century. However, the immigration of destitute Irish labourers placed considerable strain on the English Poor Law system, so the Poor Relief (Ireland) Act in 1838 made specific provision for dealing with poverty in Ireland. This followed the same principles as the English Poor Law, including setting relief below the level of the lowest wages to discourage all but the really destitute. However, the very low wages in Ireland at that time and the extent of destitution made this impossible and, instead, the main deterrent became workhouse discipline. The Great Famine of the 1840s highlighted the inadequacies of the Poor Law System so provision for 'outdoor relief' was made in 1847. The fundamental philosophy and the central provisions of the Poor Law Acts of 1838 and 1847 endured well into the 20th century.

The Workmen's Compensation Act of 1897 was similar to that in most European countries. Compensation for work-related injury took the form of a weekly payment, according to a fixed scale and with specified limits, worth about 50% of the weekly wage of a skilled worker at that time. Further Acts over the next decade extended the coverage.

The British National Insurance Act of 1911 applied also to Ireland and provided sickness and disablement benefits. The Irish Insurance Commissioners supervised the administration of the schemes which were actually run by non-profit making 'approved societies'. By 1933, there were 65 approved societies catering for approximately 474,000 insured people in Ireland. The societies were free to cater for particular groups of people, and membership ranged from 55 in one small mutual benefit society to over 100,000 in a central society covering the whole country. Some societies with highly selected membership in special situations could provide much better benefits, but others catering for poorer or disadvantaged people could be in considerable financial difficulty, which resulted in marked variation in benefit levels. The National Health Insurance Act in 1933 amalgamated all of the societies into The National Health Insurance Society.

The Department of Social Welfare was established in 1947 to co-ordinate and provide more efficient administration for the various Social Welfare Schemes. The Social Welfare Act in 1952 proposed that all employees should be treated equally and insured for all benefits and effectively provided a single co-ordinated social insurance scheme.

In 1965 a commission reported on the Workmen's Compensation Scheme. After considerable political debate, the Social Welfare (Occupational Injuries) Act of 1966 introduced an Occupational Injuries Scheme which replaced the Workmen's Compensation Scheme and provided compulsory insurance against occupational injury or disease for all employees with no age limits and no contribution conditions for entitlement.

Invalidity Pension was introduced in 1970 for people who had been in receipt of disability benefit for at least 12 months and were found on examination to be totally incapable of work and likely to remain so for at least a further 12 months. The contribution conditions were somewhat stricter than disability benefit but once people received Invalidity Pension they no longer required continued medical certification of illness.

The Social Welfare Act in 1974 removed the distinction between manual and non-manual workers and abolished the earnings limit for social insurance (in the earlier stages, certain higher-paid groups earning above a certain amount were exempt from the Social Insurance Scheme). In 1979, a completely new system of pay-related social insurance contributions was introduced, with a percentage of earnings up to a specified ceiling being collected by the taxation system. This also removed a former differential between men and women.

Overall, during the 1960s and 70s, there was considerable expansion in social welfare. Many new benefits and services were provided, their coverage and operations were extended and the real value of benefits was increased, so the living standards of welfare recipients and many of the most disadvantaged in society improved significantly.

By the mid 1980s, the range of payments provided by the Department of Social Welfare fell into four categories:

1. Social Insurance Schemes financed from pay-related NI contributions collected from employers and employees. However, the contributions were insufficient to meet the payments from the Social Insurance Fund and the deficit was paid by the State from general taxation. Entitlement to Social Insurance Benefits depended on the claimant's NI contribution record

2. The Occupational Injuries Scheme financed solely by contributions from employers with no qualifying conditions related to the claimants NI record

3. Social Assistance Schemes financed by the state and means tested
4. Children's Allowances financed by the state and paid to all families irrespective of their other income.

The *Report of the Commission on Social Welfare* (Curry 1986) provided a comprehensive review of the Irish social welfare system. The Commission did not recommend radical change in the structure of the welfare system, but did recommend some fundamental changes in its future direction and the way income support was delivered:

- The social insurance system should be extended, in terms of both coverage and benefits provided
- Social assistance, while providing a supporting role which would diminish over time as the social insurance system developed, should be made more comprehensive
- Both systems should be simplified and rationalised
- Benefit rates should be substantially improved to a minimally adequate income, especially for those on the lower payments and families in particular.

The Commission recommended that the disability and occupational injury systems should remain basically unchanged. In principle, they favoured some transfer of responsibility for sick pay to employers. They considered there was duplication between the functions of the Departments of Health and Social Welfare which should be rationalised. In particular, income maintenance, such as Disabled Person's Maintenance Allowance, should be transferred to the Department of Social Welfare.

Most of these changes to the welfare system were implemented, apart from SSP, and had profound impact on the social security structure for the next decade.

A further Commission on the Status of People with Disabilities published its report in November 1996. The main recommendations were (MISSOC 1998):

- A non-means-tested 'Disability Pension' to compensate for incapacity for full-time work or work to full potential, which would replace existing Disability Allowance, Invalidity Benefits and Blind Person's Pension
- A graduated payment to meet the additional costs associated with disability
- Changes in the financial support available to carers
- Benefit rates in real terms recommended by the earlier Commission on Social Welfare (Curry 1986) should be achieved as a matter of priority
- Responsibility for provisions for sick and disabled people to be simplified and streamlined in the Department of Social, Community and Family Affairs (1996–97).

Income support for people who are sick or disabled is now provided mainly through the various state income maintenance schemes. Other sources of income support include occupational sick pay and pension schemes, permanent health insurance and compensation through the legal system, although there is still no SSP. Social security benefits for people who are sick or disabled now include:

- The contributory schemes of Disability Benefit for people aged between 18 and 66 years who are incapacitated for work due to illness and Invalidity Pension for those who have been off work for at least 12 months and who are permanently incapable of work because of illness

- A range of Occupational Injuries Benefits for people who are incapable of work or disabled as a result of an accident at work, including in particular short-term Injury Benefit and longer-term Disablement Benefit. (Note this is a benefit for occupational injuries and quite different from the UK SDA or SDA for congenital or developmental conditions)
- Means-tested Disability Allowance for people aged between 16 and 66 years whose employment capacity is *substantially handicapped* because of a specified disability. (This is the equivalent of the UK SDA)
- Means-tested Supplementary Welfare Allowance for people whose means are insufficient to meet their needs includes a range of additional *supplementary* payments. There is no equivalent to the UK disability premiums, but there are supplements for exceptional heating expenses due to ill health and for special diet due to a medical condition
- A range of secondary benefits in kind, e.g. Free Fuel Allowance, Free Electricity, Free Travel and Free TV Licence. Entitlement is normally based on eligibility to Old Age or Disability income support payments.

In 1999 there were a total of 166,000 recipients of illness-related benefits and allowances at a cost of £IR737 million.

Eligibility for benefits for disability and incapacity depends on:

- NI contributions or means testing
- The degree and expected duration of disability or incapacity for work.

Medical assessment is in two stages (Leech 1999). The first is 'desk evaluation' which applies to the majority of claims; this is cost-effective and administratively preferable. It is also efficient and customer friendly as it is selective and refers claimants for medical examination only when necessary.

To obtain the relevant quality information required for desk evaluation, a new medical report form was introduced in 1999 for completion by treating physicians. This form considers not only impairment but also the resulting degree of disability; 100,000 such forms were issued in 1999 and a fee of £IR20 is payable for completion and early return.

The second stage is medical examination, which is necessary when desk evaluation cannot make a decision solely on the basis of the available medical information. Examinations are also carried out in all cases of occupational injury or disease, appeals, cases being assessed for the UK or other EU member states' benefits, or those countries with which Ireland has bilateral agreements, e.g. the US, Canada and Australia. The Department currently has 20 medical assessors, who evaluate approximately 100,000 medical reports and carry out 60,000 medical examinations per annum related to sickness and disability benefits.

Medical Evaluation was reformed in 1996, with changes somewhat similar to those in the UK (Leech 1999). A new composite medical report form was introduced to accommodate all the various illness-related schemes. It was designed to be easily understood by non-medical persons and to provide an evaluation which would be consistent, fair and evidence-based. It covers: the medical history; work, educational and vocational history; the patient's own account of their injury and illness, and the resultant loss of function in activities of daily living and work; a systems review and general medical evaluation; a detailed medical examination of the affected system or body part; and any medical evidence furnished. The medical examiner then evaluates the appropriate degree of disability affecting various recognised functional areas, similar to the *All Work Test* (see page 158). In reaching this evaluation, the degree of disability should in the majority of cases be consistent with the severity of impairment. If the medical assessor's evaluation is at odds or differs significantly from the claimant's report of disability, the assessor must justify his or her evaluation, e.g. if the patient's symptoms are not adequately explained by the objective clinical findings or by inconsistencies and inappropriate responses noted during examination.

Trends

Between 1947, the year the Department of Social Welfare was established, and 1985 when the report of the Commission on Social Welfare was prepared, the number of recipients of social welfare payments increased in absolute terms and as a proportion of the total population (Table 4.51). The numbers receiving old-age pensions actually fell relative to the population, while the numbers receiving unemployment benefits increased most markedly. There was also an increase in the number of recipients of long-term payments, particularly with a shift from disability benefits to invalidity pensions. There was a significant shift from assistance to insurance payments.

Table 4.52 gives more detailed statistics of the various disability benefits from 1981 to 1999.

The fall in the number of people claiming Disability Benefit between the mid 1980s and mid 90s has been attributed to a number of factors including:

- The introduction of stricter contribution conditions for eligibility
- Improvements in the Medical Assessment and Review system
- The movement of people on long-term Disability Benefit to Invalidity Pension.

The progressive increase in the number of people on long-term Invalidity Pension has been attributed to:

TABLE 4.51 Growth in social welfare 1947–1985: thousands of recipients (excluding dependents) of each benefit at the end of each calendar year

	Old-age pensions	Unemployment benefits	Disability benefits	Invalidity Pension
1947	—	18.0	24.4	—
1966	40.6	33.4	52.6	—
1971	46.5	36.6	54.4	11.6
1976	55.2	55.1	70.8	10.2
1982	70.0	77.6	63.4	20.4
1985	73.0	89.2	77.8	24.2

From Curry (1986).

TABLE 4.52   Disability, Invalidity and Occupational Injury Benefits

	Disability Benefit	Invalidity Pension	Occupational Injury Benefit	Occupational Disablement Benefit	Disability Allowance[1]	Total disability benefits
1981	68,186	18,684	n/a	4986	22,776	114,632
1982	68,079	20,395	n/a	5351	22,759	116,584
1983	69,960	20,849	687	5829	21,936	119,261
1984	73,557	21,981	637	6183	—	—
1985	79,118	24,229	725	6510	24,197	134,779
1986	79,168	26,107	774	6771	24,661	137,481
1987	71,525	28,415	737	6825	24,854	132,356
1988	61,967	29,242	573	7499	25,047	124,328
1989	55,521	30,909	525	6967	25,901	119,823
1990	52,765	34,068	577	7241	26,397	121,048
1991	49,726	36,156	951	7530	27,741	122,104
1992	47,733	36,849	765	7855	28,759	121,961
1993	43,924	38,894	725	8301	30,049	121,893
1994	41,869	40,226	740	8646	30,693	122,174
1995	41,830	42,092	658	8977	32,699	132,256
1996	42,460	43,046	690	9364	37,054	132,614
1997	43,000	43,633	720	9748	43,192	140,384
1998	43,766	44,925	746	10,182	47,126	146,751
1999	45,535	46,946	748	10,577	50,431	154,237

[1]Previously Disabled Persons Maintenance Allowance funded by Dept of Health up to August 1995.
From Department of Social, Community and Family Affairs statistics, courtesy Dr C Leech.

- An increase in the eligible population
- Measures to move people to more appropriate benefits, e.g. those on long-term Disability Benefit for a number of years.

The progressive increase in the number of people on Occupational Disablement Benefit has been attributed to changes in the eligible labour force and improved publicity to recipients of Injury Benefit about their potential entitlement to Disablement Benefit.

Table 4.53 gives the age distribution of recipients of Disability Benefit and Invalidity Pension.

Table 4.54 gives duration on benefits versus return to work.

Very limited data are available on back pain, but back and neck incapacities (of which the ratio of back:neck is approximately 15:1) is the largest single group of Disability Benefit recipients, and the number of current Disability Benefit cases increased from 4677 in October 1996 to 7429 in January 1999. The corresponding figures for Disablement Benefit were 3796 in December 1996, 4486 in December 1997, and 4985 in December 1998.

Unfortunately, there are no data on back incapacities for Invalidity Pensions or Disability Allowance, which makes it impossible to estimate the total impact of back pain.

TABLE 4.53   Age distribution of recipients of Disability Benefit and Invalidity Pension

Age	Disability Benefit	Invalidity Pension
<25	1892	5
25–29	3429	86
30–34	5487	534
35–39	6285	2051
40–44	5876	3635
45–49	5568	5522
50–54	5879	8040
55–59	5514	9776
60–64	5218	13,316
65+	387	3981

Department of Social, Community and Family Affairs statistics, courtesy Dr C Leech.

TABLE 4.54   Duration on benefits and return to work

Duration on benefit (weeks)	% returned to work	% still off work
1	9.9	90.1
2	44.1	55.9
4	65.1	34.9
8	78.6	21.4
10	82.0	18.0
20	89.2	10.8
30	92.0	8.0
40	93.2	6.8
52	94.1	5.9
104	97.0	3.0
156	97.7	2.3

Sweden

[Much of this section is based on Waddell & Norlund (2000) with permission from SBU.]

The population of Sweden is just under 9 million with one of the highest birth rates and immigration rates in the EU. Sweden has the lowest marriage rate in the EU and a relatively high divorce rate with just under half of all births outside marriage and 19% of all families with children headed by a single parent.

Nachemson (1991), Olsson et al (1993), Folkesson et al (1993), Svensson & Brorsson (1997) and Waddell & Norlund (2000) reviewed changes and trends in the Swedish social security system during the 1980s and 1990s.

In Sweden, responsibility for taxation and social services is divided between the state, the county councils and the municipalities (MISSOC 1995). The county councils and municipalities also levy income taxes. The division of responsibilities is basically:

- The state is primarily responsible for the social insurance system. It pays certain subsidies to the county councils and municipalities
- The county councils are responsible for health care
- The municipalities provide general benefits in kind (with the exception of health care), which includes some benefits for the handicapped. They also provide some social assistance to people in need, both in cash and in kind.

Traditionally, the 'Scandinavian model' of social security or 'Nordic welfare society' is based on economic prosperity and high living standards. It is generally accepted that society should and will take good care of its citizens when they are ill, unemployed, get old or are otherwise in economic need (Olsson et al 1993). The Swedish welfare system had its roots in the depressions of the 1920s and 30s, when visions developed of national welfare policies of comprehensive financial security, and the right of the entire population to social services on equal terms (Folkesson et al 1993). These concepts were developed during an almost unbroken period of social democrat government up to the mid 1970s. The main characteristics of the Swedish social insurance system are that it is statutory, universal, based on residence, not means tested, and income related. Each person is entitled individually rather than as an employee or as a member of a family.

In the early 1980s the Swedish Court of Insurance (Försäkringsdomstolen) took several decisions that had a major impact on the numbers and duration of claims for sickness and invalidity benefits. The appeal court changed the interpretation of work injury from a purely biomedical concept to an administrative and legal concept. Judgements of incapacity for work took account of the availability of work and the prospects of gaining employment, and increasing allowance was made for age (Sjuk-och 1997). In the mid 1980s sickness benefits were also improved, with abolition of the waiting day and improvement of benefit levels for short-term absence. Following these changes the number of claims for benefits increased which led to administrative delays in processing claims in the local social security offices and hence poorer control of claims and diminishing efforts at rehabilitation and re-employment. Although Swedish legislation did not set any time limit for sickness benefits, for many years it was almost an unwritten rule that they should not last more than one year, but this was gradually relaxed. The end result was an increase in the number of claims for work-related injuries (Table 4.55), in the average duration of sickness absence, and especially in the amount of long-term sickness and invalidity (Table 4.56). This led to gradually increasing numbers of invalidity pensions through the 1980s (Palme 1994). In effect, during the 1980s, sickness absence and longer-term invalidity became more or less accepted and tolerated in a time of economic prosperity and high employment. However, it is important to note that this increase was related to these various structural changes mainly affecting the earlier stages of sickness and progress to long-term disability, without any significant change in the financial level of the invalidity benefits.

Larsson & Bjornstig (1995) followed up a 1-year sample of 1785 occupational injuries from 1985–1986 in Umea, Sweden. Two years later 39% had 'persistent medical problems' (most commonly pain) and 5 years later 23% had persistent problems. Only 4% had major, definable, permanent medical impairment such as fracture or amputation. Back aches and

TABLE 4.55 Benefits for work-related injuries 1980–1998 (all types)

	Total current benefits	New benefits approved	% new claims approved
1980	189,964	22,271	66.0
1981	182,036	24,044	64.6
1982	178,022	24,226	67.4
1983	183,419	25,545	71.7
1984	203,748	28,974	73.7
1985	218,022	38,632	75.1
1986	233,828	49,551	80.4
1987	244,133	64,382	87.2
1988	260,352	73,488	88.1
1989	248,287	78,313	86.0
1990	222,961	78,447	82.9
1991	191,043	79,285	79.6
1992	155,661	67,636	72.3
1993	232,158	57,457	64.0
1994	132,634	31,917	51.9
1995	118,517	15,668	49.8
1996	113,948	9179	55.7
1997	108,334	7800	62.7
1998	110,612	n/a	n/a

RFV Statistical information.

TABLE 4.56 Total number of cases of sickness benefit lasting longer than 1 year and ongoing disability or temporary disability pensions

	Sickness benefit	Disability pension	Total		Sickness benefit	Disability pension	Total
1980	19,000	292,000	311,000	1994	47,000	422,000	469,000
1985	30,000	323,000	353,000	1995	45,000	420,000	465,000
1990	75,000	361,000	436,000	1996	47,000	419,000	466,000
1991	76,000	367,000	443,000	1997	42,000	423,000	465,000
1992	71,000	383,000	454,000	1998	40,000	422,000	462,000
1993	53,000	414,000[1]	467,000[1]				

[1] From 1993 this includes people with only a supplementary pension (ATP).
RFV Statistical information.

pains accounted for 42% of persistent problems. People in health care, social and nursing occupations were most likely to have persistent problems. Of those with persisting problems at 5 years, one in five had changed jobs and one in 10 had retired early or remained on long-term sick leave. The early retired and long-term sick had a large proportion of younger women and older men.

By the early 1990s, it was widely accepted in Sweden that the fundamental problem with the social security system was wrong incentives (Folkesson et al 1993). MISSOC (1995) gave a more detailed list of the major problems in the Swedish social security system by 1990:

- Pension systems out of line with economic growth
- Wrong incentives
- No co-ordinated administrative responsibility for prevention, benefit payments and rehabilitation
- Lack of incentives for employers to participate in prevention and rehabilitation
- Occupational injury insurance out of control
- Compensation levels different in similar schemes
- Total costs out of control because of all these problems.

These problems of the changing interpretation of work injury and increasing sickness absence led to a special council on rehabilitation (1985), and a commission on the work environment (1989). The political debate and reforms accelerated following the election of a coalition government in 1991 (Palme 1994), although the reforms had already begun and were also fuelled by the economic recession. Although there was still broad political support for Sweden's social policy in general terms, high public spending, high taxation and negative economic trends in the early 1990s led to demands for re-assessment. Folkesson et al (1993) considered at that time that the social security system in Sweden was facing significant change, from traditional institutional regulation and stability towards increased flexibility and local adaptation. There was an attempt to renew the public sector in terms of efficiency, freedom of choice, and privatisation with the aim of creating competition. The underlying aim was to deregulate public monopoly and decentralise operative responsibility. However, these changes appear to have been largely structural rather than any fundamental re-consideration of the basic principles of the Swedish social security system.

The first legislative step was to restrict early retirement pension to medical reasons alone and not labour grounds, and in practice there was increasing demand for medical reasons for all sickness and invalidity. The only acceptable grounds for sickness absenteeism and early retirement became the working capacity of the individual ('arbetslinjen'). Legislation in 1993 changed the definition of work injury or disease, which was now only accepted if the balance of probabilities was that it was the result of harmful influence at work. [Previously this rule of evidence was formulated the opposite way in a unique 'reverse' burden of proof (MISSOC 1995).]

From 1991, there were progressive cuts in the level of sickness benefit (Table 4.57) and also legislation to limit the extent of any collective agreements. In 1993, a waiting day was introduced for sickness benefits, the level of sickness benefits was cut further, and the levels of all types of pension were reduced. There was a specific further cut in the level of sickness benefit for those who were still absent after more than 1 year and inactive, i.e. not receiving medical treatment or any form of rehabilitation. Between 1991 and 1993, short-term industrial injury benefits were progressively made the same as sickness benefits, and were effectively abolished. However, if work injury led to permanent loss of working capacity of >1/15, the individual still received 100% wage replacement. Palme (1994) also reviewed proposed policy changes that were never implemented, including in particular two attempts to abolish partial pension plans that were blocked on both occasions.

TABLE 4.57 Successive changes in sickness benefits in 1990–1998 as % wage replacement rate

Days of sickness	1990	March 1991	January 1992	April 1993	July 1993	January 1996	January 1998
1	90	65	75	0	0	0	0
2–3	90	65	75	75	75	75	80
4–14	90	80	90	90	90	75	80
15–90	90	80	80	80	80	75	80
91–365	90	90	90	80	70/80	75	80
365–	90	90	90	80	70/80	75	80

The changes in the sickness benefit system in the mid 1990s, compared to the late 1980s, illustrate the impact of incentives and controls. In the 1980s, during the period of economic growth and prosperity, Sweden had very high wage replacement rates with low financial self-risk, and at the same time very weak social security controls on benefits. In the 1990s, as economic conditions deteriorated, the wage-replacement level of benefits was reduced which increased the financial self-risk for the individual. At the same time much stricter controls were introduced both by employers and by the social security system. Over this period the amount of sickness and disability rose in the 1980s when benefit levels were generous and fell from the early 1990s when benefit levels were reduced. However, it is not possible to attribute this simply to the level of benefits as there were simultaneously major changes in the structure and control mechanisms of the social security system. Allowance must also be made for the major changes which occurred in the whole economic and labour market situation in Sweden over this period. Moreover, the greatest changes in benefit levels during this period were for relatively short-term sickness absence, but the major trends were in work-related injury benefits and in long-term invalidity and early retirement. More detailed examination of these changes suggests that the structure and practice of the benefits system had the most immediate and greatest impact on the amount of different benefits paid.

There was also separate legislation in 1991 to improve the work environment and work safety to reduce the risk of work injury. The employer now had direct legal responsibility for providing a safe working environment and greater responsibility for vocational rehabilitation and work re-placement. From 1992 employers had to pay the first 2 weeks of sick benefits. The aim of all these measures was to impose a direct financial incentive and control function on employers to reduce injury and sickness.

In the 1997 budget, the Swedish government stated that the most important prerequisite for a stable welfare policy was balancing the finances. The entire social security and all benefits and allowances must be designed to support employment and reduce unemployment (MIS-SOC 1996). In 1996, a government committee report on disability and invalidity pensions called for a clearer separation of unemployment and disability benefits. The more favourable treatment of people over the age of 60 who had labour market difficulties was abolished.

Various government committees have proposed changes to improve rehabilitation, including making all the different parties involved in rehabilitation co-operate more efficiently and effectively, as this is perhaps the best way to reduce social security costs. Sweden has made a particular effort to co-ordinate the medical, social, psychological and work-related aspects to provide more holistic rehabilitation. In the 1990s there was a further drive for financial co-ordination between the different rehabilitation elements in the public sector. From 1992, each local office of the Swedish National Board of Sickness Security (RFV) was made responsible for the co-ordination of rehabilitation measures, both in general and for the individual case. Specific government funds were allocated to purchase vocational rehabilitation, although in practice these were often simply used for physiotherapy as there were few other resources available. There were a number of local projects to integrate the organisation of sickness benefits and social security at the municipality level, health care and employment.

After these reforms, official RFV statistics showed that the average time the local RFV office took to contact those on long-term sick leave decreased from 100 to 66 days, and the proportion contacted increased from 31 to 60%. For all categories of sickness the average duration of sickness absence fell from 242 to 149 days. There were fewer recurrent cases leading to long-term sickness absence, and in those who were employed the level of early retirement fell from 29 to 22%. However, for most years after 1992, the Swedish National Health Insurance Office was unable to use the budget of US$51–71 allocated for work-related rehabilitation (Jensen et al 2000). Moreover, the outcomes were not so good for musculoskeletal symptoms, of which back pain formed a major part. Official figures show that for back pain, the median number of days before any rehabilitation measures started increased from 119 to 129 days, and complete recovery fell from 85 to 81%. An independent study by Jensen (1998) showed that only 18% of those sick listed with back pain for >3 months actually got rehabilitation. Of those over 55 years of age, only 5% received any rehabilitation before they received a disability pension. Official figures also showed that, although the number receiving early retirement for back pain fell, their proportion increased from 11 to 16% of all early retirements. So the greater efforts at rehabilitation were less successful for those with musculoskeletal disorders than for other forms of sickness. Jensen et al (2000) suggested that one reason for this was that 'expert' judgements by physicians, physical therapists and social insurance officers were too unreliable to predict who would benefit from rehabilitation.

As part of the drive to improve rehabilitation, a large number of pilot projects were set up financed by public organisations. These can be divided into four groups (Table 4.58).

Unfortunately, many of these projects were poorly designed, with almost complete lack of control groups, and inadequate evaluation of the results. As one example only, Arbetslivsfonden spent >3000 million SEK on rehabilitation projects for 25,000 enterprises and public organisations. Of >3000 different projects, only two made any attempt at including a control group, and one of these was simply the previous, out-dated, and inadequate, local RFV data. The summary report on these 3000 projects has never been published by the organisation that sponsored it.

These approaches to rehabilitation in Sweden in the 1990s had lofty and laudable aims, and some reports claimed that they produced great benefits for individuals and society.

TABLE 4.58 Reports on Swedish rehabilitation projects in the 1990s

Project name	Aim of rehabilitation	Problems of evaluation
Arbetslivs-fonden	Better rehabilitation back to work. Better and safer work places	No adequate control groups. Before/after measurements of official statistics of sickness days, etc not reliable when unemployment has increased from <2 to >13%, plus great changes in sickness benefits and the control system
Dagmar	Special funding to the health care sector in order to speed up rehabilitation by cutting waiting time to treatment (mainly for persons 16–64)	No control groups (most reports) or inadequate controlgroups. No conclusions re. effects can be drawn
FINSAM	Better and faster rehabilitation from co-ordination even financially between the health care and the local sickness benefit offices (only for persons 16–64)	Control groups are questionable in many cases, e.g. the city of Stockholm compared to rural villages dominated by farmers in southern Sweden in one of the projects
SOCSAM	Better and faster rehabilitation from co-ordination even financially between health care, municipality and sickness benefit offices (total financial co-ordination)	Control groups are questionable in many cases

Unfortunately, there was lack of proper scientific evidence to support these claims which met political scepticism.

MISSOC (1998) summarised these changes through the 1990s. In the early 1990s sickness and disability insurance was changed to promote active rehabilitation and increase incentives to work. Disability pensions were more closely linked to the sickness insurance scheme, with disability pension as the final solution after every possible rehabilitation measure had been unsuccessful. Eligibility for sickness and disability benefits were tightened. There were measures to improve co-operation between the various agencies involved in supporting and rehabilitating sick and disabled people, to improve efficiency and control fraud. This trend had continued. Measures in January 1997 further tightened eligibility. Long-term disability benefits were now based on incapacity for any form of work, not only previous type of employment, and even if the alternative work was lower paid. Sickness and disability benefits were also based purely on the claimant's medical condition, without any consideration of social or labour market conditions or actual job availability.

Trends in back pain

Table 4.59–4.61 show the increase in the incidence and duration of work loss due to back pain, although this is based on limited statistics for one area that may not be representative of the whole country.

TABLE 4.59 Increase in the incidence and duration of work loss due to back pain in Göteborg

	% having time off work with back pain	Average days lost per annum
1970	1	20
1975	3	22
1980	4	25
1987	8	36
1992	8	39
1997	5	36

TABLE 4.60 Millions of days per annum of sickness benefit absence due to neck and back pain in Sweden, based on a sample from Göteborg

	Low back pain	Neck/shoulder	Combinations	Total
1987	13.4	9.3	5.3	28.0
1995	10.6	8.2	3.0	21.8
1996	4.5	9.2	4.1	17.8

TABLE 4.61 Million days per annum of sickness absence due to back pain compared to all days of sickness absence

	Back pain	All causes	% back pain
1987	28.0	107	26
1995	21.8	74	29
1996	17.8	44	40

Table 4.62 shows that the total number of early retirements for all causes remained more or less constant from the early 1970s to the mid 80s, but there was a rise about 1984–1985 and then a further rise about 1992–1993, particularly in the number of partial retirement benefits. From 1994 there was a fall in the number of early retirements for all causes, with a slightly greater fall in the number of partial retirements. Between the early 1970s and early 1990s, there was a marked increase in the number of early retirements due to back pain, particularly about 1989, and the proportion they accounted for of all early retirements rose from 7 to 22%. After 1993, the number of early retirements due to back pain progressively fell, initially as part of the general trend but then continuing so that by 1998 backs only accounted for 13% of all early retirements. There are anecdotal accounts that this reduction in early retirements was counter-balanced by an increase in long-term sickness absence, but there is no national, diagnostic-specific, data available to analyse that further.

These trends for back pain do not entirely reflect the above account of the increasing social security problems during the 1980s and the effect of the social security reforms in the early 1990s. The number of early retirements for all causes remained more or less constant from 1971 to 1985, but there was a progressive increase in the proportion due

TABLE 4.62   Early retirement and temporary disability pensions in Sweden 1971–1998

	Total early retirements (full + partial) (number of people)	Total full-time equivalents	Early retirements due to back pain (full + partial) (number of people)	Backs as % of total
1971	43,984	41,565	3070	7.0
1972	52,370	49,692	4064	7.8
1973	52,148	49,398	4785	9.2
1974	45,931	43,274	4334	9.4
1975	45,457	42,637	4738	10.4
1976	45,306	41,919	5885	13.0
1977	46,350	42,371	6589	14.2
1978	45,144	40,837	6784	15.0
1979	44,278	39,600	7094	16.0
1980	45,289	39,908	6933	15.3
1981	43,615	37,869	6123	14.0
1982	42,286	36,764	5469	12.9
1983	43,338	38,177	5872	13.5
1984	46,792	41,859	6870	14.7
1985	51,009	45,897	7703	15.1
1986	50,106	44,732	8666	17.3
1987	51,691	46,169	7255	14.0
1988	54,135	48,136	8976	16.6
1989	51,991	45,622	11,037	21.2
1990	50,493	43,382	11,253	22.2
1991	49,554	42,289	10,726	21.6
1992	58,382	49,534	12,998	22.3
1993	62,465	52,023	13,280	21.2
1994	48,531	38,536	9602	24.5
1995	39,204	30,732	8715	22.2
1996	39,245	31,009	6375	16.2
1997	41,198	33,861	6907	16.8
1998	34,489	28,180	4602	13.3

RFV Statistical information.

to back pain between 1971 and 1976. There was a more marked increase in the number of early retirements for all causes in 1984–1985 and again in 1992–1993, but the major increase in early retirements due to back pain and the proportion they accounted for of all early retirements was in 1987–1989. The initial fall in the number of early retirements due to all causes and to back pain after 1993 does fit with the social security reforms, but there was then a continuing fall in the number of early retirements due to back pain. Some of these trends were undoubtedly explained to some extent by the changes in the structure and practice of the social security system. Some probably reflect changes in the whole economic and labour market situation. However, the long-term rise in early retirements due to back pain since the early 1970s and the fall after about 1996 appeared to be more specific to back pain (see the discussion of similar trends in the UK, p 172).

There is a footnote to the above account of social security trends in Sweden (A Nachemson, personal communication, May 2002). Recent years have seen continued changes in Swedish politics and the social security system. Between 1997 and 2001, the number of sick days has doubled and is now once again approaching the levels of the late 1980s. The number of people on long-term sickness and disability for >1 year has now risen to approximately 120,000. However, there are no detailed statistics available yet on back pain.

The first report of the Swedish part of the ISSA study on Work Incapacity and Reintegration described the baseline data (Bergendorff et al 1998). A prospective cohort of 1822 employed men and women aged 18–59 who were sick listed for at least 28 days due to low back or neck pain was recruited from social security files in 1994–1995. Within this, a subset of people incapacitated for 3 months due to low back pain (LBP) formed the international comparison cohort. Questionnaires were administered at baseline (77%), 90 days (63%), 1 year (55%) and 2 years (49%). The battery included:

- Psychosocial aspects of work (Karasek-Theorell)
- Euroqol (a general quality of life index)
- Zung depression inventory
- Hannover back-related disability scale (activities of daily living)
- SF-36 (general health questionnaire)
- Pain and Disability scale (Von Korff).

The baseline questionnaires showed that 73% of the cohort had LBP and 27% neck pain; 57% were women. A majority had had back symptoms for >1 year, and two-thirds of those with back pain reported radiation to one or both legs. Two-thirds claimed they first experienced symptoms at work. Low back or neck pain was the main reason given for not working but 12% regarded a co-morbidity as another severe obstacle to returning to work. Compared to the entire population, the cohort had a higher proportion of:

- Older people
- Women
- Immigrants
- People with low education
- Blue-collar workers
- People with low income
- People who stated that they have bad working conditions, high psychological demands and low decision latitude, and low social support at work
- Smokers and people with obesity
- People with severe pain, depressive symptoms and lack of vitality
- People with low quality of life.

The Swedish study had a stronger focus on the effects of case management within the social security system. At baseline, 28 days after sick listing, 61% expected to be able to return to their usual work, 26% expected to be able to return to some form of work but not their usual work, and 13% thought they would never be able to work.

Sydsjo (1998) and Sydsjo et al (1998) reported on sick-listing due to back pain during pregnancy in Sweden. The single most common reason for sick-listing was 'back pain during pregnancy', which increased from 11% of employed pregnant women in 1978 to 29% in 1986, although by 1997 it had fallen to 17%. The average number of days sick-listing during pregnancy increased 100% between 1978 and 1987, although the corresponding increase for non-pregnant women was only 20%. There was no obstetric explanation for these findings, and it was not related to occupation or unemployment. In the 1986 data, Sydsjo (1998) also found that 75% of employed pregnant women were sick listed in Sweden compared with 48% in Norway. The increase in sick certification in Sweden from 1978 to 1986 followed the introduction of substantially improved pregnancy and parental benefits in 1980, while the slight fall between 1992 and 1997 coincided with a modest reduction in benefit levels and tightening of eligibility. Sickness rates were also higher in Sweden where benefits were more favourable than in Norway. In a questionnaire study about personal attitudes in 1995, Sydsjo (1998) found that only 4.2% of the women reported that they had suffered a clearly pregnancy-related disorder, while conversely 74% of women who had been sick listed during pregnancy nevertheless reported that they had enjoyed good or excellent health during the whole of their pregnancy. Sydsjo (1998) considered that the amount of sick-listing was not simply related to the level of maternity benefits. Rather, he suggested that the most plausible explanation of changed patterns of sick-listing during pregnancy might be 'a change in attitudes to pregnancy and its subjective consequences, together with a sensible adaptation to the prevailing conditions within the social security system'.

Norway

Norway is one of the smaller European countries with a population of 4.3 million. Similar to other Nordic countries, 44% of births are outside marriage and 19% of all families with children are headed by single parents.

The Norwegian Social Security System covers all residents, whether or not they are economically active and irrespective of contribution record. There is very little means testing. Benefits are granted to individuals more or less irrespective of the family situation with strong gender equality. They are financed by the state, employers and employees, and administered by central government. There is however a strong 'work subsidiarity principle' so that benefits should not be paid if work is possible and available.

All employees are granted 100% sickness benefits from the first day of absence for a period of up to 12 months and then transferred, either to another year of medical rehabilitation or to permanent disability pensions, both with reduced compensation. The first 2 weeks' sickness absence are paid by the employer and are not included in the National Insurance Administration (NIA) statistics.

Laerum (personal communication, 2000) reported that LBP accounts for 5% of GP consultations in Norway—600,000 per year lasting an average of 15 minutes. There are

7000 physiotherapists in 1800 institutions, about 200 of whom specialise in manual therapy. There is increasing scientific orientation of the physiotherapy profession but there is still extensive use of passive modalities. There are about 200 chiropractors in Norway and 50–80% of their practice is for LBP. Two-thirds of patients self-refer to a chiropractor and 20% are referred by their family doctor: although all patients pay privately. Chiropractors can carry out X-rays and issue sick certificates although there is no information on how much of this work they do. It is now proposed that physiotherapists might also be allowed to issue sick certificates although this is still under discussion. Secondary care of back pain is by the usual range of specialists but is fragmented and there are no data on numbers. There are about 15–20 clinics with a special interest in back pain which offer: multidisciplinary second opinion (although the professional make-up is very varied); surgery (there are about 4000 back operations per annum); and about 6–10 rehabilitation clinics, the nature of which again varies. Laerum's overall impression was of:

- Lack of co-ordination of services and lack of co-operation between services
- Many patients are confused and frustrated by conflicting advice
- Long waiting lists: 6 months to see a specialist, 3–6 months for surgery (but very variable)
- Lack of guidance (despite a consensus statement in 1995) and some reluctance and resistance to clinical guidelines
- Common beliefs: 'Do not return to work till completely pain free'; 'Better back surgery in Sweden'.

In response to these problems, a Norwegian Back Pain Network was set up in 1999 with the following objectives:

- Improve back health in Norway: better clinical management; secondary prevention of chronic pain and disability
- Research
- Information: health professional (including the development of Norwegian clinical guidelines); public education
- Inter-disciplinary collaboration.

Ploug & Kvist (1994) reviewed recent social security developments. After a long period of steady growth which had led to a gradual extension of the social security programme, in the early 1990s the Norwegian welfare system underwent the most thorough re-evaluation since the present system was set up soon after World War II. It entered a period of reform which included continued expansion in a few areas but the first signs of major cut-backs of entitlement in other areas.

In 1990 a programme was agreed which aimed to reduce the amount of sick leave by 10% in the following year. Unlike Sweden, the benefit level remained at 100% wage replacement and Norway did not introduce any cut-offs. However, in June 1993, the medical criteria defining sickness were made more restrictive. The NIA specified that problems such as grief, economic difficulties, normal ageing and marital problems did not give entitlement to sickness benefits, which was a reversal of the previous trend to liberalism. There was a shift of responsibility for determination for eligibility for sickness benefits from the claimant's own doctor to the local NIA. After the first 12 weeks of sick leave, the administration had to verify continued eligibility. The administration could also check the doctor's sick certification for benefits at an earlier stage and draw up a plan for possible rehabilitation in co-operation with the employer.

However, there were even greater changes in long-term disability benefits. After a long period of 'symptom liberalisation', much stricter criteria were introduced of what constituted disability. There were more than 20 changes in the law. In particular in 1991, the definition of disability was changed to put greater emphasis on medical criteria. Reduced capacity for work must be clearly related to medical disease, injury or defect. Prior to these reforms regional variations in employment opportunities were taken into account, but the reforms also introduced greater demands for geographical and labour market mobility. At the same time, there were some extensions of entitlement. Benefits for the congenitally disabled were increased, some supplementary benefits were made available to those with responsibility for caring for dependents and there were more lenient rules for partial disability for housewives in part-time work.

Norway also produced a green paper on rehabilitation in 1990–1991. The major change was the emphasis on activity or work orientation in place of the former passive support. Benefits were actively linked to efforts by the claimant and the authorities to become self-supporting. During the early 1990s the government also started to stress the principle of 'targeting' welfare benefits to those with greatest needs. There was increasing emphasis on incentives and the need to remove possible disincentives. In January 1992 responsibility for rehabilitation benefits were transferred from the Social Insurance Administration to the Department of Employment and changes were made in rehabilitation benefits.

The result of all the efforts to reduce the level of sick leave and the number of disability pensioners was a temporary drop in both figures. Today, with low rates of unemployment, the figures are 'back to normal'. An important part of the Norwegian situation, however, like in most Nordic countries, is the high level of work participation compared to other European countries (OECD 1997b), mainly among women and the elderly.

Hagen & Thune (1998) analysed the Norwegian NIA records of 89,190 claimants who received benefits because they had taken more than 2 weeks off work due to back pain in 1995–1996. (This analysis excluded those who returned to work within 2 weeks, who received sick pay from the employer only and were not included in the NIA statistics.) The 1-year incidence was 1.91% for men and 2.72% for women. It increased with age from 1.42% for those aged 20–24 to 2.63% for those aged 55–66. The median period on benefits was 43 calendar days. Those with radiating leg pain were on average off work for 3 weeks longer. Altogether, approximately 35% returned to work by 1 month, 70% by 3 months and 85% by 6 months, but the rate of return to work deteriorated rapidly after being on benefits for >6 weeks. After 1 year, only 6.1% were still on sick leave. Recalculating this data on the assumption from international series that about 75% of people with back pain return to work within the first 2 weeks (Waddell 1998), suggests that about 84% of Norwegians who take any time off work with back pain return to work within 6 weeks, 92.5% by 14 weeks and >96% by 6 months. Only 1.5% are still off work at 1 year.

Strand et al (2001) reviewed sick certification for back pain. In 1998, half those on long-term sick leave (9–52 weeks) had a musculoskeletal diagnosis, 31% with back pain. They reported that there is debate in the Norwegian medical literature about the basis of sick certification in primary care, and that it is suggested patients have more control over the process than general practitioners. One cited study (Lappegaard & Bruusgaard 1997) attributed decrease in sick leave in a community to close follow-up and co-operation between local physicians and the national insurance office.

In 1998, 90.9 per 1000 Norwegian inhabitants aged 16–67 years (men 77.2, women 105.1) were receiving disability pensions for all conditions. The corresponding prevalence for back conditions was 13.0 per 1000, which is 14.3% of all disability pensions. The corresponding numbers for new disability pensions in 1998 for all conditions was 12.5 (men 10.9, women 14.3) per 1000 persons at risk and for back conditions was 1.8 (men 1.6, women 2.1). Table 4.63 gives prevalence data for back conditions by gender and age. Interestingly, the prevalence of disability pensions for back conditions in Norway has not changed from 1991 to 1998 (men 11.6 to 11.3; women 14.2 to 14.8 per 1000).

TABLE 4.63   Prevalence of disability pension for back conditions in Norway 1998 according to age and gender

	16–39	40–49	50–59	60–64	65–67	Total 16–67
Men	0.6	6.6	21.8	60.0	78.6	11.3
Women	1.1	10.4	30.9	66.0	75.6	14.8

D Bruusgaard, personal communication.

In 1993, Norway introduced 'Active Sick Leave' which enabled the employee to return to modified work with individual modification of the workload (Scheel et al 2002a). All patients in Norway must attend a doctor for sick certification after 3 days sickness absence, and if they are still on sick leave after 16 days their absence must be notified to the NIA. Active Sick Leave is an optional arrangement which requires the co-operation of the GP who recommends the scheme, the employer who permits modifications at work, the NIA office which approves the arrangements, and the worker. The NIA pays 100% of the worker's wages, so there is no cost to the employer who can in theory also employ a full-time replacement. In principle, Active Sick Leave is a 'win-win-win' situation: if modified return to work is effective, the employee will recover faster; the employer can maintain production at no additional cost and fulfil his legal obligations to organise the work situation according to individual needs; the GP has an alternative to standard sick certification when the employee still has some partial capacity to work; the societal costs of sickness absence and particularly chronic incapacity will be reduced to the benefit of all. Those workers, GPs and employers who used Active Sick Leave are generally highly satisfied (Scheel et al 2002a). However, unfortunately, in 1995 only 1% of all sick workers used ASL, probably due to a combination of lack of awareness of the scheme by all workers, GPs and employers, and lack of communication between them. By 1998–1999 this had increased to 12%.

A randomised controlled trial was carried out in 1998–1999 of interventions to improve uptake of Active Sick Leave in patients on sick leave for LBP for 16 days (Scheel et al 2002b): 65 municipalities were randomised to a pro-active intervention, a passive intervention or a control group of usual practice. The passive intervention consisted of four simple administrative measures: targeted information about Active Sick Leave to all the parties, a check box on the sick certificate to remind GPs about ASL, a standard agreement between employees and employers about rehabilitation plans and Active Sick Leave (as required anyway by legislation) and a desktop summary of clinical guidelines for LBP. The pro-active intervention included all these measures plus continuing education for GPs about LBP and ASL, and a 'resource person' (an occupational physical therapist) for each region who provided support and assistance between all the parties in facilitating Active Sick Leave. Active Sick Leave is used significantly more in municipalities with the pro-active intervention (17.7%) compared with the passive intervention (10.8%) and the control group (12.4%) ($p = 0.02$). The study concluded that 'having all the players on side may be essential, but it is not sufficient to bring about action in work place strategies'. The passive intervention had no effect. The pro-active intervention did have a modest impact, improving uptake of Active Sick Leave by 7%. The authors considered the impact of the pro-active intervention was mainly through direct contact and motivating telephone calls to patients. To the extent that GPs' practice was changed, it was either patient mediated or by patients by-passing their GP.

Scheel et al (2002c) reported further on the impact of Active Sick Leave on the duration of sickness absence. Back patients who received Active Sick Leave were off work for a mean of 232 days compared with 243 days for those who did not receive it. Those who received Active Sick Leave were more likely to return to normal work within 1 year (i.e. even counting Active Sick Leave as still being on a form of social security benefits) (85.2% vs 71.9%, $p = <0.0001$). However, this could reflect self-selection rather than a direct effect of Active Sick Leave. In the randomised controlled trial of Active Sick Leave, there was no significant difference in the duration of sickness absence (again counting Active Sick Leave as being time on a form of social security benefits) or the proportion who returned to work within 1 year in either of the intervention groups (Table 4.64).

There is a footnote to this study (I Scheel, personal communication May 2002). Norwegian politicians, employers and trade unions are reluctant to accept these results but continue to believe that Active Sick Leave is 'a good thing'. 'The Confederation of Norwegian Business and Industry has decided to believe that Active Sick Leave is effective.' 'We have blind faith in the [Active Sick Leave] policy. Both the trade unions and the employers organisation will stand by it to their dying day.'

TABLE 4.64 Impact of Active Sick Leave on sickness absence

Group	Median days of sick leave	Return to work by 1 year (%)
Pro-active intervention	70	89.0
Passive intervention	68	89.5
Control	71	89.1

Based on data from Scheel et al (2002c).

Finland

Finland is one of the smaller EU countries with a population of about 5 million. The proportion of births outside marriage is just under 30% which is lower than in most other Nordic countries but higher than the EU average, and 14% of all families with children are headed by a single parent. During the 1970s and 80s, Finland had a period of high economic growth with a large increase in public expenditure and public employment as a result of developments in social policy and social services. Unemployment, which was already low at 5% in 1985, fell to about 3% in 1989. Between 1989 and 1993 the economy deteriorated rapidly and much more severely than in any other EU country due to a combination of the general European recession and the collapse of the neighbouring Russian economy. Unemployment rose rapidly to 17.7% in 1993, the highest unemployment rate in any OECD country. There was a particular problem with youth unemployment which rose to nearly 31% by 1992.

Ploug & Kvist (1994) reviewed recent developments in social security in Finland.

Finland has a Scandinavian model of welfare which provides broadly universal services and benefits to all residents. The Social Insurance Institution (SII) administers basic insurance-based sickness benefits and disability pensions, together with unemployment benefit and old-age pensions.

After 1991, when a new coalition government of the centre and conservative parties was formed, Ploug & Kvist (1994) characterised the Finish economic policy as 'attack and retreat'. Up to the end of 1993, there were no fundamental changes in the various welfare schemes and services, but rather an equal spread of minor adjustments and cuts, including cuts in the wage-replacement rate of sickness benefits.

The Finnish government which came into office in March 1995 enacted several social security reforms (MISSOC 1996). Its main goals were:

● To reduce overall costs, particularly in the long term
● To restructure the benefits schemes to favour employment rather than reliance on benefits.

From January 1996, sickness benefits were only paid to claimants with a yearly income of at least FIM 5000. Those with lower or no income received a lower, means-tested allowance for disability or illness which lasted >60 days. Those with incomes above FIM 5000 per year continued to receive income-related sickness benefit.

MISSOC (1998) stated that there had been little further change in sickness and invalidity benefits since 1996.

The Netherlands

The Netherlands is a medium-sized EU country with a population of 15 million and has the lowest number of elderly, although this will come closer to the EU average over the next 20 years.

Soeters & Prins (1985), Beljaars & Prins (1996), Aarts et al (1996) and Geurts et al (2000) provided Dutch reviews of social security in The Netherlands. The Netherlands has also been of considerable interest to all other countries because in some ways it presents an extreme example of common social security problems (Olsson et al 1993, Folkessson et al 1993, Lonsdale 1993, Lonsdale & Aylward 1993, 1996, Eardley et al 1996, Bolderson et al 1997).

Aarts et al (1996) summarised the problem. Social security provisions in The Netherlands improved dramatically in the late 1950s and 60s, with extended cover both of risks and people, and increase in the real value of benefits which rose faster than wages. There was then explosive growth in the number of people receiving sickness and disability benefits during the 1970s. This was exacerbated by the economic recessions of 1975 and 1981–1983, population ageing, increased labour force participation by women, more part-time work, changed family structure and a surge in early retirement. Despite concerted efforts by policy makers to control the system during the 1980s, both the number of people on benefits and costs continued to rise. Aarts et al (1996) attributed this to a deliberate policy of trying to use the disability system to protect workers from job loss due to economic as well as health reasons, and then the combination of loose eligibility criteria, lenient administrative control and generous benefits. The employment rate fell from almost 60% of the working age population in 1970 to about 50% between 1984 and 1994, while the number of people on social security benefits rose from 2 million in 1970 to 4.4 million in 1994. By 1990, the average Dutch worker in the private sector was sick 1.6 times per annum, each spell lasting for an average of 15 days (Beljaars & Prins 1996). By 1993, one in every 10 Dutch of working age was receiving disability benefits, and nearly 40% of those aged 55–64: four in every five of them were then expected to remain on disability benefits until they reached retirement age (Aarts et al 1996). Overall, 921,000 people were on disability benefits in a working population of 7.23 million (Beljaars & Prins 1996).

Commentators on the Dutch social security systems have argued that its origin and design owe much to the Netherlands' geographical position and geo-political history (Eardley et al 1996). It is a small but economically important trading nation 'at the cross-roads of Europe' which has been subject to considerable influence from its larger neighbours France, Germany and the UK. Although urbanisation, democratic institutions and the development of a capitalistic economy came relatively early, industrialisation and consequent modernisation came later than in other neighbouring countries and it was the last among the present members of the EU to introduce a form of national social insurance. However, between 1958 and 1967 there was rapid development of social security and welfare state provision and since this time in some respects the Netherlands regards itself as a leader in the field.

Aarts et al (1996) described the hallmarks of the Dutch social welfare system as the principle of solidarity and its legal counterpart—the constitutionally established responsibility of the state to protect its residents from poverty. This is achieved by two provisions of the system: wage-replacement and minimum income guarantees. The 'social minimum' income was defined as 'the amount of money necessary to provide for basic needs' which for a two-person family was taken to be 100% of the (high) after-tax minimum wage.

Eardley *et al* (1996) related the development of social security in the Netherlands to the pluralistic nature of the Dutch society and politics. Historically, the nation has been divided by religion between the Protestant north and the Catholic south. There have been social divisions between the early urbanised centres, which fostered a liberal commercial elite and a socialist trade union movement, and rural areas which supported farmers' organisations. These social cleavages produced what became known as 'pillarisation', in which a series of minority interest groups and ideologies were all represented in organisations or political parties close to government. This resulted in coalition and consensus politics and compromise. The new social security system reflected the influence of the Netherlands' powerful neighbours and trading partners, and the specifically Dutch political, economic and religious divisions. The polarisation of Dutch politics and society led to strong competition between the different interest groups to achieve the best possible benefits for their members. During the expansion of social security between 1958 and 1967, this had the result of increasing the cover and level of benefits and easing criteria for eligibility.

Bolderson *et al* (1997) reviewed the current social security system in the Netherlands, which is provided by three separate schemes (Table 4.65). The general scheme of national insurance is by far the largest and covers retirement pensions, widow's and orphan's pensions and child benefits. The general scheme also provides a disablement pension for the non-employed, but this is administered together with the insurance scheme for employees. This national insurance scheme was established in the 1950s and reflects a Beveridge-type universal principle. However, this was not extended to all benefits because there were still strong corporate traditions of public provision in the Netherlands. The 'Employee's Insurance Scheme' is for those in full- or part-time employment and dates from 1952. It is strongly rights-based and financed from contributions by employers and employees. It involves substantially less total expenditure than the national insurance scheme but the benefits per head are much more generous. The insurance schemes for employees are run by 19 industrial associations, each covering a specific market sector, and governed and administered jointly by equal representation of employer and employee organisations. Co-operation between the two sides of industry runs deep in Dutch coalition politics and in Dutch social

TABLE 4.65   Number of recipients of various social security benefits in 1994

National Insurance Scheme	Employees Insurance Schemes	Social Assistance Scheme
Retirement pensions 2,142,000	Unemployment benefits 435,000	Unemployment 326,000
	Sickness benefits (ZW) 171,000	Income provision for older 21,000
Disability pensions (AAW) 240,000	Disability benefits (WAO) 660,000	And partially disabled people 6000
		General assistance 190,000

Population: 15 million; working population 7.3 million.
Based on Bolderson *et al* (1997).

organisations. The Social Assistance Scheme is the smallest of the three schemes. It is largely financed by central government but administered by local authorities which occupy an important position in Dutch democratic government and have a long tradition of welfare provision for the poor.

Short-term sickness is covered by the Sickness Benefits Act of 1930 (ZW) which now covers *all* short-term sickness, irrespective of cause, including sickness, industrial injury and maternity. The Netherlands is unique in having abolished the distinction between occupational and non-occupational injury or illness in 1967. Since this time, there has been no financial advantage for work-related injury and the question of causality does not arise. However, this occurred at the same time as the introduction of more readily available and more generous benefits in either case, so it is not possible to assess the effect of removing causality alone.

The two main longer-term invalidity benefits are WAO and AAW. WAO benefits were introduced in 1967 and are compulsory insurance benefits for employees only. WAO covers approximately three-quarters of all disability beneficiaries. AAW benefits were introduced in 1976 to extend cover to the self-employed and those who became disabled before taking up employment, with married women also becoming eligible in 1980. The basic rules of entitlement to both benefits are incapacity for work for at least 52 weeks. 'Incapacity' means not being able to earn the same wage as a healthy person in suitable work. 'Work' means that which someone can reasonably expect to do, in the light of their training and former occupation. People on WAO or AAW are allowed to have some earned income, but they have to inform the authorities of this and their benefit might be reviewed if it is thought this indicates a capacity for more permanent employment.

Olsson *et al* (1993) hypothesised that the development of the Netherlands' labour market was heavily dependent on the legal, financial and administrative structure of the corporate sickness insurance and invalidity benefits and the incentives these produced. Legislatively, the industrial insurance boards were independent of the state, and employers and employees jointly financed and administered sickness benefits. In practice, employers and employees also handled the operational definition of sickness between them, which made it possible for them to broaden the definition within the framework of the law. They jointly made up the executive level of the industrial insurance board, with equal say in the decisions. At the individual level, they often had a shared interest in moving workers from sickness benefits to invalidity benefits. Trade unions could protect the income of their members by supporting invalidity decisions, instead of unemployment. Once an employee had been sick for months, employers often feared that a brief return to work would be expensive because it postponed a final dismissal, so the incentive for employers was to hasten early retirement and settle the necessary costs. This system could create perverse incentives and processes for the individual, the employer and the state. If a sick employee with an uncertain prognosis and some desire to end his or her working career is assessed by a non-public authority with a vested interest in moving the employee into the invalidity system, then employee and employer incentives might be crucial in the growth of disability benefits. The employee might get early retirement and a reasonable financial package. The employer might regard paying 1 year's sickness benefit and supplementing the first year or two on disability pension as cheaper than maintaining a potentially sick employee on the regular payroll until normal retirement age. Under this system, the employers and trade unions administratively and in practice largely controlled the sickness and invalidity benefit systems and early retirement pensions. The state and the tax payer had little say in these decisions, but in the long run had to bear the bulk of the costs. Neither employers nor workers were confronted with the economic consequences of high sickness and disability rates.

Moreover, in the Netherlands, there were also other financial mechanisms of leaving the labour market. Early retirement schemes were particularly important. Many large firms organised their own schemes, while smaller firms used more than 100 pre-retirement private foundations. All civil servants and about 70% of private employees were covered by such schemes with the minimum age gradually declining to 60 years. In 1980, 9% of men aged 60–64 on social security benefits were on early retirement benefits compared with 78% on disability benefits. By 1989, 41% of male beneficiaries aged 60–64 were on early retirement benefits, 46% on disability benefits and 13% on unemployment benefits (Aarts et al 1996). These pensions were arranged by employers and, as noted above, were completely outwith government control.

Evaluation for permanent disability was by a multidisciplinary team consisting of a social security physician, a labour consultant and a judicial expert, so medical input into the decisions was quite modest (Beljaars & Prins 1996). The government had much less control or influence than in many other countries. Collective bargaining agreements carried much of the force of government legislation and determined the real economic effects on labour supply and demand, social expenditure on sickness and invalidity, and early retirement. The advantages of this model of collective agreements for social security included effective cost control and balanced budgets, and macro-economic efficiency. However, it also had major weaknesses. The complex process of consensus and decision making and the vested interests of the various parties made it very difficult to change the system. The influence of government was weak and it was difficult for the state to control the balance and incentives between the sickness and invalidity benefit system and other public, national and economic priorities.

Recent trends and social security reforms

In the 1960s the number of days lost through sickness in the Netherlands doubled (Table 4.66). The introduction of the Disability Security Act on 1 July 1967 was followed by a rapid increase in the number of recipients of long-term disability benefits. By 1978–1981, the earliest date for which comparable international data are available, the Netherlands had the highest levels of short- and long-term sickness in Europe (Soeters & Prins 1985).

Between the late 1960s and early 80s there was a massive outflow of people and financial resources from the labour market into the social security system with increasing social consequences. By 1993, the ratio of people receiving benefits to those who were working had risen to 0.82 which meant that for every worker paying taxes there were 0.82 persons

TABLE 4.66 Numbers of people receiving the main social security benefits (thousands)

Benefit	1960	1970	1980	1985	1990
Unemployment	—	52	233	646	575
Sickness (ZW)	93	205	269	225	292
Disability (WAO/AAW)	161	295	696	772	862
Old-age pension	927	1213	1504	2025	2043
General assistance	—	292	280	217	215

depending on benefits. Some analyses suggested that 30–50% of disability payments were covering hidden unemployment rather than true disability. Other surveys of benefit recipients suggested the true proportion might be even higher.

Sickness absence and long-term disability became a subject of concern to policy makers and researchers in the Netherlands in the 1960s and 70s (Soeters & Prins 1985). At first, research concentrated on the causes of sickness and disability, such as the quality of working conditions, style of personnel management, the influence of new technologies, etc. From the mid 1970s, however, there was increasing focus on the functioning of the social security and health-care systems and how they might influence each other.

It might be hypothesised naively that improved health care would lead to improved health and so reduce the amount of short-term sickness and the number of people going on to long-term incapacity. By the late 1970s and the early 80s there was increasing evidence this was not true. Instead, increased health resources led to increased health-care consumption but not to any commensurate improvement in the health of the nation. On the contrary, Soeters & Prins (1985) suggested that certain characteristics of the health-care delivery system might actually be contributing to prolonged sickness absence.

After 1967, health care and social security became quite separate. Attendant physicians refused to certify work incapacity because this gate-keeping task might harm the doctor–patient relationship. Sick certification was left entirely to the patient, whose doctor might not even be aware of it. Nor was the caring physician under any statutory obligation to provide medical information to the Social Security Administration. So, because of clinical confidentiality, the social security physicians who were responsible for checking claims were generally unable to get access to the necessary medical information. Soeters & Prins (1985) identified this lack of communication and co-ordination between the health care and social security system as one of the fundamental problems in the Netherlands. Soeters & Prins (1985) also reviewed evidence that delays in the delivery of health care were associated with longer sickness absence. These included delays between reporting sick and the first consultation with the family doctor, delays awaiting referral to a therapist or specialist, and inactive periods during which very little treatment was taking place, in the last instance particularly for claimants with musculoskeletal or psychosocial complaints. They estimated that these delays might account for about 20% of all sickness absence days and were particularly common in claimants who subsequently went on to long-term invalidity. Soeters & Prins' (1985) discussion at this time appears to have assumed this was a question of delays in the health-care system *causing* increased sickness absence and they do not appear to have considered that these delays in health care and longer sickness absence might both be aspects of claimant/patient behaviour.

The first international comparison between various EU countries was carried out by Prins (1983) and various colleagues. In all other EU countries, unlike the Netherlands, the attending physician had to issue a sick certificate to the patient's employer and the Social Security System. However, Soeters & Prins (1985) questioned how effective this was in practice because of patient pressure on doctors to supply certificates and because doctors had difficulty separating medical and economic considerations. This had already been recognised as a problem in Belgium, France and Germany. In the UK, Sweden and Denmark, the social security system did have statutory access to the medical information about the claimant's clinical condition, treatment, progress and prognosis. This was partly a control mechanism, but also aimed to reduce delays in treatment. Unfortunately, there was little evidence this was effective. Attempts in Germany to give the social security physician a more active influence on the treatment and rehabilitation of long-term illness were considered not to have been very satisfactory. This was variously attributed to lack of co-operation by the treating physicians who saw their clinical freedom threatened, to problems of communication and to lack of co-ordination amongst the various social security services. Soeters & Prins (1985) further commented that in most of these countries there was a marked contrast between sickness benefits and industrial injury benefits. These problems were common to all sickness benefit systems but in most countries there appeared to be relatively little structural problem to administering industrial injury benefits.

Soeters & Prins (1985) main recommendations for the Netherlands at that time were for reconsideration of the question of medical certification of sickness and the need to improve communication between the caring physician and social security doctor, although they recognised the possible professional and political barriers to this.

Growing concern about social security costs in the Netherlands then led to a period of policy and institutional change (Lonsdale 1993), although these developments need to be viewed against more general changes in Dutch public services. Through the 1980s there were cutbacks throughout the public sector, applied especially to the municipalities, with increasing application of modern business management techniques. Contrary to the centralisation which had accompanied the crumbling of the old order of the 'pillars', there were moves to decentralisation. There was re-organisation and attempted cut-backs of the civil service and some privatisation.

The first attempts to control the growth of long-term sickness and invalidity benefits were proposals in 1976 to tighten eligibility criteria and reduce the level of benefits, but these had little effect (Lonsdale 1993). This was followed by a more fundamental review by the coalition government in the 1980s which tried progressively to lower the financial incentives for the individual. Between 1980 and 1983 benefits were progressively liable to tax. In 1984, the statutory earnings base was reduced, and the statutory minimum wage and contributions were reduced by 3%. In 1985 the wage-replacement level of benefits was reduced from 80% to 70% (although most employers replaced this with an extra 10%)

and automatic indexation was abolished. Overall, the net wage-replacement rate of disability benefits fell from 87% in 1980 to 70% in 1990. Aarts et al (1996) reported that as a result of these reduced financial incentives, although possibly also because of more stringent gate-keeping, the incidence rate of new disability awards fell from 20 to 14 per 1000 between 1980 and 1994. However, presumably because of an even greater fall in outflow, the total number of disability benefit recipients continued to rise from 657,000 to 921,000 over the same period while disability expenditures remained about 4.1% of GDP.

Lonsdale (1993) commented again that long-term sickness and disability benefits in the Netherlands had long been characterised by extreme generosity and leniency in assessing eligibility. The generosity was related to the political emphasis on providing a 'social minimum' income. Leniency was due to taking account of *labour market considerations* in assessing eligibility for benefits. The Disability Insurance (WAO) Act (1967) made provision for the risk of unemployment as a result of partial disability to be taken into account in assessing the degree of disability. From 1973, this began to be interpreted in such a way that poor employment opportunities were always assumed to result from employer discrimination, unless it could be proved otherwise. Although this interpretation was judged incorrect by the Court of Appeal, the practice of awarding a full disability benefit to claimants with more than 15% disability became the norm.

At least up to 1987, the definition of incapacity for work was radically different in the Netherlands and in UK (Lonsdale & Aylward 1993, 1996). Incapacity in the Netherlands was for 'commensurate work', i.e. the person's normal type of work or something very similar, which enabled unemployed, partially disabled people to claim a full disability pension. This only applied in the UK for short-term illness, whereas long-term invalidity had to be for any form of alternative work in addition to the claimant's normal work, even if there was still flexibility in judging when someone should start looking for a different type of work. In the UK, inability to get work was not, of itself, considered grounds for entitlement to sickness or invalidity benefits. However, these were the official positions based on legislation and appeal decisions which did not always trickle down to medical practice. In practice, many UK doctors did take account of availability of jobs both in a generalised and specific way when issuing certificates, which suggested that a labour market consideration may not necessarily have to be enshrined in legislation.

In 1987 the Netherlands changed the legislation to restrict eligibility to medical grounds alone and the 'labour market consideration was abolished, but this apparently made little difference in practice. A more active labour market policy for disabled people was introduced at the same time. Despite political fanfare, these 1987 system reforms failed to stop programme growth (Aarts et al 1996) and British experience appeared to reinforce the Dutch explanation for the lack of effect in practice. Gatekeepers may be unable to ignore the state of the labour market, and this illustrates the general difficulty of separating labour market considerations when assessing a person's capacity for work or earning capacity. This is likely to be even more difficult with certain disorders such as psychological disorders or degenerative conditions with fluctuating symptoms, which accounted for an increasing proportion of benefit recipients in the Netherlands, as in the UK.

The government then promised a period of social security stability but in view of the continuing problems this did not occur.

Beljaars & Prins (1996) identified four main ways in which Dutch arrangements for work incapacity due to sickness and disability differed from the social security arrangements of most other west European countries up to 1993–94:

- They ignored the issue of causality (i.e. whether work-related)
- Sickness benefits were provided by insurance schemes, separately from general health insurance. Disability benefits were considered a follow-on from sickness, separate from the general pension schemes
- Sickness and disability schemes had a highly collective character, run by employers and employees, although neither was confronted with the economic consequences of high sickness and disability rates
- Legislation, judicial decisions and operational guideline allowed the sick worker a major say in decisions about sickness absence and long-term disability, with medical evidence playing a modest role.

The major structural problem of the sickness and invalidity benefit system in the Netherlands up to the early 1990s was generally regarded as wrong incentives (Eardley et al 1996). Olsson et al (1993) considered this was probably the same as in other European countries, but the severity and complexity of the problem was greater. The various incentive problems reduced equity, cost control and macro-economic efficiency. Like most other EU countries, sickness insurance in the Netherlands was based on the labour market. It was a combination of a state insurance guarantee of 70% wage replacement for 1 year, and supplementary benefits from employment contracts which generally gave 100% compensation. These were financed by employers, based on collective bargaining with the very strong labour-market organisations. After 52 weeks of sickness benefits, the state invalidity benefit system gave 70% wage replacement up to retirement. However, most companies again topped this up to 100% wage replacement for a least a second year, or even longer. There was also a minimum guaranteed level of benefit which depended on the household situation. Invalidity benefits were financed completely by a percentage wage contribution from employees, but employers refunded this payment. Financing was unrelated to any risk and not dependent on the level of sickness absence.

By the early 1990s, Groen (1994) identified the main problems of social security in the Netherlands as:

- The social security system over-emphasised guaranteed income replacement at the expense of prevention and reintegration
- Access to a social security system was too easy and incentives to resume employment were too weak
- The system was open to fraud and misuse.

The political starting point for attempted welfare reform in 1990 was an agreement between the government, employers and unions to combat sickness absence and disability, and the government then introduced proposals to change the disability benefit arrangements, their administration and the role of occupational health services (Beljaars & Prins 1996). The government also suggested that benefit levels should be cut but this created major political controversy. In September 1991 nearly 1 million people demonstrated against the proposed benefit cuts which was probably one of the greatest political protests in Dutch history. Despite this, the 70% wage-replacement rate of long-term invalidity benefits was reduced after claimants had been receiving them for a number of years. The benefit level also fell slightly for older workers and much more for younger workers.

The Coalition Agreements of the new government in August 1994 signalled a profound re-orientation of political thinking about social security in the Netherlands (MISSOC 1994). They suggested that social security policy should be based on and encourage the individual's own responsibility for earning income rather than collective responsibility and income protection. Over recent years there had been a number of measures to improve labour conditions and reduce sick leave and it was suggested that the rights to benefits should be more selective and conditionally granted. In 1996 the government stated that one of its main aims was to stimulate new employment. To achieve this it was necessary, among other things, to reduce the cost of social security either by reducing the number of people on benefits and/or by more effective control over improper use of social benefits and frauds (MISSOC 1996).

Groen (1994) suggested that the roles of the state, employers, employee organisations and the market (private insurance companies) for the guarantee and supply of cash benefits needed to be reconsidered and reformed. A Parliamentary Enquiry Committee for Social Insurances (unemployment, sickness and disability) published its report in September 1993. Every political party was represented on the committee and the final report was presented unanimously by all members of the committee, which may explain why it was less political and more pragmatic. This report suggested three crucial conditions for future reform:

- Improved incentives for employers and employees to increase labour market participation rather than claims for benefit .
- A clear relationship within the social security system between:
  - rights and obligations in the various regulations
  - the role of government and employers' and employees' organisations
- Reconsideration of the responsibility of government to guarantee a minimum or income-related benefit, and the responsibility of employers and employees to arrange supplementary benefits.

The report recommended that responsibility for the provision of sickness benefits should be transferred from the state to employers for 1 year. Longer-term disability benefit should remain the responsibility of the state but only for those who were 'really' disabled, which required a narrower definition of disablement. These reforms would place increased financial responsibility for sickness and disability on employers. The level of employers' contribution under the sickness benefit act should vary with whether their sickness absenteeism rate was higher or lower than the average. The employer should receive 50% of the gross annual salary for 1 year of a partially disabled worker whom he or she employed and pay a similar penalty if he or she did not retain an existing employee who became disabled. State responsibility should only be for a basic level of disability benefit.

Practical changes in 1993 shifted the focus of disability assessment to ability/inability to earn income. Incapacity was to be determined purely on 'objective' medically-caused conditions and excluded any social factors. A wider definition was given to 'suitable' employment which became 'generally accepted employment'. The duration of earning-related benefits was also made dependent on a person's age. These rules were then applied to existing pensioners and beneficiaries below the age of 49.

From January 1994 employers became responsible for the full cost of paying an employee a minimum of 70% of his or her wage for the first 2 weeks of sickness (ZW) in the case of a small employer and 6 weeks in the case of a large employer. The employer was also made responsible for sick-leave inspection visits and for counselling aimed at encouraging employees to return to work. Assessment of the sick worker was carried out by the occupational health services and after 3 months of sickness absence a rehabilitation plan (signed by both the worker and the employer) had to be sent to the social insurance administration. From March 1996, the employer had to pay the first 52 weeks.

The focus of the main changes in the 1990s was to force employers and workers to confront the economic consequences of high sickness and disability rates. Employers were made responsible for providing sick pay and encouraged to take measures to control or reduce sickness absence and costs (Beljaars & Prins 1996). The scope of the state sickness benefit scheme was limited. Effectively, the sickness insurance organisations and benefits for 85% of sickness absence were privatised. Further, employers progressively had to take on some of the costs of long-term disability, with a system of incentives and penalties to encourage them to reduce sickness and return disabled employees to work. Disability benefit levels and duration were reduced, eligibility criteria tightened and more frequent reassessment was introduced (Prins & Meijerink 1997).

Over the next few years there was a progressive shift of responsibility for social insurance for sickness and disability to employers (MISSOC 1998). The last stage of this was in January 1998, when employers became fully responsible for contributions to WAO. The employer's contributions varied with the number of employees who became disabled and were no longer employed. Alternatively, the employer might bear the full costs of invalidity benefits for 5 years after disablement. The Work Disabled Act (REA) in 1998 also provided financial incentives and guarantees for employers who employed disabled persons or rehabilitated disabled employees. It indemnified employers for the financial risks of illness or increased disablement among employees who were already disabled when first employed. If 3–5% of the wage bill was spent on disabled employees, the employer' WAO contributions were reduced.

From the description by Bolderson et al (1997), the actual claim process in the Netherlands remained relatively straightforward, with limited information required from the claimant, ready acceptance of sick certification and until recently very little checking. However, in view of the continuing problems of rising costs and the need for cost containment, increasing attention was gradually given to checking this information. Knepper (Assessment of disability in the Netherlands. Unpublished report, Amsterdam 1998. P Stiddolph, personal communication) gave a detailed description of the medical assessment system in the Netherlands at that time.

The European Framework Directive on Health and Safety 1989 stimulated national governments to create healthier work places and the Netherlands introduced a series of amendments culminating in a completely new version of the Netherlands Working Act in November 1999 to promote safer and healthier work places, and defining the roles of employers, employees and various government agencies.

Government attention also focused on improved occupational health schemes and re-integration into the work force and the Netherlands Working Act provided a legal basis for the duties and certification of occupational health services (paid for by employers and generally provided from the private sector). From January 1998 all employers were obliged to provide basic occupational safety and health services for their workers with both preventative and case-management roles. This was then expanded into organisation and support for work resumption, including vocational rehabilitation, training, counselling, job search and job placement (Prins & Meijerink 1997, Thornton 1998). A *Dutch Reintegration Act* was passed in July 1998, to enhance the participation of people with disabilities into the labour force. It aimed to integrate and streamline existing services including vocational rehabilitation, training and education, job search and sheltered employment, and to make them more accessible, utilised, efficient and competitive. This was coupled with further adjustments to benefit levels, eligibility criteria and the introduction of regular assessments.

Geurts *et al* (2000) reviewed more recent criticisms of the occupational health services. Employers felt they were too slow and that medical examinations should be stricter. Trade unions felt they were too passive in the crucial early weeks of sickness, were too 'medical', failed to provide adequate support to the sick person in the work situation, and had failed to manage sickness absence, work re-integration and disability properly. They argued that medical examinations during the first year of sickness absence and associated work resumption plans should be taken over by public bodies. Government proposals were that medical examinations after 1 year of sickness should be more frequent with stricter and more objective criteria, and that there should be a 'second opinion'. In January 2000, the government set up a task force on work-related mental health problems. Various further ideas included disciplinary measures against employees who obstructed or were too passive in attempts to return to work; reduced bureaucracy for all; or a re-division of decisions on eligibility for disability benefits in public hands but private occupational health services actually providing re-integration services, and legal supervision and quality control of these services.

Bolderson *et al* (1997) stated that these various measures finally led to a reduction in new claims for disability benefit, lower assessments of degree of disability and a fall in the number of people on disability benefits in the Netherlands. There were a number of anecdotal accounts at international meetings in 1998–1999 that social security statistics showed a fall in the number of people on long-term disability benefits and an increase in the number of workers with disabilities returning to work.

Closer examination leads to more pessimistic conclusions. Aarts et al (1996) reviewed the impact of the 1987 and 1993–1994 social welfare reforms. The national social insurance programme was supported by all political parties and social partners, but proposed cutbacks led to divisions and disability policy has been a source of conflict ever since. Left-wing parties and trade unions had supported solidarity and defended the status quo while right wing parties and employer organisations had sought containment of steadily rising and seemingly uncontrollable disability benefit costs. Years of public debate and consultation with experts followed. Aarts et al (1996) concluded that the 1987 reforms did not affect the fundamental and institutional characteristics of the Dutch social welfare system. The principle of solidarity and the way the system was administered survived intact. Legal, political and administrative barriers to change prevented any real impact. Based on very limited, preliminary figures for 1994, Aarts et al (1996) were more optimistic that the 1993–1994 reforms had produced a fall in the number of new disability awards, the total number of recipients and costs.

Geurts et al (2000) provided a more recent overview. Between 1988 and 1998 the working population of the Netherlands increased from 5.8 to 6.9 million, while the employment rate rose from about 50% of the working-age population to 62%. By 1997, the unemployment rate had fallen to 5.2%. Industrial disputes were rare with only 0.1% working days lost due to strikes, although self-reported 'occupational stress' was high. However, Table 4.67 shows that the initial improvement in the disability statistics after the 1993–1994 reforms was not maintained and by 1999 disability benefit levels had more or less returned to the 1993 levels. (The apparent fall in sickness absence levels is probably at least partly due to more individuals being excluded in official statistics.) Mental health problems now accounted for a higher proportion of disability benefit recipients than musculoskeletal conditions (30% cf 28% in 1998).

Geurts et al (2000) suggested that the reforms through the 1990s not only failed to have a lasting impact, but the shift in financial responsibility from the government to employers had had some undesirable side-effects. Rather than taking advantage of the financial incentives for preventive and re-integration measures, employers seemed to be adopting structural avoidance tactics:

- Stricter pre-placement assessment to exclude high-risk employees
- Less permissive regimes and tighter controls on sickness absence

TABLE 4.67 Sickness absence, disability rate and disability benefit levels, 1993–1999

	1993	1994	1995	1996	1997	1998	1999
Sickness absence (% working days)	6.2	4.9	4.9	4.6	4.6	5.0	5.3
New disability benefit awards (thousands)	104	79	73	83	88	120	107
Total disability benefit recipients (thousands)	921	894	860	855	865	905	924
Disability rate (per 1000 workers)	16.5%	12.3%	11.2%	12.6%	13.2%	14.2%	14.6%

- Lower wage replacement rates
- Temporary contracts or hiring through agencies.

These were more likely in small- and medium-sized businesses which could not afford the costs of sickness and disability.

Geurts et al (2000) also commented on the perspectives of the various social partners on sickness absence and work disability policies in the Netherlands in the late 1990s. Responsibility, including financial responsibility, for working conditions, sickness absence and disability had shifted more and more from government to employers, on the principle that 'the polluter pays'. Quite unique to the Netherlands was that the legislation includes emphasis on psychosocial aspects of work with an explicit link between companies' policy on working conditions and their policies on sickness absence and work disability. Employers generally supported work-place actions to prevent accidents, and to prevent and reduce sickness absence and work disability, although with a bias to procedural and person-oriented activities rather than work-oriented measures. However, employers now questioned whether work pressure was the major cause of sickness and disability and pointed to personal, family and extra-work factors. So they felt it was unfair that they were held responsible for sickness absence and disabilities beyond their control. Trade unions emphasised the employer's responsibility to improve working conditions and support early rehabilitation, rather than focusing on workers' behaviour. They fought for the best possible financial deal for their members, were opposed to workers bearing any more financial responsibility for sickness absence and supported employees in their claims for compensation. The government encouraged both employers and trade unions to undertake a combination of work- and person-oriented preventive measures, rehabilitation and re-integration measures, and procedural measures.

Disability benefit reform and the political debate in the Netherlands continues. By June 2001 there were 950,000 disability benefit recipients (approximately 13% of the working population) and this figure was continuing to rise. Despite all the previous reforms, entitlement is still based on the degree of earning (in)capacity linked to the availability of appropriate work. Calculation of the financial level of benefit includes age, last earned salary and degree of incapacity. Entry into disability is automatic after 1 year on sickness benefit. Although some previous reforms temporarily reduced the inflow to disability benefits, this was more than offset by larger demographic and economic trends and continued very low levels of outflow. The latest cross-party Donner Commission was set up in 2000 and issued its Report in June 2001. It recommended a complete re-structuring of the entire system of social benefits for incapacity. There would be two new benefits. People with severe physical handicaps or 'anyone whose psychological difficulties were judged to render them permanently unsuitable for work' would be categorised as totally incapable of any work (100%) and receive a full disability benefit (possibly enhanced) until retirement age. It estimated that about 70% of current beneficiaries might be eligible for this full pension. Everyone else (possibly 500,000–700,000) would be categorised as partially disabled and receive a different new benefit at a lower rate, which would only be payable for 2 years. During this period, the employee would be under stronger pressure for rehabilitation and return to work, while employers would be under stronger pressure to help re-integration. After 2 years they would be re-categorised as unemployed, with the more effective social security sanctions of conditionality and job-seeking measures. However, in typical Dutch manner, the Donner Report now has to be passed back and forwards between the various social partners, government committees and political parties and it appears highly unlikely these proposals will receive universal approval. The saga seems set to continue.

Table 4.68 shows the proportion of disability beneficiaries with musculoskeletal conditions (Aarts et al 1996). In contrast, Prins et al (1998) suggested there was little change in the proportion of disability benefits accounted for by musculoskeletal disorders in the Netherlands between 1980 and the early 1990s and then a slight fall by 1995 (Waddell & Norlund 2000). It has not been possible to obtain any data on social security benefits for back pain from the Netherlands.

TABLE 4.68 Distribution of diagnoses among disability benefit recipients

	Musculoskeletal conditions (%)		Mental health conditions (%)	
	Private employees	Public employees	Private employees	Public employees
1970	26		17	
1980	29	20	21	32
1990	31	24	28	45
1993	34	22	28	43

Denmark

Denmark is one of the smallest EU countries with a population of around 5 million. It has one of the lowest birth rates, one of the highest divorce rates in the EU and the highest proportion of children born outside marriage; 18% of families with children are headed by a lone parent.

Unlike most other European countries, the first Danish social legislation for old-age pensions was financed from taxation rather than linked to contributions. Ploug & Kvist (1996) suggested this was because in Denmark there was a certain distaste for class-determined legislation. Denmark also rejected the complexity of the new German social insurance schemes run by independent insurance companies and instead came to rely on local government both administratively and financially, which maintained a direct link from the previous poor relief legislation. Social protection against industrial injury, sickness and unemployment was introduced early in Denmark between 1891 and 1907. These were generally statutory rights, unlike means-tested, social assistance benefits which remained at the discretion of municipalities (Eardley et al 1996).

In Denmark the first social democratic government came into office in 1924 and the most influential social policy changes came from the Steincke Social Reform of 1933. This was an extensive and judicious tidying up of many existing social policy acts which were consolidated into four national insurance laws. It was generally according to a Scandinavian welfare model and again reinforced the principle of universal eligibility. Welfare policy in Denmark was and still is seen as an integral element of society, and concepts like security and promoting good living conditions are highly valued (Folkesson et al 1993). The aim is to achieve good living conditions for the entire population, and most public services are provided free. There was a deliberate attempt at economic redistribution to offset the injustices of a purely market economy. After the World War II, the most important change was that old-age and invalidity pensions should be independent of other income. The 1960s also saw the introduction of the rehabilitation principle which aimed to promote self-reliance through (short-term) benefits and social services (Eardley et al 1996).

Ploug & Kvist (1996) and Bolderson et al (1997) considered that the distinctive feature of the Danish social security system, unlike all other European countries including the other Nordic countries, is that it is still almost exclusively financed by general taxation with an absence of insurance-based benefits.

Plough & Kvist (1996) considered there was very little change in the welfare system in Denmark from the mid 1970s through the early 90s—in contrast to most other EU countries.

Aarts et al (1996) characterised the Danish social security system as having generous unemployment and strict disability programmes, and suggested this was why Denmark has considerably higher unemployment expenditure and much lower disability expenditure than the Netherlands (Table 4.69).

Current arrangements

The first 2 weeks of sickness benefits are paid and administered by employers, and then by the municipalities. At this point sick certification from the patient's doctor is required. Sickness benefits last for up to 1 year. Thereafter, if the person is still sick but has the potential to get better, they may receive a rehabilitation allowance for up to 5 years. If the

TABLE 4.69   Total number of social security recipients in Denmark in 1994[1]

100% state funded		Shared financing under national rules		Shared financing with some local discretion	
Old-age pension	739,000			Social assistance	272,000
		Sickness benefits	185,000		
Fortidspension	120,000	Disability benefits	146,000	Training, rehabilitation and wage subsidies	66,000
Unemployment benefit	545,000				
Efterlon	101,000				

Population: 5 million.

[1]This is the total number of people who received benefits at some time during the year, not the number at one point in time, which particularly inflates the figures for sickness and social assistance.

From Bolderson et al (1997).

claimant or the case worker considers that the incapacity is 'stable and lasting' an application for a disability pension can be made. When the case worker finds that a person is no longer sick, or if applications for rehabilitation allowance or disability pensions are refused at 12 months, benefits may be terminated. At this stage the claimant may be eligible for social assistance (*efterlon*) but these are means tested and accompanied by compulsory 'activation' via training and employment projects.

Early retirement in Denmark is facilitated by several measures. Disability pensions are called *fortidspension*, which translates as 'anticipatory pension' or 'before-time pension'. The lowest level of general invalidity pension can be awarded on the basis of labour market conditions as well as medical conditions. For those aged over 60 this is payable at the same rate and on similar terms to the old-age pension which does not start 'till age 67. Central government finances this for those aged over 60, while the cost is split equally between central government and the municipality for those under 60. Another route into early retirement is provided by membership of an employment insurance fund with various benefits available for those over 60 or even over 50 who become unemployed. The higher rates of disability pension depend on more stringent medical tests of disability.

Recent developments

Ploug & Kvist (1994) reviewed developments of social security in Denmark in the early 1990s. There was a government commission on the Danish welfare state from 1991 to 1993. The first report on young people under 25 years of age stressed that long-term support should be avoided whenever possible, and made recommendations to improve the educational system, the job offer and activation systems, and to reduce unemployment benefits. On the whole, these aimed to improve the potential and incentives for education and seeking work. The second report on people between 25–60 years of age aimed to reduce the polarisation of society, exclusion from the labour market and social marginalisation. It adjusted the relative value of benefits compared with wages, to make it always worthwhile to work instead of being unemployed. It made further recommendations to reduce structural unemployment. The third report on people aged 60 years and over recommended changes to introduce a more flexible pension age and altered conditions of voluntary retirement to encourage people to continue working longer. It apparently did not deal with the particular problem of early retirement under the age of 60 on health grounds. From 1992, the state only refunded 50% (previously 75%) of municipalities' sickness benefit costs. The municipalities were given responsibility for deciding ordinary early retirement pensions at the lowest of three levels, but the state then only paid 50% of the costs (previously 100%) while the municipalities had to bear the other 50%.

Folkesson *et al* (1993) considered that developments in Denmark in the early 1990s were tending to move away from institutional regulations and towards greater decentralisation of responsibility and authority to municipal and county councils and towards more flexible solutions. There was increasing use of private and market-oriented mechanisms for financing and the organisation of treatment and care.

In 1994–1995 there was a considerable fall in the number of people on unemployment benefit, but a rise in hidden unemployment, including in particular an increase in the 'transitional allowance' (which is early retirement for the unemployed aged 50–59) which was 12,000 in the last few months of 1994 and 15,000 in the first 3 months of 1995 (MISSOC 1995).

The structure for adjudication on disability pensions is under reform at present. Adjudication on all disability pensions, including higher-level disability pensions, is being devolved to the municipalities, which will also have to pay 50% of their costs. It is hoped that this arrangement will improve efficiency, increase administrative and financial responsibility, and that the municipalities will be best positioned to relate this to rehabilitation facilities.

From 1 April 1997, once someone was absent from work for 8 weeks due to sickness, the local authority had to assess their situation and determine whether they required further medical care or rehabilitation/retraining (MISSOC 1998). This had to be monitored every 8 weeks and by 6 months at the latest the local authority had to produce an action plan.

Disability pensions and illness behaviour

Becker et al (1998) analysed socio-demographic predictors of clinical outcome in chronic pain patients treated in a multidisciplinary pain centre in Denmark. Most of the patients were already permanently out of work and on some form of long-term social security benefit. Disability Pension status was the most powerful single factor predicting pain, psychological status, social functioning and health-related quality of life, even after controlling for other influences. All 26 patient who were applying for Disability Pension failed to improve, while patients who were not receiving Disability Pension and those who were already granted Disability Pension showed moderate improvement. The effect was greatest in those applicants who were on time-limited sickness or unemployment benefits. They concluded that the multidimensional problems experienced by patients applying for Disability Pension were dominated by socio-economic factors. They also suggested that it was the process of applying for benefits rather than the receipt of benefits that influenced the outcome.

Becker et al (1998) suggested that there were several characteristics of the Danish Disability Pension system which promoted economic insecurity and illness behaviour among applicants for Disability Pensions:

- There are three levels of Disability Pension, but only the highest level provides a reasonable standard of living without supplementary income from other sources
- Often private disability insurance is not awarded unless the claimant is already on the middle or higher level of Disability Pension
- Only patients with objective evidence of a specific physical or mental disease may qualify for the middle or higher levels of Disability Pension.

Hojsted et al (1999) studied 144 patients with chronic non-malignant pain (106 musculoskeletal) who applied to the Copenhagen Rehabilitation and Pension Board in 1989–1990 for a disability pension. They analysed their health care utilisation in the year before, during consideration of their claim, and the following year. Those patients who were awarded Disability Pension had significantly less health care utilisation for their pain in the following year. Those whose claim was rejected, those who were not satisfied with the level of their award and particularly those who were appealing the decision continued to have a high level of health care utilisation for their pain. The authors concluded that lack of or insufficient financial compensation from the social security system contributed to pain behaviour.

Belgium

Belgium is a moderate-sized country in European terms with a population of about 10 million. The population is relatively homogeneous although there is some cultural division between the French- and Flemish-speaking areas.

Belgian social security has traditionally been based on the Bismarkian social insurance principle. Sickness, maternity and invalidity benefits are paid through different insurance funds (mutual insurance companies affiliated to one of five national associations, regional offices of the Auxiliary Sickness and Invalidity Fund or the Health Care Fund of the Belgium National Railway Company). Almost the entire Belgian work force is legally covered by sickness and invalidity insurance, but individuals, apart from railway employees, can choose which fund they join. The largest fund covers about 45% of all those legally insured. The National Institute for Sickness and Invalidity within the National Social Security Office distributes financial resources between the different insurance funds (MISSOC 1998). A 'general administrative body' was established on 1 January 1995 to enhance the transparency and efficiency of the financing of social security (MISSOC 1995). At the same time, a Royal Decree on the financial responsibility of the insurance funds (Mutual Benefit Societies) came into force, which attempted to improve the financial distribution between the funds according to the risks of their members. It increased financial incentives and responsibilities for the funds with either a bonus or malus, and also introduced bonuses and fines to modify physicians' prescribing habits. (It has not been possible to get any information on whether the bonus or malus scheme had any impact.)

Aarts et al (1996) again characterised the Belgian social security system (like the Danish system) as having generous unemployment and strict disability programmes compared with other European countries and suggested this was why Belgium had considerably higher unemployment expenditure and much lower disability expenditure than the Netherlands.

Disability Allowance has three elements—income replacement, integration allowance and care allowance for older persons—and for the first 6 months is based on the claimant's previous work and then for 'all the occupations he or she may have access to, according to his or her professional career and education'. The number of recipients of disability allowance rose from 98,000 in 1980 to 189,000 in 1994, faster than any other form of social assistance. Most Belgian social security statistics do not include any diagnostic coding, so there are no national statistics on trends for back disabilities.

Donceel & Du Bois (1998) studied return to work after lumbar disc surgery in nearly 4000 cases from the largest Belgian sickness fund. The outcome measure was the medical adviser's assessment of incapacity for work and continued social security benefits. About 70% of patients with standard discectomy but only 45% of those with lumbar fusion were assessed as fit to return to work within 12 months of surgery. Logistic regression showed that failure to return to work was associated with longer hospital stay (which might be related to more complex conditions, procedures or complications) but all the other factors were social: >6 months off work pre-operatively, age over 40 years, *low* daily compensation benefits, manual work, and unemployment.

Donceel et al (1999) then carried out a prospective randomised controlled trial of a social security intervention. All 710 insured patients undergoing discectomy for disc prolapse between October 1996 and June 1997 were included in the study, provided only that they had not been off work for >12 months. They were examined by medical advisers from the Sickness Fund starting 6 weeks after surgery. Half the medical advisers were randomly allocated to the experimental rehabilitation oriented approach ($n = 30$), while the control group continued their usual claims-based practice. The experimental advisers were instructed to base their claims management on a rehabilitation protocol for early mobilisation and early return to work. It included advice and guidance to motivate the patient and the treating physician towards social and occupational re-integration. In practice, it focused on information, partial or gradual return to work, stimulating early mobilisation, and contact and case discussion between the social security medical adviser, the treating physician and the occupational physician. At 52 weeks, 90% of the patients in the experimental group had returned to work compared with 82% in the control group ($p = <0.01$). It appears from this study that independent medical advisers from the social security system *can* have a beneficial influence on clinical management and outcomes.

France

France is the third largest country in the EU with a population of almost 58 million. It has the lowest marriage rate in the EU, a relatively high divorce rate, and the second highest rate of births outside marriage after Denmark.

Folkesson et al (1993) reviewed the social security system in France. France has a well-developed system to guarantee the social welfare of its citizens, with wide freedom of choice. It differs considerably from the UK and Scandinavian systems in that it is:

- Less uniform, which gives the individual greater freedom of choice
- More complex in its organisation and financing
- Less automated and therefore more demanding for the individual, with greater risk of social exclusion.

The compulsory social insurance scheme is divided into various parts, including sickness, industrial injury and pensions, and each part contains a number of insurance funds for different categories of workers. These funds are administered and managed by representatives of the employers and employees without state intervention. Social policy and legislation governing the operation and financing of the funds are decided by the government, but the actual arrangements and benefits may vary, particularly those related to sickness and pensions.

Bolderson et al (1997) gave a detailed description of the social security arrangements in France. Most elements in the current structure date from 1945 when an attempt was made to unify the previously extremely fragmented social security structure. However, many groups had already established better provisions and terms, and these were allowed to continue. The entire system was based on the principle of 'democratic management'. This meant that the system should be:

- Managed by those with an interest in it
- Decentralised, with small, local accessible offices
- Independent, subject to only limited supervision by the state.

However, progressively rising coasts, the need for the government to support budget deficits (including the independent schemes), and the need for cost-containment meant that by the late 1990s the government had to exert increasing leverage. The independence of the administration from parliamentary scrutiny is now seen as a source of some of the problems and is under reform.

The National Health Insurance Scheme for salaried workers covers approximately 28 million workers. For sickness insurance and subsequent (after 3 years) invalidity pension, the main test is an inability to earn two-thirds of previous wage. Invalidity pensions stop at the state retirement age of 60. The claim form is mainly concerned with the diagnostic category of the disability but since 1993 the disability scale has been based on a test of functional limitations. Processing the applications can take up to 6 months and often involves assessment by a doctor and a psychologist. Bolderson et al (1997) considered there was no fixed pattern for review of sickness and invalidity benefits, although Hadler (1989, 1997) commented on continuing review of the clinical decision process by social security doctors and also occupational physicians with the goal from the outset of return to work if possible.

The Allocation aux Adult Handicapes (AAH) was introduced in 1975 for people aged 20–60 who have a permanent disability of at least 80% or a disability of at least 50% who are also classified as incapable of work. They must not be in receipt of invalidity benefit and AAH is means tested. Once people are recognised as handicapped, they are eligible for a number of other benefits. AAH is payable for 5 years at a time and there is a medical test prior to renewal. Expenditure on AAH increased six-fold in real terms between 1978 and 1993.

Eardley et al (1996) commented that it is true in principle that social insurance has been extended since 1978 to cover all French citizens. However, much of the system is based on employment and on the family, and people who are not in paid employment or who do not belong to a family in which one person is employed have to take steps themselves to join an insurance scheme. If they lack the financial means to pay contributions these can be paid through social assistance, but the individual still has to make the arrangements.

Entry to the funds and claiming every type of benefit depends on detailed rules and the individual often has to produce a number of different documents and certificates. The most vulnerable groups inevitably have difficulty coping with this administrative process, and consequently do not get access to the support to which they are entitled in principle. In practice, long-term unemployment can effectively result in an individual being excluded from the welfare system if they are not married to a working spouse. Folkesson et al (1993) considered that in practice the French have gradually distanced themselves from the basic concept that social support from society should be based on need rather than income, and that increasing numbers of French people were being excluded from the system. If there is one major weakness to the French system, it is the vulnerability of the most disadvantaged groups. Society only guarantees what is really a minimum level—no more and no less. The basic allowance for disabled people or the state old-age pension for workers hardly makes it possible to live a reasonable life (Eardley et al 1996).

However, the French population enthusiastically defends their present social security system (Eardley et al 1996). All attempts to reform it in the direction of a more uniform system or towards a fairer distribution of contributions and benefits have met with solid public and political resistance. Despite the constantly recurring financial crises in the social security system, there is a reluctance to allow the state increased control. Even though it is the government who legislate the social security system, the population feels that the system is or should be autonomous. Each professional group defends the rights it has managed to negotiate for itself. The trade unions have greater influence on the boards of the funds than their actual membership in France, so they resist any reforms that might change the current division of responsibility.

Weill et al (1998) reviewed the epidemiology, present knowledge, current practice and costs of back pain in France. They concluded that although there is limited epidemiological data available, the prevalence appeared comparable to other European countries. Guidelines for the management of acute LBP were comparable to other international guidelines. Three different surveys of health-care consumption suggested that back pain accounted for about 3.4% of all general practitioner and 1% of all specialist consultations, higher for men than for women, for those aged 40–62, and highest for industrial workers. The average time between onset of an acute attack and consulting a physician was 3.5 days and 80% had a previous history. Each patient was seen on average 1.7 times per episode. About one-third had an X-ray and 1005 were prescribed drug(s)—98% anti-inflammatory for an average of 10 days, 59% muscle relaxants and 55% analgesics. In a study in 1991, 59% were prescribed strict bed rest and in 1994–1995 93% were prescribed some form of rest; 55% and 82% respectively of working patients were prescribed sick leave from work for an average of 8–9 days.

Lafuma et al (1998) reviewed the management of a representative national sample of 2406 patients aged 18–65 treated in primary care in France during the winter of 1994–1995 for acute LBP of <48 hours duration. The average age was 43 years, 60% were men and 80% were economically active. Management consisted primarily of rest (32% bed rest, 61% rest at home) and analgesics (mean 3.2 drugs per patient). Among economically-active patients,

82% were put on sick leave for an average of 8.4 ± 4 days, with average sickness payments of 421FF per patient.

Two surveys from the CNAMTS Medical Board in 1993 and 1995 found that LBP accounted for 11.6% of all sickness absence, 13.9% of sickness absence due to accidents at work, and 6% of all new cases of permanent invalidity pensions. The total costs of back pain in France was of the order of 15.5–34.8 billion FF per annum, or 2.2–5% of all health-care expenditure.

The French social security system does not have fully computerised national statistics, at least to the mid 1990s. Pender *et al* (1993) analysed what data were available from Medical Service examinations for the Health Insurance Scheme in 1991: 7000 persons claimed daily sickness benefits for >6 months due to back incapacities, about a third of which were first claims. Back incapacities accounted for 11.7% of all claims lasting >6 months. A further 5600 people had consolidation of benefits for back injuries at work, and 8300 were accepted as relapses of accidents at work, which was about 15% of all industrial accident benefits. This is a total annual incidence of about 0.25 long-term sickness benefits and 2 long-term industrial accident benefits per 1000 insured workers for back pain.

There are some anecdotal accounts that because of the rules of the French social security system few people get disability pensions for back pain, but this is not consistent with the data quoted above and other French witnesses state that chronic back disability is comparable to other European countries. Unfortunately, the French social security does not routinely record any diagnostic data, so there are no national statistics available on back pain. However, back pain is sufficient of a problem that the social security system plans a major data collection on back pain within the next few years. (The two previous such investigations were on diabetes and hypertension.)

Germany

Germany is the largest country in the EU with a population of about 81 million (including the former German Democratic Republic). It has one of the lowest birth rates in the EU, but one of the highest levels of net immigration. Germany has the third highest percentage of lone parents in the EU.

Germany is unique in that it achieved a steady decline in the number of recipients of disability pensions from 1985 through the early 1990s, which has evoked considerable interest from other countries.

Olsson *et al* (1993), Folkesson *et al* (1993) and Bolderson *et al* (1997) have reviewed the German social security system, which is still largely a social insurance system and generally more dependent on contributions than in other countries. There is also a strong link between earmarked contributions and social security expenditure. Tax legislation and social security benefits are based on the family and not the individual, which has significant marginal tax effects. Marital status therefore has a major effect and the increasing number of divorces creates a particular problem of entitlement to benefits for former non-working wives. Also, with increasing numbers of people living together outwith marriage, each needs to get their own entitlement.

Under labour law (not social law) employers must pay full wages for the first 6 weeks of sickness. Health care and further social security are provided through a complex bureaucracy of funds covering different regions, firms and branches. About 90% of the population is compulsory or voluntarily insured in the public-regulated sickness insurance funds. About 25% have private insurance either to supplement this or as their only form of insurance. Only 0.4% of the population are not covered by any sickness insurance but they are ultimately protected by social assistance. In 1993, there were 1200 different sickness insurance funds, mainly concerned with providing and paying for health-care provision. These funds are also responsible for paying sickness benefits after the first 6 weeks at 80% of gross earnings subject to a ceiling. In total, sickness benefits are paid for up to 78 weeks within a 3-year period. Nevertheless, these wage protection elements only account for 4–6% of the sickness funds' expenditures, most of which goes on health care. Thereafter, incapacity pensions are paid through the pension institutions, at two levels. Full incapacity pension is paid to people who are unable to pursue any kind of work in the foreseeable future and is paid at the same rate as retirement pension. Partial disability pension is paid to people who have >50% loss of earning capacity in their normal occupation. There has been a marked rise in sickness benefit expenditure by the sickness insurance funds which they attribute to delay by the pension institutions accepting sick people who will clearly be in need of long-term disability pensions. Bolderson et al (1997) considered this to be part of the 'pass-the parcel' syndrome which is a feature of the German institutional structure.

The employer initiates this entire system on a medical certificate provided by the employee's own doctor. If the person is still sick after 5 weeks, the doctor sends a medical diagnosis to the sickness insurance fund and the employee is not allowed to see this diagnosis. Depending on the nature of the illness, but particularly if it is likely to require an incapacity pension, the sickness insurance fund arranges a further medical examination. Invalidity pensions are only paid after assessment and provision of medical and vocational rehabilitation services.

Legislation was passed in 1957 to assist older workers faced with unemployment who had little chance of returning to work. These workers could get their pension at age 60 if they had fulfilled the working criteria and had been unemployed for at least a year. Invalidity benefits were also used as a means of leaving the labour force early. Prior to 1969, the criteria were purely medical, but by the early 1990s just under a quarter of all disability pensions included a labour market criteria. This was due to Federal Social Court decisions in 1969 and 1976 which meant in practice that someone could only be awarded partial pension if they were offered a suitable part-time job as well. With the limited availability of jobs, this had the effect of increasing the proportion of people eligible for the full pension. In addition, people over the age of 50 receiving disability pension automatically got the full rate. By the early 1980s Germany had similar structural problems to the Netherlands with early retirement and disability pensions. Employers and trade unions had a shared interest to give early retirement to workers with a poor sickness record, high risk of illness or long-term health problems.

Like most EU countries, Germany experienced growing financial problems in the social security system during the 1980s, although its relatively good economic situation eased the pressure. From the mid 1980s, the German government took various steps to try to reverse the increasing trend of early retirement (Lonsdale 1993). The Pre-retirement Act of 1984 meant that employers had to bear the cost of early retirement but this scheme was not successful and was abandoned after 3 years. In 1985, eligibility for disability benefits was tightened by a requirement that claimants must have worked in 3 of the preceding 5 years to be eligible for incapacity benefits. This had a much more dramatic effect, particularly on women. In 1993, the Federal government proposed various changes in the public system of invalidity and early retirement pension to discourage individuals and firms from using this exit from the labour market but this was generally unsuccessful because of political opposition and legal blocking. Up to the early 1990s, however, Germany did not need to face up to any fundamental question about its social security model, and the underlying structural problems, and instead concentrated on careful, long-term adjustments to the levels of contributions and benefits. Germany showed some scepticism about the large social experiments planned and implemented in the UK, the Netherlands and France, and appeared willing to leave these risky social experiments to others while waiting to see the outcomes. However, the underlying structural problems and political discussion about public finance have accelerated since the pressures of re-unification.

Folkesson et al (1993) considered that the insurance institutions in West Germany gave strength to the system, but had also created inertia which resisted change. The social security system still had paternalistic and even feudal characteristics from the Bismarck era. The German situation was further complicated by the constitutional supreme court, consensus politics and the division of responsibility between the Lander and the Federal state. Bolderson et al (1997) reviewed the literature on German government and suggested that Germany was 'a state without a centre'. Policy and institutional configurations were very stable because of the need to negotiate any change between multiple centres of policy making. German institutions were also relatively reluctant to change their management style. Overall, there was resistance to change because of the stalemating effects of diffuse policy making, dispersed power, legal regulation, and institutional and employees' interests. This stemmed from the nature of law and bureaucracy in Germany, the demarcations between institutions, the way in which self-administration was perceived, and the effects of decentralisation. As one example, the institutional demarcation between pension institutions, the sickness insurance funds and the Federal Employment Institute might cause difficulties dealing with people with multiple problems. There were difficulties categorising people as either incapacitated or long-term unemployed, as employable and therefore recipients of unemployment benefits, or as 'unemployable' requiring social assistance.

Bolderson et al (1997) considered their analysis showed that:

- There was little central direction of social security provision from the Federal Executive
- The institutions which delivered the benefits were effectively also involved in policy making and there was no clear division of responsibility between policy and implementation
- Policy information was exercised by multiple institutions and was diffuse.

The Federal system produced a 'layered democracy' with interlocking representation and responsibility between the various tiers of government.

Olsson et al (1993) characterised the major problem in the German system as stemming from market failure, which created the traditional insurance problems of creaming, adverse selection and free-riders. The mix of public and collective responsibility had not been sufficiently strong to achieve cost containment. Market failures had led to growing concern about inefficiency and injustice. The insurance model provided little control over rising costs and might have a perverse effect of increasing demand for better types and levels of insurance. It was generally agreed that the relatively high wage replacement level in Germany did not create much unnecessary sickness absence, which might reflect other, more complex, German attitudes to work. The expensive state sickness insurance legislation in Germany left relatively little place for supplementary collective agreements on the labour market. However, the German state had long argued that levels of social security should be set by a partnership between employers and employees. During the 1980s there was an intensive debate about contribution and benefit levels. Employer organisations argued that contributions were too high and damaging to the competitiveness of German firms. The administration was complicated by the large number of different funds and institutions. Officially, this only accounted for 5% of the total budget in administrative cost, but Olsson et al (1993) claimed that unofficially it was often admitted that the system could be cumbersome and expensive. The Federal government tried on at least two occasions to introduce structural reforms in the sickness insurance system but this had been blocked politically.

Perhaps surprisingly in view of these criticisms, but perhaps reflecting a more complacent view of the German social security system, Gutberlet's (1994) review of current and likely future social security problems and reforms in Germany made no mention of sickness or invalidity benefits.

From 1 January 1997, expenditure on rehabilitation benefits was substantially reduced in Germany (Kuptsch & Zeitzer 2001). In-patient rehabilitation was limited to a maximum of 3 weeks, repeated courses of rehabilitation were only allowed after 4 years unless there was an urgent medical reason, and people on early retirement benefits no longer received rehabilitation benefits. As a result, the number of claims for rehabilitation decreased significantly in 1997, and the approval rate also fell: overall the number of rehabilitation benefits paid fell 43% from 1995 to 1997.

The Pension Reform Act (1999) completely revised disability pensions, with the declared intent of limiting contributions and costs, and acknowledging the failure of earlier reforms in 1992 to do so (Kuptsch & Zeitzer 2001). It remained insurance based, and replaced the previous system with a uniform but graded pension system for long-term reduced earning capacity (MISSOC 1998). It effectively removed the previous categories of partial incapacity based on previous occupation or earnings, and future pensions will depend on incapacity for all forms of work on the general labour market. To receive a full pension, the disabled person must be unable to work >3 hours per day. Those able to work 3–6 hours per day will receive a 50% pension. Those able to work 6 or more hours a day in any job will receive no disability pension. Assessment of earning capacity will be based solely on the state of health of the injured person and will not take any account of the labour market or the availability or prospect of jobs. There are new limits on how disability pensions can be combined with further earnings. The value of disability pensions will be aligned with old-age pensions drawn early, effectively meaning that claimants aged 60+ will receive a reduced old-age pension and there will be no financial benefit to a disability pension. Disability pensions will be temporary rather than permanent awards and subject to review, unless the medical condition and incapacity is likely to be irreversible. Disability pensions will only be paid 6 months after onset of disability, effectively transferring the first 6 months of costs to the sickness funds.

In recent decades, Germany has often been held up as a good social security example for incapacity and rehabilitation. This reputation appears to be based on:

- The Prussian model in the 19th century was the international starting point for all other workers' compensation and social security systems
- Historically, the German system has always had more emphasis, legislation and infra-structure for rehabilitation, especially compared with the UK but also with most other European countries
- In the 1980s, Germany was unique in reporting no increase or even a fall in the number of people on sickness and invalidity benefits (although in retrospect this was largely for the structural reasons discussed above).

It has always been extremely difficult to get any hard social security statistics about trends of sickness and invalidity benefits in Germany and it was not possible to obtain any German social security statistics on LBP. However, some relevant German statistics have appeared throughout this review which may be collated here. Germans have the highest prevalence of self-reported low back symptoms and disability and have been characterised as 'the hypochondriacs of Europe' (page 2, Tables 1.1, 1.2, 3.1). There is conflicting evidence from various international comparisons whether German rates of sickness and invalidity, disability pensions and social security expenditure really are lower than the European average (Tables 3.2–3.6, 3.12–3.14), but even if they are this appears to hide a particular problem of older workers leaving the work force through early retirement, unemployment or on grounds of ill health (Tables 3.7, 5.2, 5.3, 5.5, 5.6). The ISSA study of people off work 3 months with low back pain (Bloch & Prins 2001, Tables 2.13, 2.14) showed that Germany actually delivers (one of) the lowest levels of rehabilitation and vocational interventions in Europe. Germany had by far the lowest return to work rates at 2 years and the highest rate of early retirement. The German cohort were significantly older (38% >55 years of age), less educated (70% primary education only) and included more blue-collar workers than any of the other countries. Of the German cohort 32% predicted at 3 months they would never be able to return to work (higher than for any other country). German return to work rates were still lower even for comparable age groups and education levels.

Eich (personal communication 2001) described rehabilitation in Germany from the perspective of a large re-insurance company. Germany (together with Austria and

Switzerland) is the only major European country that still has a workers' compensation system. (All other European countries apart from the Netherlands do provide industrial injury benefits, but none has separate medical or rehabilitation services for work-related injuries or illnesses.) All insurance companies in Germany report increases in high-cost, long-duration claims and greatly increasing costs for personal injury. They share the common problems of assessment of incapacity associated with 'minor' injuries. Although there are many 'rehabilitation centres' these vary greatly in their resources, the services they provide and their effectiveness. Despite legislation to have a rehabilitation plan, in practice 'everyone does their own thing'. Too often, injured workers get what is available rather than what they need. There is lack of communication and co-ordination between insurance companies, health-care and rehabilitation providers, and delays, which are so bad the re-insurance company is developing case-management services.

The VdK (Association of the Victims of War and Military Service, the Disabled and Pensioners in Germany) represents injured workers. It now has 1.1 million contributing members with 9000 local offices throughout Germany and 85,000 regular and voluntary workers. It provides information, advice and legal representation and represents its members in society and at a political level. It also runs its own sanatoria and vocational rehabilitation centres, 'taking an holistic approach to promoting re-integration into work' which previously claimed an 80% success rate although this has now fallen to 60% because of the deteriorating labour market.

All of this casts doubt on whether the German system for work-related incapacity really is more successful or a good example for other countries to follow, at least until better evidence is available.

The United States

The US is the largest country in the OECD with a population of 256 million but a relatively low density/square kilometre. Population growth up to the 1980s was high because of a high birth rate and high rate of immigration. The US is ethnically and culturally very heterogeneous: the 1990 census showed the population to consisit of 209.2 million white, 30.6 million black and 22.6 million Hispanic. The divorce rate is the highest in the OECD: marriage and re-marriage rates and the proportion of families headed by a single parent are comparatively high. The proportion aged 65+ is below the OECD average and the proportion of elderly people living with their children is relatively low. The US is the largest single economy in the world and at purchasing power parity has the highest per capita income.

Bixby et al (1993) provided an exhaustive and authoritative description of current US Social Security programmes in the early 1990s. Bixby et al (1993), Nelson (1994), Rupp & Stapleton (1995, 1998) and SSA (1996b) considered trends in US disability benefits while Osterweis et al (1987), Mashaw & Reno (1996), Steuerle & Bakija (1997) and Kingson & Schulz (1997) considered the theoretical basis for future developments.

Both the US and Japan took a more independent approach to the social reforms which swept Europe in the late 19th and early 20th centuries.

Bixby *et al* (1993), Berkowitz (1997) and Kingson & Schulz (1997) provided detailed accounts of the development of social security in the US, and the Social Security Administration (SSA) website provides additional historical material (www.ssa.gov/history). Social security programmes in the US have been shaped by its geographical size, ethnic diversity, and a tradition of self-reliance fostered by the frontier ethos (Bixby *et al* 1993). This has had several effects. The development of social welfare programmes in the US was pragmatic and incremental to meet specific needs as they were identified, rather than according to any planned national agenda. The state system has always been very decentralised with division of responsibility between federal, state and local government. The private sector has played a large role in the provision of health care, in social welfare and in the administration and provision of government programmes.

The original aim of the US social security was a combination of social assistance and insurance, i.e. a 'progressive' system to establish a 'floor' (or safety net) to protect the poorest and at the same time to allow greater benefits for those who had made greater contribution. There has always been a strong political conviction that it is not only economically impossible to provide full wage replacement, but actually undesirable because of the 'moral hazard' of removing any incentive to work. Eardley *et al* (1996) characterised the US as the archetypal 'liberal' welfare regime with residual public assistance benefits alongside extensive private provision. Berkowitz (1997) characterised the the US social security response to industrialisation as 'privileging veterans over civilians, local over national government, and private over public sector'. US expenditure on disability benefits is lower than in Europe (Table 4.70).

TABLE 4.70 Disability benefits in 1991

	% GDP
US	1.3[1]
UK	1.9
Germany	2.0
Sweden	3.3

[1]Including workers' compensation.
From Mashaw & Reno (1996).

Berkowitz (1997) described four distinct periods in the development of the the US SSA:

- Pre 1935: the struggle to gain legitimacy
- 1935–1950: the struggle to survive against competing programmes
- 1951–1972: expansion
- Post 1972: increasing costs, fiscal crisis and political criticism.

Re-distributive social programmes and collective arrangements for social security have always met strong political opposition in the US, and disability insurance for the general population came relatively late compared with European countries. Disability pensions for veterans began soon after the Civil War. The first Workers' Compensation statute became law in New York in 1911, in all but four states by 1929, but not in the last state (Mississippi) until 1949. Railroad workers and federal, state and municipal employees typically had early and generous cover. Professionals and white collar workers could and generally did obtain commercial insurance policies from the 1920s on. Yet the average person who was not in one of these groups and who was disabled by any reason other than a work accident suffered devastating loss of income. Only the Great Depression drove home that the economic security of many US workers was almost totally at the mercy of economic forces outwith their individual control and that only federal resources were sufficient to provide adequate cover. This led to the passage of the Social Security Act in 1935, which provided old-age pensions and unemployment insurance for workers and their dependents. In its 1935 Report to the President, the Committee on Economic Security recognised the financial hardship workers and their families could face during periods of disability (DHHS 1992), but because of political opposition disability insurance was still not included in the 1935 Social Security Act. At the time of the New Deal in the 1930s, the US might have regarded itself as a leader in welfare thinking but this was very slow to be put into practice for disability. Over the next 20 years, numerous reports and congressional debates highlighted this serious gap in welfare provision but practicalities delayed any implementation (DHHS 1992). There was long and heated debate about the definition of disability and the limitations of medical evaluation of disability, and this debate about medical evaluation and the role of the medical practitioner continues to this day (e.g. Hadler 1978, 1984, 1996, 1997, 2001). There was great concern about how to control the likely costs. Berkowitz (1997) noted that even before the introduction of Social Security Disability Insurance (SSDI), this concern about the definition of disability (unlike old-age pensions or poverty which are much easier to define) led to recognition that 'disability' might become an elastic concept which would respond to other socio-economic influences such as unemployment and provide an alternative route to early retirement from the labour force. The end result was that it was not until 1956 that amendments to the Social Security Act finally established SSDI.

SSDI was finally set up in 1956, but even then:

- Initially only for workers aged 50–64 years (subsequently in 1960 extended to workers of all ages and in 1967 to widows and widowers over age 50)
- With a separate insurance fund so that it could be monitored [regarded by Berkowitz (1997) as effective]
- With a strong disability determination service [regarded by Berkowitz (1997) as effective]
- With strong links to vocational rehabilitation [regarded by Berkowitz (1997) as never effective].

Eardley et al (1996) summarised the view of many experts that the current US welfare state is distinguished by a dichotomy between relatively generous social insurance provisions and a comparatively weak set of targeted programmes for the poor. This is overlaid by a strong moral distinction in public debate between 'social security' which is desirable and 'welfare' which is undesirable and which has considerable social stigma. Another major feature is that the US is still the only OECD country without a comprehensive national system of health care or health insurance, and access to expensive health care may depend on receiving other social security or workers' compensation benefits. This provides a very strong incentive for claiming and staying on social security benefits, even apart from immediate financial benefit. It may form a particular barrier to welfare recipients coming off benefits because they can generally only get low-paid jobs, many of which do not carry health cover.

There is no federal sickness benefit entitlement in the US and only five of the 50 states regulate income protection for short periods of sickness and incapacity (with the exception of workers' compensation for work-related injury or occupational disease). Short-term sickness cover in the US generally comes from employment-related arrangements or private insurance plans.

The SSA administers two disability compensation systems. The SSDI programme covers workers (i.e. those with a recent work history in SSA-covered employment) and their dependants. The disability portion of the Supplemental Security Income (SSI) programme provides social assistance for those who do not have the necessary work history or entitlement for SSDI. SSA benefit levels are generally low and comparable to old-age retirement pensions.

The purpose of SSDI is to provide disability insurance for workers and their families against long-term incapacity for work. With minor exceptions, SSDI is universal and compulsory and covers about 95% of jobs in the US. A worker's entitlement is based on employment and contributions of earmarked Social Security taxes. There is a 5-month waiting period after disability commences before benefits are paid. For workers whose earnings are average or above, SSDI wage-replacement rates range from 43% for an income of $25,000 per annum to 26% for an income of $60,000. At lower earning levels, SSDI benefits plus supplements may amount to 50–60% of earnings, but still fall below the poverty level.

SSI is intended to provide a basic minimum income below which no American should have to live if he or she is elderly or has a severe work disability. It is a means-tested, federally-administered, income assistance programme for needy, older and disabled people, which replaced the earlier federal-state matching grant programme in 1973. All but nine states now provide optional supplements to the federal payment. To qualify for SSI a claimant must be a US citizen and also a resident of the US. There is no time limit on SSI. SSI benefit levels are low: the federal benefit rate in 1993 was $650 per month for a couple which was about the official poverty level, and in 1996 was $470 for an individual which was only about 70% of the poverty level. Various states add anything up to about $100 per month. Receipt of SSI may lead to eligibility for other benefits, by far the most important of which is entitlement to health care through Medicaid which may be the only means for many of these people to get health-care cover.

Claimants may apply for both SSDI and SSI concurrently, although generally once they start to receive SSDI they then exceed the income ceiling for SSI.

A third source of disability insurance is Workers' Compensation which is legislated and administered at state level. It provides much more specific insurance for work injuries and occupational diseases, and now covers about 88% of all US employees. Workers' Compensation is now the exclusive remedy for work-related injuries and precludes civil litigation. It provides health care, sickness benefits and disability pensions, and provision for physical rehabilitation. Wage-replacement levels are variable but at about two-thirds are significantly higher than social security benefits.

Mashaw & Reno (1996) provided an overview of the various sources of financial support for disability in the US in 1992–1994 (Table 4.71). They estimated that about half the 30 million Americans with some sort of impairment or work disability were receiving benefits while about half were working despite their functional limitations.

TABLE 4.71   Relative size of disability programmes

Programme	$ billions
Federal	
SSDI (3.5 million beneficiaries)	37.7
SSI (4.1 million beneficiaries)	14.7
Workers' compensation (2 million[1])	42.9
Private	
Short-term sickness and disability benefits	14.6
State mandatory temporary disability insurance	4.0
Long-term disability insurance benefits	3.1

[1]With days away from work.
From Mashaw & Reno (1996), Bolderson et al (1997).

Both SSDI and SSI use similar definitions and methods of assessing disability. Only total disability is accepted, which is defined as the 'inability to engage in any substantially gainful activity' because of a 'medically determinable physical or mental impairment' which is expected to last for at least 12 months or to result in death. Further, such impairments must be 'demonstrable by medically acceptable clinical and laboratory diagnostic techniques'. The SSA has established a set of medical 'listing of impairments' and the procedures for application and adjudication are complex. The result is much more restrictive criteria for severe physical or mental disability than in any European social security system or the US Worker' Compensation system, which reflects the dominant US work ethic and minimal social support. Workers' Compensation generally provides for temporary or permanent, and for partial or total disability. The definition and determination of disability is still focused on objective impairment but is less stringent than that of the SSA, with the main additional element that it is necessary to prove that the injury or illness 'arises out of and in the course of employment'.

Osterweis et al (1987) compared disability evaluation at that time in the US and certain European countries. In practice, SSDI operationalised disability as the inability to earn a fixed amount (about $300 in 1985 dollars) in *any job that exists in substantial numbers in the entire national economy*, irrespective of whether there was a suitable job the person could do in their community or whether they would be hired. In comparison, Germany defined disability as an inability to earn a fixed amount of money (much higher than the US amount) by doing one's previous job or any other job that corresponded to one's education and capabilities *and that does not entail a significant decline in social status.* This definition recognised that work provides both income and social status. In the Netherlands, disability was *inability to earn what similarly trained healthy people earn in the same community* by working *at the place where the person last worked or in a similar place.* This definition expressed the ideas that what mattered was standard of living relative to others, and that people had legitimate roots in their community.

There are a number of measures to assist or encourage a disabled person to return to work in the US and disability benefits may be terminated for a recipient who refuses vocational rehabilitation without good grounds. Benefits may be continued for up to 9 months of trial work. Impairment-related expenses of return to work are discounted in assessing earnings. There is a special insurance fund to cover re-injury if a worker is re-employed. Medicare cover is continued for at least 3 years after return to work.

Eardley *et al* (1996) discussed social stigma within the US benefit system. Public opinion surveys in the US showed general sympathy for the poor but very little sympathy for public assistance recipients. Help for poor children, preferably in kind, was popular but financial aid for their parents was not. Recipients of locally-administered social assistance were particularly stigmatised, the worst at that time being single mothers and their children. However, after SSI was federalised in 1973 it came to be viewed by many people as a form of 'social security' which therefore did not carry the same stigma and was often regarded as a form of 'pension'. In contrast, in more recent years, the increasing number of disabled and the increasing number of claimants whose disability was caused by alcohol or drugs has caused some increased stigma.

Table 4.72 provides the raw data for new awards of SSDI and SSI, while Figures 4.6 and 4.7 give visual presentations of the trends. Table 4.73 shows the total number of recipients of SSDI and SSI benefits and Table 4.74 shows the claims/award *rate.* Figure 4.8 shows the termination rate of SSDI disability benefits. Figures 4.7 and 4.8 relate the award and termination rates to the economic cycle.

The numbers receiving SSDI and SSI benefits have risen steadily ever since their respective introductions (Table 4.73). There were particularly rapid increases in SSDI in the early–mid 1960s, SSDI and SSI in the mid 70s, SSI in the late 80s, and both SSDI and SSI throughout the 90s. However, during much of this period the US population of working age (18–64 years) was increasing, so the *percentage* of the insured population receiving SSA disability benefits actually fell slightly from 3.37% in 1978 to 2.93% in 1983, and then rose to 5.3% by 2000. Overall, the number of new awards of both SSDI and SSI has tended to rise (Table 4.72), although allowance must be made for the increasing population and there were falls in the number of new awards of SSDI in 1961–1964, SSDI and SSI in 1977–1982 and SSI in 1993–1997 (see also Figures 4.7 and 4.8). The claims/award *rate* for SSDI has fluctuated but with a particular reduction in the late 1970s to early 80s and a gradual rise ever since (Table 4.74). However, any falls in awards have never been sufficient to counter

TABLE 4.72 Number of new awards of Social Security Administration disability payments to Americans of working age (18–64) (thousands)

Year	SSDI	SSI	Year	SSDI	SSI
	Founded		1978	464	365
1957	179		1979	417	332
1958	131		1980	397	333
1959	178		1981	352	281
1960	208		1982	297	232
1961	280		1983	312	298
1962	251		1984	362	361
1963	224		1985	377	364
1964	208		1986	417	436
1965	254		1987	416	415
1966	278		1988	410	403
1967	301		1989	426	434
1968	323		1990	468	512
1969	345		1991	536	625
1970	350		1992	637	851
1971	416		1993	635	861
1972	455		1994	632	780
		Federalised	1995	646	745
1973	492	1312	1996	624	668
1974	536	558	1997	587	575
1975	592	569	1998	608	624
1976	552	445	1999	620	631
1977	569	421	2000	622	n/a

From SSA Annual Statistical Supplements.

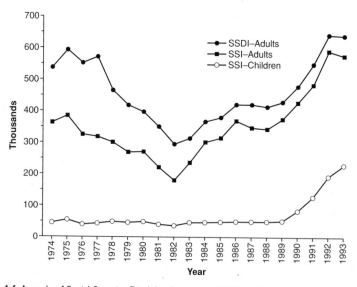

Figure 4.6 Awards of Social Security Disability Insurance (SSDI) and Supplemental Security Income (SSI) disability awards 1974–1993

Reproduced with permission from Rupp & Stapleton (1995)

TABLE 4.73 Number of Americans of working age (18–64) in receipt of Social Security Administration disability payments (thousands)

Year	SSDI	SSI	Year	SSDI	SSI
	Founded		1979	2871	1727
1957	150		1980	2858	1731
1958	238		1981	2776	1703
1959	334		1982	2603	1655
1960	455		1983	2569	1700
1961	618		1984	2596	1780
1962	740		1985	2656	1879
1963	827		1986	2728	2010
1964	894		1987	2786	2119
1965	988		1988	2830	2203
1966	1097		1989	2895	2302
1967	1193		1990	3011	2450
1968	1295		1991	3195	2642
1969	1394		1992	3468	2910
1970	1493		1993	3729	3148
1971	1648		1994	3967	3335
1972	1833		1995	4187	3482
1973	2017	Federalised	1996	4385	3568
1974	2237	1503	1997	4508	3562
1975	2489	1699	1998	4698	3646
1976	2670	1714	1999	4879	3691
1977	2837	1737	2000	5042	n/a
1978	2879	1747			

From SSA Annual Statistical Supplements.

TABLE 4.74 Claims/award rate of Social Security Disability Insurance benefits

Year	Awards as % of claims	Year	Awards as % of claims	Year	Awards as % of claims	Year	Awards as % of claims
1965	47.9	1974	40.3	1983	30.6	1992	47.7
1966	51.1	1975	46.1	1984	34.9	1993	44.6
1967	52.6	1976	44.8	1985	35.4	1994	43.8
1968	44.9	1977	46.1	1986	37.3	1995	48.3
1969	47.5	1978	39.2	1987	37.5	1996	48.8
1970	40.3	1979	35.1	1988	40.2	1997	49.8
1971	45.0	1980	31.4	1989	43.2	1998	52.0
1972	48.1	1981	30.3	1990	43.8	1999	51.7
1973	46.1	1982	29.1	1991	44.4		

From SSA Annual Statistical Supplement (2000).

the low and falling outflow (Figure 4.8) so the number of recipients has continued to rise inexorably, particularly in the 1990s when recipients of SSDI increased by two-thirds and of SSI by a half (Table 4.73). The group receiving both SSDI and SSI concurrently has risen most since 1984. This group is disproportionately female, young and in poverty, which reflects population factors. There was also a marked increase in the number of widows

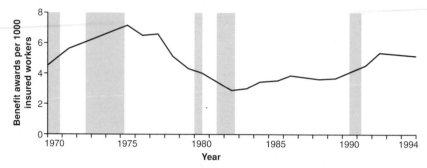

Figure 4.7 Award rates of Social Security Disability Insurance 1970–1994 with shaded areas showing economic recessions

Reproduced with permission from Mashaw & Reno (1996)

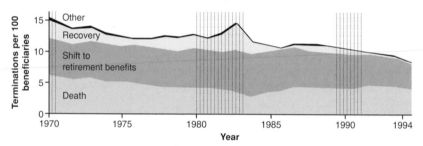

Figure 4.8 Termination rates of Social Security Disability Insurance by cause 1970–1994 with lined areas showing economic recessions

Reproduced with permission from Mashaw & Reno (1996)

and widowers aged 50+ receiving SSI for disability from 97,000 in 1990 to 141,000 in 1993 which was attributed to a slight relaxation in the definition of 'gainful activity' (Nelson 1994). The average age of those receiving SSDI awards fell from 59 years in 1957–1959 to 54.5 years in 1960 and then gradually to 50.1 years in 1985, since when it has remained more or less constant (SSA Annual Statistical Supplement 2000). Overall, on these crude total data, there is no obvious relationship to the economic cycle.

These statistics and trends must be interpreted against the legislative background over this period.

The Medicare and Medicaid bills of 1965 introduced the current US health-care arrangements, but also liberalised the definition of disability, began a programme of rehabilitation services for people on disability insurance, and made it easier for social security recipients to work without losing their benefits. Minor liberalising adjustments were made in 1967, 1969, 1971 and 1972. In particular, the definition of disability was changed from 'can be expected to result in death or to be of long-continued and indefinite duration' to the less restrictive 'can be expected to result in death or which has lasted or can be expected to last for a continuous period of not less than 12 months'. During this period the real value of SSDI benefits were also increased, by 15% in 1970, 10% in 1971 and 20% in 1972. When SSDI was first introduced public awareness was limited and the growth in beneficiaries was slower than expected. Following the legislative changes in the 1960s there was a dramatic upswing in the number of workers applying for and receiving benefits and particularly in the pool of continuing recipients.

Title XVI of the Social Security Act was passed in 1972 and over a few years imposed the rules and bureaucracy for administering SSDI on the state welfare systems. At about the same time the older state grant-in-aid programme was federalised into the SSI programme. Increasing pressure was put on both programmes by the major economic shocks and rising unemployment in the early–mid 1970s. The rapidly rising number of claimants coupled with declining termination rates led to a dramatic increase in the numbers and costs of disabled Americans receiving various forms of social security, increasing from 1 million in 1966 to 3 million in 1976 (Autor & Duggan 2001). During the 1970s, the total number of SSA disability recipients for adults aged 18–64 years doubled despite what some physicians regarded as a strict test of disability (Osterweis *et al* 1987). The sheer volume led to a decline in administrative control and a dramatic decrease in federal supervision leading to further increases (DHHS 1992). DHHS (1992) concluded that these rising trends during the 1970s were due to a combination of the introduction of SSI; easing of entitlement, weakening of administrative controls by the SSA and higher benefit levels; and the economic recession of 1974–1975.

In response to concerns that these increased benefits were now going to many recipients who were not really disabled, in 1979 the SSA tightened medical eligibility and exercised firmer control over how the state boards interpreted the rules. New regulations and directives emphasised the use of 'objective criteria' when making disability awards. As a result, the proportion of SSDI applicants who were awarded benefits fell from 46% in 1975 to 29% in 1982, with a slightly greater fall in SSI award rates (Mashaw 1997, Autor & Duggan 2001). Augmenting this administrative action, Congress passed legislation PL96-265 in 1980 which required the SSA to carry out regular reviews of benefit recipients with the aim of purging the rolls of those who had recovered sufficiently to return to work. In 1980–1981 the SSA intensified these 'continuing reviews' of disability cases and tightened the medical eligibility criteria. The result was termination of benefits for nearly half of those reviewed, with people in chronic pain believed to be particularly affected (Osterweis *et al* 1987).

These dramatic reductions in the numbers awarded benefits, occurring during the deepest US depression since World War II, and the perceived consequences on the disabled, led to public and political criticism of the SSA (Autor & Duggan 2001). 'The horrible personal costs, including a number of suicides, that were associated with the aggressive terminations in the late 1970s and early 1980s illustrate just how crucial entitlement security is for persons with disabilities' (Mashaw 1997). There followed several years of appeals and litigation, and more than half of those who appealed had their benefits restored. By 1983–1984, 17 states refused to implement the disability review process and the federal administration placed a moratorium on benefit termination and on denial of certain categories of benefits until new policies were developed. In response, congress passed legislation in 1984 which profoundly altered the application process for both SSDI and SSI, with a more expansive definition of disability, and more recognition of the voice of the applicant and their medical providers. In particular (Autor & Duggan 2001), the SSA was required to:

1. Relax its strict screening of mental illness by placing less weight on diagnostic and medical factors and more on functional factors
2. Give most weight to the evidence supplied by the applicant's own health-care provider rather than the SSA's consultant
3. Give more consideration to pain and related factors
4. Allow more for the cumulative effect of multiple, less severe impairments as constituting a disability
5. Only terminate benefits if the SSA could demonstrate compelling evidence of health improvement
6. Continue terminated benefits while termination was under appeal
7. Suspend Continuing Disability Reviews for mental impairments and pain until appropriate guidelines could be developed (which are still under discussion and dispute).

Following the 1984 liberalisation, there was a dramatic increase in the claims/award rate and the number of awards, and from 1984–1999 the number of recipients of SSDI and SSI has grown at an average rate of 4.6% per annum.

This episode also led to disagreement and tension between the SSA and the federal courts about chronic pain. There were similar tensions in regard to Workers' Compensation, with particular administrative and legal debate about whether LBP occurring as a result of an everyday activity such as lifting in the course of work was actually an 'accident' and caused by work and so constituted a compensable injury. In practice, the US courts have tended to expand the original legislative intent of disability insurance, which has led to further legislative changes which attempt to redress the balance. The 1967 Age Discrimination in Employment Act which protects individuals who are 40 years of age or older and the 1990 Americans with Disabilities Act have strengthened the legal rights of people with disabilities and opened new areas of litigation, although it is difficult to determine what, if any, impact they have had on people with a condition like back pain returning to work. The intent of The Age Discrimination in Employment Act was that the declining work capacity of older workers could not be taken into account in assessing capacity for work but, in practice, there was actually some increase in the number of older workers receiving benefits. Osterweis et al. (1987) discussed the tensions between congress and the SSA; among physicians, claimants and SSA administrators; between administrators and appeal judges; and between the SSA and the federal courts, which all provide a set of checks and balances [see Hadler (1978, 1984, 1997)]. DHHS (1992) provides further discussion of the SSA administrative responses to trends in the 1960s–early 90s.

In response to these problems, the 1984 amendment to the Social Security Act included the first statutory consideration of pain. The section concerning the evaluation of symptoms was amended to include specific mention of pain as a symptom to be considered and evaluated in the determination of disability. It accepted that pain (and other symptoms) could be the basis for disability, but only when 'medical diagnosis and findings showed a medical condition that could be expected to produce the pain'. In other words, there was still an emphasis on some medical confirmation of the claimant's subjective report, although it also opened the possibility of then considering evidence from the patient, health professionals or others about the disability caused by the pain.

These problems also led to a Commission on the Evaluation of Pain (Foley 1986) which was followed by a major report by the Institute of Medicine Committee on Pain, Disability, and Chronic Pain Behaviour (Osterweis et al 1987). This report used LBP as an example because there was most epidemiological, clinical and administrative data available for it, it was the most common SSA 'problem case' and it might illustrate the issues surrounding assessment and management of chronic pain in general. The review stressed that chronic pain, especially musculoskeletal pain, is a common health problem affecting a substantial proportion of adults. Pain is inherently subjective; there are no reliable ways to measure it; and the correlation between severity of pain and level of dysfunction is imperfect, yet it interferes with every aspect of life. The course of chronic pain and disability is inextricably intertwined with social, psychological, economic and cultural factors. As a clinical problem, chronic pain is often elusive and intractable. As a public policy problem, it is difficult to determine in an efficient, fair and reliable manner whether claimants whose pain and dysfunction are not accounted for by objective clinical findings are really disabled for work. The Commission also identified a number of tensions within the system:

- Medical diagnosis and findings versus functional concepts
- Income support versus rehabilitation
- Physicians' role as health carer versus gatekeeper for social security
- Social security assessment of claims versus judicial appeal.

The Commission and Committee made several recommendations:

1. Pain should be considered in disability evaluation
2. Disability benefits never have been and should not be awarded on the basis of self-reported pain entirely uncorroborated by objective findings
3. Significant pain, even in the absence of clinical findings to account for it, should trigger a functional assessment of capacity to work. This should also consider serious functional limitations and the effect of pain on the individual's life
4. Neither 'chronic pain syndrome' nor 'illness behaviour' should be added to the regulatory list of impairments as the basis for SSA disability evaluation. Although these terms are of value in certain clinical contexts, there is no basis for a single chronic pain syndrome and, similarly, illness behaviour is neither a disease nor a diagnosis
5. Chronic pain is not a psychiatric disorder.

They also recommended better data recording, better training of health professionals in the management of pain, and further research into the assessment and early rehabilitation of chronic pain patients.

There is extensive further US and Canadian medical literature, workers' compensation legislation and case-law on chronic pain and disability evaluation which is beyond the scope of the present review. However, Hadler (1997) has commented that neither the Institute of Medicine Committee nor any other official body seem willing to try to replace impairment rating for disability evaluation and they seem afraid of the alternatives.

Rupp & Stapleton (1995) made an econometric analysis of determinants of the growth of SSA disability programmes using time-series data from 1988–1993, and comparing different states. Earlier analyses in the mid 1970s had shown a relationship to the business cycle. Rupp & Stapleton (1995) considered a wide range of demographic, epidemiological, economic and structural factors that might influence applying for and staying on disability benefits. The size of the population working and eligible for SSA benefits was obviously important and accounted for an average rise of 1.2% per annum from 1975–1992. This was due to growth in total population, increasing labour force and increasing number of working and insured women. Between 1980 and 1994 the number of insured men rose 15% and the number of insured women rose 45%. The age structure of the population and poverty levels had relatively minor effects, but there was a significant effect from the increasing number of single parent families. The rising number of immigrants was not reflected in SSA disability recipients. There was no evidence that the rise was due to health trends, apart from a modest rise attributable to drug abuse, HIV and AIDS. The strongest relationship demonstrated in Rupp & Stapleton's (1995) analysis was the effect of the business cycle as measured by unemployment rates. The actual level or wage replacement rate of disability benefits appeared to have a relatively weak effect, although the relative value of alternative or complementary benefits was more significant. Rupp & Stapleton (1995) found it very difficult to demonstrate any effect of the structure of the benefits system (e.g. changing definitions and criteria for disability) in their econometric analysis. Table 4.72 and Figure 4.6 show that the fall in the number of disability new awards and total recipients of both SSDI and SSI between about 1977 and 1982 actually preceded rather than followed the tightening of the criteria and administration of disability in about 1980–1981, despite political claims. The problem was that there is always a delay in obtaining data so political changes always lag behind the trend.

Rupp & Stapleton (1995) concluded that the increasing number of applications and awards between 1988 and 1992 was largely attributable to the 1990–1991 recession; cuts in general assistance programmes and other efforts by states to shift welfare recipients to SSI and outreach programmes by SSA itself to enrol eligible persons; and a variety of supply factors which expanded eligibility for disability benefits. The increased number of people who moved on to disability benefits as a result of these pressures were then likely to remain on benefits even when these factors reversed. However, these effects should be self-limiting and when these factors reversed the rate of growth in disability recipients should diminish again.

Rupp & Stapleton (1998) provided a more extensive discussion of research between about 1992 and 1995 into the growth in SSA disability benefits, most of which was presented to a conference in 1995. Fisher & Upp (1998) concluded that by 1995:

- Application and award rates had peaked and were now in decline
- Changes in the characteristics of those applying for and being awarded benefits were leading to beneficiaries spending longer on the benefit roles
- The resultant decline in the termination rate might well be the most important driver of programme growth for the next two decades or so.

Batavia (1995) argued, as a person with a disability who was also a policy maker, that the growth in SSA disability programmes was unsustainable and that the system was fundamentally flawed in principle because it 'convinces people with disabilities, and particularly children with disabilities, that they are too disabled ever to work' and had built-in disincentives to work. Instead, 'we must fix the programmes to ensure that the people who rely on them will receive the benefits that they need, but in a manner that encourages and empowers them to be more independent and productive... Adults with disabilities must be given the expectations, opportunities and incentives to seek and obtain gainful employment'.

In response to a request from congress, the National Academy of Social Insurance set up a Disability Policy Panel from 1993 to 1996 to propose, evaluate and recommend changes to the US programmes for people with disabilities (Mashaw & Reno 1996). The panel's fundamental belief was that the primary goal of the national disability programme should be the re-integration of people with disabilities into American society. Reforms should improve work outcomes for people with disabilities while maintaining basic income security for those who cannot work. Their success should be judged by the balance between these two aims.

The Disability Policy Panel's basic finding was that the SSA disability programmes did not pose strong incentives for Americans with disabilities to seek benefits in lieu of working. Rather, the strict and frugal design of these programmes made remaining at work preferable to benefits for those who were able to work. SSA benefits were very much a refuge of last resort. The Panel commented that although SSA was sometimes criticised for making applicants 'prove their disability', this was a fundamental and unavoidable requirement of any disability insurance. They made structural proposals for financial vouchers for vocational rehabilitation, disabled worker tax credits, and improved medical cover on return to work. They considered that the most important way to improve work incentives in the SSA programmes was to implement them effectively, and proposed a number of organisational changes. They stressed that adequate SSA administrative resources were essential. They suggested that medical and vocational criteria for disability should be reviewed and kept up-to-date, with a particular focus on common and increasing problems such as mental impairments and pain.

Equally interesting are the proposals that the Disability Policy Panel considered but recommended against:

- Disability evaluation based purely on impairment irrespective of its impact on ability to work. This would eliminate questions of effort or motivation. Moreover, it was estimated that it would lead to a doubling of the number receiving benefits

- Disability evaluation based on an occupational test of ability to perform one's own occupation. This might be regarded as more 'worker friendly' but would lead to substantial increase in the number eligible for benefits
- Partial benefits for partial incapacity or partial loss of earning capacity. Disability is obviously a continuum and not 'all or nothing'. They cited the experience of the US Workers' Compensation system and other countries' experience that this is difficult in practice and costly
- Partial benefit offset, reducing SSDI benefits by $1 for each $2 of earnings as recipients return to work (as already done with SSI benefits). It was concluded that this was also likely to increase costs more than encourage people back to work.

The Panel recognised and accepted that current SSDI and SSI programmes had a very strict test of work disability. Rather than changing this, it was considered that the proposal for a disabled worker tax credit was a more targeted, effective and equitable way to encourage work when impairments limited but did not preclude work. The final dilemma, to which the Panel did not have any good answer, was what to do about the large number of claimants who did not meet the disability criteria and were denied disability benefits but remained unable to obtain work.

The SSA subsequently reported to congress (SSA 1996a,b) on the growth in SSDI recipients from 1989. It considered that long-term growth appeared to be due partly to the gradual increase in the insured population, but also to the increasing number of appeals and the increasing success rate of these appeals. Short-term growth was also sensitive to factors such as poor economic conditions, changing public awareness and perceptions about benefits. The characteristics of disability recipients were changing—becoming younger, more female, poorer, and with more mental impairments, all of which were associated with greater likelihood of remaining on benefits longer. It reiterated most of the conclusions of Rupp & Stapleton (1995) but added that the placing of greater emphasis on pain and other symptoms in disability evaluation had also played a part.

Mashaw & Reno (1996) reviewed the ways in which people came off disability benefits (Figure 4.7):

- 4.5–5% of SSDI recipients died each year. This rate had remained stable
- At age 65 they moved to retirement pensions. This proportion was declining because the average age of those receiving disability benefits was falling
- They recovered medically or returned to work despite their continuing impairment. This number had always been small but was now at an all time low.

The number coming off disability benefits had always been more stable than the number starting benefits, falling slightly from about 12% per annum in 1986–1988 to about 9.5% per annum in 1994. The SSA report (SSA 1996a–c) attributed this to:

- Decreased average age of disability recipients (and therefore stay on benefit longer until retirement)
- Decreased number of continuing disability reviews in 1990–1992

- SSA legislation and regulations and court decisions. In practice, a new standard of requiring proof of medical improvement before disability benefits could be terminated (in contrast to proof of continued disability to continue benefits)
- Work incentive programmes had proven to be largely ineffective in encouraging return to work
- Increasing legal representation, appeals, successful appeals and successful court decisions.

The SSA response (1996b,c) was to increase the number of reviews of continuing disability to ensure that only those eligible remained on benefit and to increase vocational rehabilitation efforts (i.e. trying to increase the termination rate). It set up a major study into why some people with disability continued to work while others did not. It also proposed a fundamental reconsideration of the disability evaluation process which is still on-going with little sign of any satisfactory conclusion.

Autor & Duggan (2001) analysed the more recent rise in disability benefit recipients in the US. Following liberalisation of the SSA programme in 1984, the screening process for disability benefits rapidly became much more lenient and an interaction between growing wage inequality and a progressive benefits formula gradually produced higher wage replacement rate, particularly for less skilled workers. Between 1984 and 2000, the proportion of adults of working age receiving SSDI and SSI rose from 3.1 to 5.3%. Disability benefit recipients became younger, and the award rate of benefits increased most for those under 40 years of age. The mortality rate fell and substantially more had conditions like musculoskeletal disorders, pain and mental disorders. The increase was greatest for those with lower educational levels, especially high-school drop-outs. Finally, in keeping with trends to gender equality, the proportion of women gradually rose.

Kearney (1997) reported baseline data from the US portion of the ISSA *Work Incapacity and Reintegration Study* (Table 4.75). A total of 924 employed people aged 59 or younger who had been off work for at least 3 months due to a back disorder were included in four cohorts:

- New Jersey Temporary Disability Insurance (TDI) beneficiaries
- California Temporary Disability Insurance (TDI) beneficiaries

TABLE 4.75 Characteristics of disability benefit recipients who had been off work for >3 months with back pain

	New Jersey TDI	California TDI	SSDI	SSI
Average age (years)	43	44	54	52
Male (%)	39	48	67	50
Other chronic diseases (%)[1]	51	55	75	77
Median previous monthly income ($)	1600	1724	1800	1000
Median income on monthly benefits ($)	1066	1100	1499	581
Returned to work by time of interview (%)	69	33	3.4	1.5

[1]Most commonly headaches, other musculoskeletal disorders and rheumatism.
From ISSA Work Incapacity and Reintegration Study. Kearney (1997).

- SSDI beneficiaries
- SSI beneficiaries.

SSDI and SSI recipients were older than the TDI recipients (85% of SSDI and 67% of SSI recipients being aged 50–59), had less education, had heavier jobs and described their health as poorer. The most frequent investigations and treatments received (in 1995–1996) were X-rays, analgesics, bed rest, heat or cold, and external supports. Virtually none of the SSDI or SSI recipients had returned to work by the time of interview, in marked contrast to the TDI recipients.

Hadler (1997) summarised the current US disability system as an unwieldy, inefficient, heavily bureaucratised version of the Prussian system, which still fails to provide health insurance for the working population. Nevertheless, these disability schemes may be the best or even the only medical and financial recourse for anyone who cannot work, for anyone who will not work, or even for anyone who can and wishes to work but is unable to gain employment.

SSA only routinely publishes statistics for broad diagnostic groups such as musculoskeletal disorders (Tables 4.76 and 4.77).

TABLE 4.76   Awards of Social Security Disability Insurance (SSDI) for musculoskeletal disorders (as % of total awards)

	SSDI awards % musculoskeletal		SSDI awards % musculoskeletal
1990	15.9	1995	22.0
1991	17.7	1996	22.9
1992	15.2	1997	23.1
1993	14.8	1998	23.4
1994	13.4	1999	23.7

From SSA Annual Statistical Supplements.

TABLE 4.77   Current recipients of Social Security Administration disability benefits for musculoskeletal disorders (as % of all conditions)

	SSDI	SSI		SSDI	SSI
1990	19.1	7.5	1995	21.3	6.6
1991	19.4	7.6	1996	21.6	6.8
1992	20.0	7.1	1997	22.4	7.5
1993	20.5	6.9	1998	22.4	7.7
1994	20.9	6.7	1999	22.8	7.9

From SSA Annual Statistical Supplements.

The proportion of SSDI benefits paid for musculoskeletal conditions has risen gradually from 19 to almost 23% over the past decade, while that of SSI benefits has remained relatively constant at about 7–8%. However, there was a particular jump from 14 to 22% in the proportion of new awards of SSDI for musculoskeletal conditions in 1994–1995 for which there does not appear to be any obvious explanation.

Most international social security data suggest that back disorders account for about half the total musculoskeletal disorders, but there are very limited SSA data available on back conditions. Many authors have quoted a 2680% rise in SSDI benefits for back pain between 1957 and 1975 (SSA Annual Statistical Supplement 1979) but this figure gives a very false impression. It referred to the specific diagnosis of 'displacement of the intervertebral disc' and reflected medical diagnostic practice and fashion rather than the total impact of back pain. There was a subsequent fall of 42% from 1977 to 1984 which few authors quote (Waddell 1998).

It has been incredibly difficult to get current SSA data on back pain through many attempted channels, even under the Freedom of Information Act. However, Volinn (personal communication 2000) finally succeeded and kindly shared the following data. He is presently analysing US National Health Interview Survey data from 1987 to 1996, which showed that self-reported chronic back pain causing inability to go to work or school increased from approximately 1 million in 1987 to 1.5 million in 1993 and then decreased significantly from 1993–1996. Table 4.78 shows the total number of initial claims for SSDI and SSI benefits by adults of working age with 'back disorders' (SSA code 7240) from 1990 to 2000. This SSA code 'closely parallels' but is 'not identical' to ICD-9 code 724 which is 'other and unspecified disorders of the back'. It has not been possible to get any SSA data on the various other ICD codes for back disorders, particularly code 722 'intervertebral disc disorders' or the various codes for 'sprains and strains'. The data in Table 4.78 only account for about 4–5% of total new awards of SSDI (Table 4.72) and a quarter of awards for musculoskeletal disorders (Table 4.76), which is almost certainly a (possibly gross) underestimate. Nor are there any data on the total number of recipients on SSA benefits for back disorders. Unless the SSA produces any better data, it is therefore impossible to assess overall US social security benefit trends for back pain and disability.

TABLE 4.78 Initial awards of Social Security Disability Insurance and Supplemental Security Income disability benefits for 'back conditions' to adults of working age

	New awards for SSA code 7240		New awards for SSA code 7240
1990	18,704	1996	23,654
1991	27,066	1997	24,867
1992	34,215	1998	30,337
1993	27,609	1999	35,351
1994	24,592	2000	20,402[1]
1995	23,792		

[1]Provisional figure issued within a month of the end of the statistical year, which is likely to be an under-estimate.
Data supplied by SSA. E Volinn, personal communication August 2000.

Workers' compensation

Workers' compensation laws in every state require employers to provide cash benefits, medical care and rehabilitation services to their employees for injury or illness arising out of and in the course of employment (Butler 2000). Provision of cover is mandatory in 48 states. In the other two states (New Jersey and Texas), employers who opt out of workers' compensation retain unlimited liability for civil litigation, so in practice most employers join the workers' compensation system voluntarily. The 'no-fault' trade off is that employers provide insurance cover for work-related injury or illness in exchange for which workers agree to forgo the right to civil litigation for such injuries or illness. Typically, after so many waiting days, wage replacement is about two-thirds between specified minimum and maximum amounts, and all of these are determined at state level.

Ballantyne (1999) is an excellent resource on informal dispute resolution process as well as formal dispute adjudication in US workers' compensation systems.

Lampman & Hutchens (1988) pointed out that the history of workers' compensation has not been one of steady growth. During several of its first seven decades it languished or stagnated. Then in the 1970s, it 'exhibited a vibrant capacity to grow' which they attributed to 'pointed prodding by the federal government'. From the 1960s, and particularly in the 1970s, there was little change in the incidence of serious work-place injuries, but a rapid rise in the number of claims for work-related injuries leading to time off work (Worrall 1983). Between 1971 and 1991 the number of workers who had time off work for all work-related injuries and illnesses increased from 3.3 to 4 per 100 workers per annum, whereas the amount of time lost increased from 48 to 90 days per 100 workers per annum (Hadler et al 1995). Costs also rose greatly (Table 4.79).

However, in more recent decades other social security provisions for disability have risen much more spectacularly (Table 4.73) and this may have taken some of the pressure for growth off the workers' compensation system. Table 4.80 shows that there has been a fall in the number of workers' compensation cases in the last decade.

Because workers' compensation is basically a state responsibility or funded by private insurers, there is no national database and it has not been possible to get any official, national statistics on workers' compensation trends for back pain. Nevertheless, some data are available from various representative samples.

Nearly all earlier studies of US workers' compensation, at least up to the late 1980s, reported a large increase in the number of back-injury claims over several decades. The most

TABLE 4.79   Costs of workers' compensation programmes (US$ millions)

	Expenditure		Expenditure
1940	256	1975	6598
1950	615	1980	13,562
1955	916	1985	22,472
1960	1295	1986	24,613
1965	1814	1990	38,238
1970	3031		

From Bixby et al (1993).

TABLE 4.80 Number of occupational injuries and illnesses with days off work

	Number of cases (millions)	Incidence per 100 full-time workers
1987	2.5	3.4
1988	2.6	3.5
1989	2.6	3.4
1990	2.6	3.4
1991	2.6	3.2
1992	2.3	3.0
1993	2.3	2.9
1994	2.2	2.8
1995	2.0	2.5
1996	1.9	2.2
1997	1.8	2.1
1998	1.7	2.0

From Bureau of Labor Statistics. www.nasi.org/workcomp/1997-98Data.

comprehensive data from the National Council for Compensation Insurance (NCCI) showed an 80% increase in the number of claims during the 1980s and a marked shift towards soft tissue injuries such as sprains, strains and low back claims, although the *proportion* of low back injuries actually only increased marginally from 29.2 to 31.8% between 1981 and 1990 (NCCI 1992). Lampman & Hutchens (1988) considered that part of the growth in workers' compensation expenditure between 1950 and 1980 was due to a doubling of the work force and quadrupling of earnings. However, changes in coverage and benefits had also doubled expenditure. Butler et al (1996) analysed the earlier rise and suggested that much of it was due to the 'moral hazard' of altered claims behaviour.

Gluck & Oleinick (1998) analysed a retrospective cohort of 24,000 workers' compensation claims for low back injuries leading to >7 days off work in Michigan in 1986 and 1987, which was probably representative of the picture for the US at that time. The average back injury claim rate was 0.39% per annum, with a male:female ratio of 1.4. The claim rate in men peaked at age 25–34 while in women it was more evenly spread between 25 and 44 years. The claim rate was highest for men in blue-collar and women in white-collar occupations. However, although the nature of the occupation had a considerable effect on the incidence of low back injury claims, paradoxically it appeared to have very little effect on return to work. Heavier and more physically demanding jobs might have more back injury claims but did not appear to act as barriers to return to work. Rather, during both the acute and chronic stages, the strongest predictor of delayed return to work was increasing age. They estimated that the total working life-time risk of a workers' compensation back injury claim was about 15%.

There is now evidence that the earlier rising trend of workers' compensation claims may have reversed. Hashemi et al (1998) analysed claims data for 1988–1996 from a large workers' compensation provider covering approximately 10% of the privately insured labour force. Over this period they reported a 40.6% fall in the number of low back injury claims, comparable to a 37.3% decrease in non-back injury claims. The average duration of back injury claims fell 60.9% from 156 to 61 days, while that of non-back injury claims fell 60.5% from 76 to 30 days. The percentage of back injury claims lasting <1 week increased from 65 to 75% while those lasting >1 year decreased from 8.8 to 4.6%. Low back injury costs fell 65% compared with 28.5% for non-back injury costs, with a decrease in both medical and indemnity costs. The proportion of all workers' compensation claim costs accounted for by back injuries fell from 38.4 to 22.7%, mainly due to the fall in the number of long-duration, high-cost, back injury claims.

Murphy & Volinn (1999) independently analysed the same claims database from 1987 to 1995 and also verified the findings on Washington State Department of Labor and Industries claims data from 1991–1995 and US Bureau of Labor statistics from 1992–1995. Most of the their analysis produced similar conclusions to Hashemi et al (1998) with minor and unimportant variations in percentages because of the slightly different years analysed. Murphy & Volinn (1999) estimated that the annual back injury claim *rate* decreased 34% between 1987 and 1995. Back injury claims lasting >3 months fell by 12%, particularly since 1990. Annual compensation costs for all back injury claims fell by 58% and those lasting >3 months by 65%. The trends were confirmed on the other two data sets. Murphy & Volinn (1999) estimated that in 1995, the latest year for which they had data, there were 1.8 back injury claims per 100 workers, of which 29% were compensable, and total US workers' compensation costs for back pain were $8.8 billion.

As a relatively minor point based on two time points in a table, Murphy & Volinn (1999) suggested that while the back injury claim rate fell, the non-back injury claim *rate* remained more or less constant. This is completely contrary to Hashemi et al's (1998) analysis of the same database. Murphy & Volinn's (1999) method of calculating *rates* involved various assumptions about the population at risk, but this was presumably the same for both back and non-back injuries. The original data show clearly that overall trends were similar for back and non-back injuries (Table 4.81). The Washington State data also showed that the incidence rate for back claims decreased 24% from 1989 to 1996 while all claims decreased 27% (Silverstein & Kalat 1998).

TABLE 4.81   Back and non-back injury claims

	Back injury claims	Non-back injury claims	All claims
1988	148,917	818,077	966,994
1990	131,102	693,439	824,541
1992	106,961	504,245	611,206
1994	105,333	514,273	619,606
1996	88,766[1]	513,059	601,825
% fall 1988–1996	40.4[1]	37.3	37.8

[1]Corrected from published article.

Raw data for Hashemi et al (1998). Data supplied by Webster (personal communication 2001).

O'Grady (2000) summarised Canadian data on accepted time-loss workers' compensation claim rates from 1983 to 1997. These peaked in 1986 since when they had fallen >40%. This varied between provinces, falling about that amount in Ontario and Quebec but only 18% in British Columbia. However, earlier data on back injury claims in British Columbia (Waddell 1987) showed these peaked in 1980 and had already fallen by 1983, so that overall the fall was probably comparable to the other provinces.

All of these data suggest there has been a general decrease in all North American workers' compensation injury claims since the late 1980s or early 90s. Despite some conflict about how the evidence is analysed, it appears that the earlier rise and the more recent fall in back injury claims very largely reflects general workers' compensation trends. However, there does appear to be a recent, very specific and precipitous fall in longer duration back claims and in back claim costs.

Hashemi et al (1998), Murphy & Volinn (1999) and an accompanying commentary by Shekelle (1999) have speculated about the causes of these recent trends. During this period there were many changes implemented by workers' compensation systems, insurance carriers and employers with a deliberate attempt to control claims and costs. These included medical fee schedules, utilisation review procedures, managed care, and schemes for modified work and early return to work. These interventions were directed to all work injuries, although they could have had a differential effect on back injuries. There was a major increase in the number of employers with back injury prevention and rehabilitation schemes, reaching about one-third by 1992. During the latter part of this period there was a major change in advised clinical management of back pain (Bigos et al 1994), although there is little evidence on how much this has influenced routine practice. In any event, these trends probably pre-dated any significant change in clinical practice. O'Grady (2000) commented that between 1983 and 1997 there was considerable strengthening of legislative and administrative support for joint health and safety committees of workers' representatives and local managers in Ontario and Quebec but not in British Columbia, which might be related to the relative falls. However, if it were simply a matter of timing in the different provinces, this conclusion may not be justified. It is likely that all of these and other unidentified factors had a cumulative effect. It is not clear if there has been some more specific shift in patient–provider–purchaser behaviour about long-duration, high-cost, back injury claims.

It should be emphasised that all of these trends are about injury reporting and workers' compensation claims and do not necessarily reflect any change in the prevalence of back pain or actual 'injury' rates.

Moreover, all of the above discussion is focused on specific influences within the workers' compensation or health-care systems. Hager (1997) suggested that in reality the economy may be the single largest factor impacting on workers' compensation claim rates and costs, and predicted that now the economic boom of the 1990s is over and the US economy enters recession the recent workers' compensation trends will once more reverse.

Australia

Australia is geographically a very large country, with a relatively small population of about 19 million and a young age structure with only 11% aged 65+ years. Australia has had high levels of immigration for many years, rising to a peak in the late 1980s and about a third of the population are first- or second-generation immigrants. A much higher proportion of immigrant men are in manual jobs and there is a higher proportion of working immigrant women than men. Most Australians have access to a family doctor who acts as a gatekeeper for referral to specialists. Australians visit their physicians frequently—at an average of almost 10 times per annum.

Depending on the cause, sickness and incapacity are covered by:

- Workers' compensation for work-related accidents
- Third-party insurance for road traffic accidents (both with variation in the legislation, administration and benefits in each state) or
- Social security, which is the same across the country.

Social security

Lonsdale (1993) pointed out that Australia differs from all European countries in that all social security benefits are means tested on income and assets and this is still true. Sickness Benefit (SB) was originally designed for short-term incapacity for work due to illness. However, by 1987, nearly half of all men and one-third of all women aged 45 or more who were receiving SB had been on benefit for >2 years. One study in 1983 found that more than half the recipients of SB had transferred from unemployment benefit, from special benefits, or had never been employed. SB was increasingly becoming a form of long-term support for the unemployed or marginally employable.

Australia introduced a Disability Reform Package in 1990 (Lonsdale 1993). The main thrust was to stop assuming that people on long-term sickness and invalidity benefits were permanently incapable of work and actively to promote their re-integration into the labour force. Various projects focused on barriers to employment and active rehabilitation as ways of improving placement and referral procedures. In December 1994, the government laid out its *Commonwealth Disability Strategy: A ten year framework for Commonwealth departments and agencies* (www.facs.gov.au/disability/ood/cds.htm) which dealt with access and equality issues and was comparable to anti-discrimination legislation in other countries.

In November 1991 SB was replaced by Sickness Allowance which is paid to people between 16 and 65 years who are temporarily unable to work due to illness or injury. To be eligible, however, the person must have a job or study to which they can return. People who receive sick pay from their employer do not qualify for SA. Since March 1996, if someone becomes incapacitated while unemployed they receive a different Newstart Allowance. The other main change in November 1991 was the introduction of a 12-month time limit after which the long-term incapacitated were transferred to Disability Support Pension (DSP).

At the same time, in 1991, Invalidity Pension was replaced with DSP. Previously, Invalidity Pension was payable to people who were permanently at least 85% incapacitated for work. DSP provides income support and assistance for people aged 16 or over with a physical, intellectual or psychiatric impairment of at least 20% as measured by impairment tables, who are assessed as being unable to work for at least 30 hours per week at full wages, or to be retrained for such work, and whose incapacity is expected to last at least 2 years. DSP is paid at the same rates as Age Pension and the same income and asset tests apply to all DSP applicants, except for blind people for whom there is no means test. Youth rates for those under 21 were introduced at the same time. DSP recipients and other disabled people are eligible for rehabilitation, training, labour market programmes and labour force re-entry assistance.

From October 1991, all applicants for a DSP were assessed more rigorously in terms of their medical condition only, with a minimum impairment threshold of 20% and limitation of the range of non-medical factors that could be taken into account. People who were considered likely to benefit from rehabilitation and training or assistance also had vocational assessment. They were then placed in an 'active category' of DSP and required to undergo rehabilitation and seek employment as a condition of receiving benefit. The earnings limit that was allowed was also increased. DSP rates for those under age 21 were the same as other levels of income support to avoid any incentive to claim disability benefits. These reforms to the benefit and pension system were accompanied by a Workforce Transition package to assist disabled people to re-enter the labour market, which included a range of incentives, increased training schemes, additional accommodation places in the community for the disabled, rehabilitation programmes and other support programmes. From April to May 1998, revised impairment tables were introduced and supplemented by Work Ability Tables to assist assessment of whether there is 'continuing inability to work'. The structure and function of the income test, the interaction of the tax, superannuation and social security provisions, and the delivery of information and customer services are all designed 'to encourage customers .... to maximise their labour force participation' (Australian Department of Social Security Annual Report 1997–1998). There is continuing debate and piloting of methods of assessing impairment, particularly for more subjective complaints like back injuries and chronic pain.

The continuing policy objectives of the social security system are laid out on the Commonwealth Department of Family and Community Services website (www.facs.gov.au):

Objective: to ensure that people with a disability, their carers and those temporarily incapacitated for work have adequate levels of income. As part of this, the project aims to:

- Ensure that payments are made only to those who are entitled and are targeted to those most in need
- Provide maximum opportunities for these people to participate in the economic and social life of the community.

Disability Support Pension: to provide income support for people with disabilities who do not have adequate levels of income and to provide maximum opportunities to participate in society.

Table 4.82 shows the growth in social security disability benefits over the past 20 years. Throughout, men have received about twice as many of both benefits, gradually falling over this period from 77 to 69% for Sickness Allowance and from 69 to 65% for DSP.

TABLE 4.82   Number of recipients of social security benefits for sickness and disability in June each year from 1980 to 2001

	Sickness Allowance	Disability Support Pension[1]		Sickness Allowance	Disability Support Pension[1]
1980	40,191	229,219	1991	71,399	334,234
1981	48,875	221,951	1992	44,172	378,558
1982	50,350	216,649	1993	46,579	406,572
1983	62,668	220,289	1994	47,132	436,234
1984	62,501	240,574	1995	47,311	464,430
1985	62,030	259,162	1996	33,215	499,235
1986	64,136	273,810	1997	15,759	527,514
1987	70,232	289,050	1998	16,285	553,336
1988	75,189	296,913	1999	11,724	577,682
1989	79,001	307,795	2000	10,733	602,393
1990	79,195	306,713	2001	10,942	623,926

[1]Invalidity Pension prior to 1991.
From Australian Department of Social Security and subsequently Commonwealth Department of Family and Community Services Annual Reports.

Table 4.83 shows the age distribution of DSP is heavily skewed to older recipients (see also more detailed age breakdown in Australian Commonwealth Department of Family and Community Services Annual Report 2000–2001).

TABLE 4.83   Age distribution of Disability Support Pensioners in 1998

Age	Number	% increase 1995–1998
16–19	13,178	28
20–39	124,712	18
40–59	311,398	22
60+	104,048	11

The Australian Commonwealth Department of Family and Community Services, *Customers: Statistical Overview* (1998) considered that the dramatic fall in Sickness Allowance between 1990 and 1992, after the peak in 1990, was due to intensified review activities and better assessment of claims. People who were removed from Sickness Allowance at that time were transferred to Job Search Allowance or DSP, and hence the rise in the numbers on DSP which in fact more than out-weighed the fall in SA. The marked decline in the numbers on Sickness Allowance between 1996 and 1997 was attributed to the change from March 1996, when unemployed people who became ill no longer transferred to Sickness Allowance after 13 weeks incapacity but remained on Job Search Allowance.

DSP has continued to rise inexorably by 87% in the 10 years since the Disability Reform Package implemented in 1991. The Australian Department of Social Security Annual Report 1997–1998 suggested that the continued growth in DSP reflected:

- Demographic changes, with an ageing working population and associated increase in disability
- Reduced access to other forms of social security benefits and income support, while there was a delay introducing the revised impairment tables for DSP
- Structural changes in the labour market leading to decreased availability of some forms of work, particularly for those aged over 55 years.

In 1999, 31% of DSP beneficiaries had musculoskeletal conditions and 20% had psychological/psychiatric conditions. Unfortunately, the Department of Family and Community Services do not record any separate statistics on DSP for LBP (personal communication 1999).

The Australian Department of Family and Community Services (previously the Department of Social Security) is the principal policy formulation and advisory body with responsibility for ensuring that the government's social security policies are implemented. In July 2000, the Department of Family and Community Services issued a Final Report on *Welfare Reform* (www.facs.gov.au/welfare_reform_final/part1_1.htm) which dealt mainly with demographic and labour market changes, economic and social disadvantage, and welfare trends. In 1997–1998, however, service delivery was formally separated in the largest purchaser–provider arrangement of its type in Australian government history (Australian Department of Social Security Annual Report 1997–1998). Running costs are now about 3.4% of social security expenditure. In recent years there have been structural developments in both Australia and New Zealand, comparable to recent social security developments in the UK (P Wright, personal communication 2001):

- Merging their equivalents of the Benefit Agency and the Employment Service, forming Centrelink in Australia in 1997
- Introducing purchaser–provider splits, private sector service suppliers with outcome based payments, and competition
- Australia's recent budget announced extended services for their welfare-to-work programme (Australians Working Together), including a number of proposals for people with disabilities:
  - A central gate-way and assessment process
  - Centrelink Personal Advisers
  - 'Disability Co-ordination Officers'
  - 'Independent assessment and advice about rehabilitation and work options'
  - There will be three types of programmes, with streaming into appropriate levels of assistance: 'Job Search Support' for those who are job ready; 'Intensive Support' for those at risk of long-term unemployment; 'Personal Support' which supplements 'Intensive Support
  - Personal Support will help people with severe or multiple obstacles to finding

employment, e.g. homelessness, drug or alcohol addiction, mental illness and domestic violence
- Working Credit allows those on benefit to accumulate credits which can be cashed against tax on earnings when they return to work
- The 'better deal for people with disabilities' will provide 'an internationally accredited system to make sure disability employment assistance services deliver quality outcomes'
- Emphasis on the 'mutual obligations' of welfare recipients deemed capable of work and who are 'in appropriate circumstances' to try to find work.

In the 2001 Budget, the government announced a new initiative *Australians Working Together – A Better Deal for People with Disabilities*. One part of this will be enhanced assessment arrangements. 'The measure focuses on what people can do rather than what they cannot do, and on encouraging people to be active and to get involved.' People claiming DSP will continue to provide details about their medical conditions(s) and work ability as part of the claims process. Treating doctors will continue to provide reports on the person's medical condition or disability but will no longer be required to comment on (in)capacity for work. Impairment and work (in)capacity assessments will be contracted to external assessors. A Discussion Paper on *Better Assessment and Early Intervention* was issued and comments invited (office-disability@facs.gov.au).

Victoria WorkCover

The situation in the state of Victoria is described in detail because it is one of the most innovative and interesting workers' compensation systems in the world and for which most information and data are available. Victoria has a population of 4.7 million and labour force of 2.4 million (November 1999). However, although Victoria is one of the larger states with about a quarter of the Australian population, it is only one of 10 Workers' Compensation Authorities in Australia. What has happened in Victoria is not necessarily representative of the situation in other states.

Workers' compensation in Australia is an employer-financed, no-fault, occupational disability programme for work-related injury and disease (Heads of Workers' Compensation Authorities 1998). There are substantial similarities but also some differences between workers, compensation systems in Australia and those in North America (Hunt *et al* 1997). Under the legislation, an Australian worker is entitled to compensation if there is an injury 'arising out of or in the course of employment' and also if the worker's employment was 'a significant contributing factor to the injury'. Compensation includes medical benefits, wage replacement benefits, physical, psychological and occupational rehabilitation, and benefits for permanent disabilities. In North America workers' compensation has from an early stage been the sole remedy, while in Australia until recently workers could also pursue common law claims. All Australian schemes operate on wage-loss principles, although with considerable variation between states on duration and capitalisation into a lump sum payment. However, unlike the US, scheduled disability principles based on impairment rating do not apply to wage-loss payments although they do to lump-sum payments.

The Workers' Compensation Act (Victoria) 1914 established a no-fault system of compensation for work-related injury or disease. However, recipients still had the right to civil litigation for work-related injury provided their injury met the definition of 'serious', and also depended on establishing negligence. The present system largely dates from the Accident Compensation Act 1985. Once an injury is accepted as being work related, the employer pays the first 10 days of wage replacement and the first $426 of medical costs, and WorkCover then provides medical expenses, compensation for loss of wages and lump-sum payments for permanent incapacity. Total or partial incapacity is based on a general medical assessment of fitness for some form of work. Permanent impairment is assessed according to a *Table of Maims*, based on the American Medical Association Guide to impairment rating.

Victoria WorkCover now has approximately 30,000 claims per annum, of which about a quarter are for back injuries (Table 4.84). Back injuries account for a higher proportion of 'serious' and long-term claims and nearly 45% of the cost of all claims. However, Table 4.84 shows that there has been a progressive reduction in the number of claims since the late 1980s, with a more marked fall between 1991–1992 and 1994–1995, since when they have more or less plateaued. Throughout most of this period, back pain has reflected the general trends although since 1996–1997 there has been a more marked fall which appears to be specific to back pain.

TABLE 4.84 Victoria WorkCover 'standard' claims

	All claims	Back claims	% of total
1985–1986[1]	43,207	11,614	26.9
1986–1987	63,603	17,117	26.9
1987–1988	59,327	16,267	27.4
1988–1989	59,407	16,511	27.8
1989–1990	54,179	14,880	27.5
1990–1991	55,956	15,531	27.8
1991–1992	54,255	14,788	27.3
1992–1993	47,110	11,859	25.2
1993–1994	37,777	8352	22.1
1994–1995	32,684	8662	26.5
1995–1996	33,227	8796	26.5
1996–1997	32,367	8802	27.2
1997–1998	30,639	7978	26.0
1998–1999	31,605	7991	25.3
1999–2000	31,561	7618	24.1

[1] 10 months.

'Standard' claims exclude small claims with medical payments below a certain threshold and <10 days' compensation. They also exclude 'journey to work' claims which are now the responsibility of the Transport Accident Commission.

From Victoria WorkCover Authority 1999–2000 Statistical Report.

Table 4.85 shows that the vast majority of back injuries are simple strains.

TABLE 4.85 Diagnostic classification of Victoria WorkCover back injuries

Sprains and strains	97.2%
Contusions	2.2%
Fractures	0.6%

From Victoria WorkCover Authority 1999–2000 Statistical Report.

The distribution is remarkably even between 20–50 years of age and declines sharply after age 55, although there is no information on a possible 'healthy worker' effect (Table 4.86).

TABLE 4.86 Age distribution of Victoria WorkCover back claims

Age	Men (%)	Women (%)	Age	Men (%)	Women (%)
Under 20	3.3	3.8	45–49	11.1	14.1
20–24	10.5	12.0	50–54	9.6	9.6
25–29	13.3	12.1	55–59	7.3	4.3
30–34	14.4	12.1	60–64	3.7	1.0
35–39	13.7	15.0	65+	0.2	0.1
40–44	12.8	15.8			

From Victoria WorkCover Authority 1997–1998 Statistical Report.

Back injury claims tend to be of longer duration than any other common type of injury (Table 4.87). Of those who take time off work because of back injuries, about 17% are still off work after 1 year (Table 4.88). The rate of return to work has deteriorated slightly over the years.

TABLE 4.87 Median claim duration (days) by condition (open long-term claims)

Back injuries	956
Other sprains/strains	668
Repetitive strain injury	661
Stress	692
Other	727

From Victoria WorkCover Authority 1997–1998 Statistical Report.

These patterns once again need to be interpreted against the legislative background. Hunt et al (1997) provided a detailed history of the development of Victoria WorkCover since 1914 and commented that statutory changes over the past two decades effectively constituted a grand policy experiment. Prior to 1985 Victoria operated a privately underwritten workers' compensation system, from 1985 to 1992 a public monopoly system, and from 1992 a mixed model.

TABLE 4.88   Duration of work loss for Victoria WorkCover back claims

Weeks off work	% returned to work	% still off work[1]
1	26.9	73.1
2	41.2	58.8
3	49.2	50.8
4	54.3	45.7
8	64.6	35.4
13	69.5	30.5
26	76.4	23.6
39	80.0	20.0
52	83.0	17.0
104	88.8	11.2
156	92.7	6.3
208	95.2	4.8

[1] As % of those who take any time off work; 29.7% of total back claims do not take any time off work.
Recalculated data from Victoria WorkCover Authority 1995–1996 Statistical Report.

Politicians claim that a fundamental objective of the Accident Compensation Act 1985 was to reduce the incidence of accidents and diseases in the work place, and attribute the downward trend in the number of WorkCover claims to a combination of legislative changes, education and advertising campaigns, and premium incentives (The Victoria WorkCover Authority 1995–1996 Statistical Report). The 1996–1997 and 1997–1998 Statistical Reports provided more detailed summaries of changes in the WorkCover system over the years.

1985–1986	Accident Compensation Act (1995) came into effect
	Average levy on employers set at 2.4%, ranging from 0.57 to 3.8%
1986–1987	Changes to remuneration of claims agents
1988–1989	Bonus and penalty system introduced for employers
	Average levy increased to 3.3%
	Weekly compensation payments reduced for workers on benefits >12 months and impairments <15%
1989–1990	Bonus and penalty system expanded
1990–1991	Removal of statutory minimum level of weekly compensation
	Maximum compensation set at 80% of pre-injury earnings, excluding overtime
1992–1993	Liberal and National Coalition Accident Compensation Act amended and WorkCover set up in December 1992
	Weekly benefits for first 26 weeks increased to 95% of basic weekly earnings, excluding overtime. After 26 weeks, reduced to 90, 70 or 60%
	Partial incapacity benefits cease at 2 years
	Right to civil litigation restricted to workers with serious injuries (>30% impairment) and capped (although 'serious' has never been defined by statute and the practical definition has varied over time)

	Claims require *employment to be a significant contributing factor to the injury*
	Employers must offer suitable alternative employment within 12 months of injury
	Major return to work, multi-media advertising campaign
1993–1994	Employers excess increased to 10 days
	Rehabilitation based in work place
	Credibility adjusted experience-rated premium system introduced
	Average premium reduced to 2.25%
	Major safety awareness, start of multi-media advertising campaigns
1994–1995	Increased incentives for return to work
	Additional lump-sum payments for pain and suffering introduced
	Major safety awareness, multi-media advertising campaigns
1995–1996	Average premium reduced to 1.98%
	Safety campaigns continue
1996–1997	Average premium reduced to 1.8%
	Serious injury determinations for civil litigation changed to require minimum of 30% impairment
	Definition of serious injury claims changed to exclude psychological overlay in impairment rating
	However, a 'narrative system' was also introduced in parallel which included psychological overlay and eventually covered up to 80% of claims
	Health and Safety Organisation and WorkCover merged
	Safety campaigns continue
1997–1998	Multimedia advertising campaigns targeting specific accident types
Nov 1997	Major amendments to Accident Compensation Act
	Right to civil litigation for new work-related accidents abolished
	Common law claims fell from a peak of 5000 in 1991–1992 to nil by 1997–1998
	Injuries must be notified within 30 days
	Table of maims replaced by assessment based on whole body impairment and AMA *Guides* 4th Edition. However, psychiatric assessments did not use the AMA *Guides* but retained WorkCover's own method of assessment
	Threshold for permanent disability lump-sum claims reduced to 10% impairment for physical injuries, 30% for psychiatric injuries
	Focus on work capacity rather than injury or incapacity
	New long-term benefits to support partially incapacitated workers back to work
	Employer bears costs for first 10 days. Compensation rate for first 13 weeks' incapacity 95% of pre-injury ordinary time weekly earnings up to approximately Au$900. After 13 weeks, wage replacement reduced to 75% if total incapacity for work or 60% with a partial incapacity or 'current work capacity'. Compensation ceased at 104 weeks unless totally permanently incapacitated for work

October 1999   Labour government re-introduced right to common law litigation
               Increased benefits for lower levels of impairment
               Attempt to tighten up on the 'narrative system'

During the early–mid 1990s, Victoria WorkCover had a particular problem of secondary psychological complaints. In 1993–1994, 12% of serious injuries had a 'psychiatric component' but by 1995–1996 this rose to 26%. This secondary psychiatric element has effectively now been disallowed and only primary psychiatric disorders are accepted.

Anonymous senior legal comment was that over this 15-year period:

● There had been constant changes and political tinkering with the legislation which has produced increasing complexity
● This had been driven mainly by cost containment
● The changes had generally been oppressive and often unfair
● The changes led to many more legal disputes and appeals.

From the opposite perspective, it may be argued these legislative changes had been in reaction to and countering:

● Escalating claims and costs
● Legal decisions which had generally broadened claims and awards for disability and incapacity.

As in any system, these changes reflect the balance between attempting to get the legislation right (based on medical principles) and the delivery system (which depends on key senior people):

● Legislation: political reality
● Delivery system: structural
● Outcome: assessment/decisions, which depend on data.

The comprehensive Upjohn Report (Hunt et al 1997)—which was 'independent' but commissioned by the Authority—on the state of the Victoria WorkCover Authority compared it with other Australian and North American workers' compensation systems. It considered that Victoria WorkCover had achieved an 'amazing transformation in just a few short years' from a system characterised by a 'compo' philosophy, uncontrolled claims incidence, excessive durations of disability and runaway costs to 'one that appears to be sustaining a level of performance that would have been unimaginable 5 years ago'. The Report particularly singled out 'cultural change through media….We are not aware of any other workers' compensation system in the world that has used media more aggressively or more effectively than has the VWA. Their use of the power of the media to effect a reversal in the 'compo' culture that characterised Victoria's workers' compensation system previously is unprecedented, and a valuable model for other systems around the world'.

Occupational rehabilitation was a relatively late component of Australian workers' compensation systems (as part of the legacy of their British rather than German system origins) (Hunt et al 1997). Through the 1970s and early 80s there was increasing recognition of the need for better rehabilitation, although early initiatives by private insurers were initially met by suspicion from the union movement who saw them as being a form of benefit control. One of the distinguishing features of the Victoria Workcare scheme in 1985 was the emphasis placed on rehabilitation. This was an enormous challenge to start from virtually nothing and develop one of the most advanced occupational rehabilitation systems in the world, and problems were inevitable. To overcome earlier union suspicions and with tepid support from employers under the business/labour compact, a largely independent Victorian Accident Rehabilitation Council (VARC) was set up as gatekeeper and regulator of rehabilitation services, although the actual services were from approved private providers. From 1986, providers had to submit an individual rehabilitation plan for each worker to a central authority. Bureaucratic delays were inevitable while the diversity of providers and the sheer volume of cases limited the amount of 'process' monitoring that could be done. So in 1991 the VARC set up a Rehabilitation Case Management Strategy to attempt to improve quality control. Despite some individually successful rehabilitation providers, the enduring impression and legacy of the VARC over its 7-year existence were strong and negative. VARC staff, health-care providers, unions and employers had very different and conflicting philosophies of rehabilitation. The concept of rehabilitation was now strongly supported by the union movement, but employer groups felt little sense of ownership or participation and came to be regard 'rehabilitation' and the VARC as dirty words. The scene was set by 1992 for wholesale replacement of the VARC system with a narrower concept of rehabilitation as, primarily, a focus on the final goal of (early) return to work. Since 1992, Victoria WorkCover has achieved a dramatic shift in perceptions of rehabilitation which was applauded in The Upjohn Report (Hunt *et al* 1997): 'The VWA's success in changing expectations of both workers and employers towards early return to work is remarkable. The VWA has been highly effective in getting this key message across in its policies, its media campaigns, and its dealings with stakeholders. They have achieved a return-to-work focus second to none'. The Upjohn Report also concluded that: 'In many ways, the policies of the VWA have operationalised the ideals of the disability management movement. Employers in Victoria (now) generally accept that they are responsible for returning workers to their employment' although the Report recognised that small- and medium-sized enterprises would need additional assistance. The key features of occupational rehabilitation under the present Victoria WorkCover are:

- Injured workers have certain entitlements under the general themes of rehabilitation and return to work
- The worker must 'make every reasonable effort to return to work' in 'suitable employment'
- The scheme mandates a high level of responsibility on employers
- The insurer's role is supportive and facilitative to the employer's ultimate responsibility
- Within 30 days of injury, the employer must prepare a written return to work plan, with the injured worker's written agreement and a nominated return-to-work co-ordinator. Within 120 days, the employer must establish an occupational rehabilitation programme
- The worker has a right to re-employment within 12 months in 'suitable employment'.

However, the debate about rehabilitation is not fully settled. In the last few years, questions have again been raised about the wide diversity of services provided in the name of 'rehabilitation' and Tito (2000) cautioned against simply 'throwing money at rehabilitation'. Everyone subscribes to the principle of rehabilitation but there is great variation in what that means in practice and the key question is whether it is effective.

Table 4.89 shows that Victoria's workers' compensation system has the lowest claims rates of any large Australian state. However, Victoria's rehabilitation statistics support the above doubts about the claimed emphasis on rehabilitation. The return to work rate is also about the national average, although it may be argued that is reasonable if there is possible case selection from the low claims rate.

TABLE 4.89 Comparison of workers' compensation claim rates and outcomes in different Australian states

	Claims 1998–1999 as % of workers covered	% who had a return to work plan	% who received rehabilitation	% who returned to work	% durable return to work (still at work after 8 months)
Victoria	1.9	40	35	81	71
New South Wales	2.4	45	32	86	76
South Australia	4.6	60	64	79	67
Western Australia	3.7	—	—	—	—
Queensland	5.7	31	17	84	75
National average	—	43	33	84	74

From Heads of Workers' Compensation Authorities (2000).

Nationally in 1995–1996, 30% of all workers' compensation injuries were to the back (Labour Ministers' Council 1998). Of all the main states, Victoria had the lowest annual incidence of all injuries causing 5 or more days compensation, while New South Wales and South Australia had the highest. For all injuries causing >60 days off work, Victoria was just below the national average, while New South Wales and South Australia were again highest. Victoria had the lowest incidence of back injuries causing 5 or more days compensation (just over 5 per 1000) of all the main states, while New South Wales and South Australia had the highest (almost 7 per 1000). By May 1997, 42% of all Australian injured workers had a return to work plan developed for them: 74% of workers found these plans helpful and 60% actually received help to do what was recommended in the plan; 65% returned to alternative duties but this made little difference to long-term remaining at work.

No detailed statistics from WorkCover New South Wales have been analysed for this review, but the situation was summarised by Molloy et al (1999). In 1996–1997, back injuries accounted for 31% of the 44,654 work-place injuries and WorkCover claims: 96% of these were 'sprains and strains' yet at 6 months only 73% of them had returned to work; 16% of male and 15% of female back injury claims went on to permanent disability. This proportion was surprisingly similar for different occupational groups, e.g. 16% in 'managers and administrators' and 17.5% in 'labourers and related workers'. Unlike Victoria, there was a continuing dramatic rise in the number going on to permanent disability pensions, increasing 2.5 fold between 1991–1992 and 1996–1997.

Cohen et al (2000) analysed the medical assessment and management of a selected sample of workers' compensation patients with spinal injuries in 1991–1993, although the study had a low participation rate of 31% of those contacted. There was little difference in medical status between those with persisting pain who were working and those with persisting pain who were not, but there was poor agreement between the probable retrospective diagnosis and the original file diagnosis in those with persisting pain up to 2 years post injury, suggesting problems with diagnosis. Despite evidence of psychosocial disturbance, medical assessments were overwhelmingly somatic, diagnostic labelling almost exclusively structurally based, and treatments mainly passive. (In fairness, this was no different from other countries at that time.) Perhaps in response to this kind of situation, the South Australia WorkCover Authority (1993) and the Victoria WorkCover Authority (1996) played leading roles in the development of clinical guidelines for acute LBP (Burton & Waddell 1998). The workers' compensation setting led to a much stronger emphasis on return-to-work issues than other international guidelines at that time. There are no data on whether these earlier guidelines had any direct impact on health care or claims. More recently, McGuirk et al (2001) made a case-control study of new, national, evidence-based guidelines for the management of acute LBP (awaiting endorsement by the National Health and Medical Research Council of Australia). Special clinics were set up with trained medical practitioners and compared with usual care by the family doctor. Twelve-month follow-up was only 58% but nevertheless this evidence-based management produced more full recovery at 6 and 12 months, less chronic pain, fewer patients requiring continuing care, lower costs and higher patient satisfaction.

Most innovative and interesting, however, are Australian developments in public education about back pain. From 1997, the Victoria WorkCover Authority ran a multi-media public health campaign aiming to change community attitudes, behaviours and outcomes about back pain, which was the first such public campaign in the world. It commenced in September 1997, ran through most of 1998, and there was a booster campaign in 1999. The whole campaign was based on the biopsychosocial model and the messages from The Back Book (Roland et al 1996), and targeted at the working population and doctors who treated workers' compensation patients. The main media was a series of about 20 television commercials, supported by radio, outdoor and print advertisements, posters, seminars, workplace visits, publicity articles and publications. Clinical guidelines for the management of workers with work-related back injuries were introduced at the same time, and copies of The Back Book (translated into 13 languages) provided to insurers and treating practitioners for distribution to injured workers.

Evaluation of the back pain public health campaign included:

- A telephone survey of three cross-sectional random samples of the employed population before and approximately 18–24 months after the start of the campaign, using a quasi-experimental before/after study design with a concurrent New South Wales control group

- A mailed self-administered survey of random samples of general practioners prior to the start of the study, compared with a concurrent New South Wales control group
- Statistical analysis of trends in Victoria WorkCover data on back pain claims, time off work for back pain and health-care costs before and after the intervention, and compared with non-back claims.

The baseline general practitioner questionnaire (M Wyatt, personal communication, 1999) showed very similar patterns of management and treatment with X-rays, medication and physiotherapy in Victoria and New South Wales. However, there were statistically significant differences in advice about return to work, e.g. about whether patients needed to be almost pain free before returning to work. It was not clear whether this was related to previous Victoria WorkCover advertisements encouraging general practitioners to return patients to work or to differences in the benefit structure.

Follow-up at 18–24 months showed that the campaign produced a significant improvement in back pain beliefs over time in Victoria, while there was no change in New South Wales (Buchbinder et al 2001a). Victorian general practitioners reported significant shifts in their management of acute and subacute LBP: ordering fewer tests and X-rays, prescribing less bed rest and advising more work modification (Buchbinder et al 2001a). In Victoria the number of workers' compensation claims decreased 15%, and the rates of days compensated and medical payments for claims for back pain declined, in contrast to claims for non-back conditions in Victoria and in contrast to New South Wales (Buchbinder et al 2001b).

However, there is a footnote to this account (G Sullivan, personal communication, Nov 2001, M Wyatt, personal communication, May 2002). There was an unexpected change in government in October 1999, resulting in a major re-shuffle of senior management in the Victoria WorkCover Authority. They have now 'moved on', dropped the entire previous educational campaign, and are not even interested in hearing about the results. Instead, they have imported a much more traditional 'accident prevention' and manual handling approach from Canada (www.workcover.vic.gov.au/dir090/vwa/home.nsf/pages/so_sprains). The new campaign is focused on employers and portrays the back pain sufferer as a passive victim. Some of the previous staff are already predicting the most recent advertisements will undo all the earlier good work and that back claims will increase again. This will form a natural experiment, although this will depend on willingness to analyse the impact of these successive policy initiatives.

New Zealand

New Zealand is a small and geographically isolated country with a population of around 3.7 million. Its age structure is significantly younger than most of the other countries considered in this review, with only 11% aged 65+ years.

New Zealand has long been regarded as a pioneer in social reform (Eardley et al 1996). It was the first country in the world to introduce universal female suffrage in 1893, one of the first to introduce old-age pensions in 1898, and it established one of the first comprehensive welfare systems in 1938 with the introduction of a national health service, retirement pensions and a comprehensive range of income-related benefits. The scope and generosity of benefits was further extended in the mid 1970s with the introduction of a universal national pension from the age of 65 and a no-fault accident compensation scheme.

Social security

The New Zealand social security system is broadly similar to the Australian system but differs from nearly all other developed countries in that it has virtually no social insurance features but is funded entirely from general taxation revenue. Sickness Benefit (SB) is for people aged 16 years and over who are incapacitated from working by illness or injury and who have lost income as a result. Invalidity Benefit (IVB) is for people aged 16 or over who are permanently incapacitated from working. Eligibility is through medical assessment.

For most of the period between the 1940s and 1980s New Zealand had a relatively young population, very low levels of unemployment and relatively high GDP, which permitted generous social security benefits but relatively low percentage GDP expenditure on social security. There has, however, been a long-term decline in New Zealand's economic position since the 1970s and the unemployment rate rose from <1 to almost 10% by the early 1990s. By 1995 it had fallen to 6.9% and then remained relatively stable.

Table 4.90 shows the continuing increase in both SB and IVB, although the numbers on these disability benefits have always remained much lower than unemployment. The most dramatic increase in the 1980s was in unemployment benefits, largely because of rising unemployment although partly also because of expanded eligibility for benefits and the increasing number of lone parents.

There were successive social security reform reviews in the mid–late 1980s. The Labour government elected in 1984 introduced sweeping changes in economic policy but social programmes were left relatively unscathed. In 1986, at a time of major taxation reform, all social security benefits were made taxable. In 1988, a Royal Commission on Social Policy reformed the tax system and the social security system. The national government elected in 1990 instituted a further range of social policy changes. The main thrust of many of the proposals was to simplify and standardise benefits and at the same time the level of benefits were reduced, although they remained generous compared to other countries. As a result, expenditure on social security, which had risen from 6.9% GDP in 1979 to 11.5% in 1985 and 13.4% in 1991 subsequently fell to 11.9% in 1993–1994.

Eardley et al (1996) summarised the main advantages of the New Zealand social security system:

- The system provides comprehensive cover, national uniformity and extensive review and appeal procedures
- Benefit levels for many groups remain relatively generous

TABLE 4.90 Recipients of social security benefits, 1980–1998

Year (end)	Unemployment and training	Sickness	Invalidity
1980	20,850	7504	15,647
1981	35,666	7104	16,961
1982	32,596	7177	17,891
1983	50,744	7669	18,757
1984	50,136	9452	20,187
1985	38,419	9627	21,464
1986	42,405	9517	21,993
1987	63,922	11,116	23,087
1988	86,782	13,132	24,379
1989	123,565	16,021	26,260
1990	149,178	19,511	27,824
1991	160,742	20,147	30,746
1992	178,224	24,093	31,831
1993	181,236	28,729	34,957
1994	170,016	31,535	37,030
1995	151,642	34,037	39,686
1996	145,522	33,386	42,450
1997	152,195	34,371	46,099
1998	162,689	35,172	49,419

Note these are raw data, and are not adjusted for population, or the numbers in the work force.

- The system is efficient in terms of the time taken to deal with claims and make decisions.

The major limitations reflect the deteriorating economic position of New Zealand and high unemployment levels which raise doubts about whether New Zealand can continue to fund such a generous social security system.

As already noted, there were complementary structural developments in both Australia and New Zealand (P Wright, personal communication, 2001):

- New Zealand merged the equivalents of the Benefit Agency and the Employment Service, forming Work and Income New Zealand in 1998
- New Zealand moved to privatise its comprehensive civil no-fault compensation scheme run by the Accident Rehabilitation and Compensation Corporation (ACC), but reverted to ACC being the single public sector supplier
- New Zealand introduced purchaser–provider splits, private sector service suppliers with outcome-based payments, and competition
- New Zealand introduced a single flat-rate benefit for both unemployed and disabled workers in 1999 (the Community Wage), but reverted to separate Unemployment Benefit and Invalids Benefit on 1 July 2001.

Accident Compensation Corporation

New Zealand also provides one of the most radical social policy experiments for accidents (Hadler 1986). By the 1960s, there was extensive cover for injuries causing work incapacity, but it was fragmentary and inefficient. After a Royal Commission and several years of debate, the Accident Compensation Act was passed in 1972 and the ACC set up in 1974. The basic principle was to provide a single, national, 24 hours per day, 7 days a week, no-fault insurance system for all citizens, which covered all medical expenses and lost wages resulting from accidental injury, irrespective of where the accident occurred and whether or not it was work-related, i.e. a 'no-fault system'. The traditional workers' compensation scheme and the right to sue under civil litigation were abolished despite opposition from the legal profession. Benefits under ACC were comprehensive. There was a schedule of lump-sum benefits for permanent partial incapacity assessed according to the American Medical Association Guides, and a further lump-sum payment for pain and suffering. There was also cover for loss of wages. For the first week the employer paid wages for a work injury and if the injured person was unable to work they received compensation of 80% earnings replacement. If a worker initially returned to work part-time or if they remained restricted to part-time work, their wages were topped up to the 80% level. Non-work injury such as motor vehicle or sport injury could also result in payment of earnings-related compensation under ACC if the worker was unable to work at their current job. ACC paid sickness benefit for non-work injury. Thereafter, benefits for total incapacity continued at 80% of previous earnings until recovery or age retirement pension.

Under this system, the average duration of benefits was >9 years. Between 1975 and 1984, total ACC claims rose from about 105,000 to 150,000 (from a total population of 3 million) but the cost of earnings-related benefits escalated nearly 10-fold. LBP was the most common reason for claims, especially those that became chronic and ongoing. By the early 1990s, chronic LBP claims accounted for >20% of the total ACC budget.

The benefits payable under the ACC scheme have, since the outset, provided for:

1. Medical fees—the costs of assessment (including investigations, radiology, etc) and treatment. Over time, the range of treatments paid for has steadily expanded, e.g. for back pain it has grown to include chiropractors, occupational therapists, clinical psychologists, and osteopaths (in addition to medical practitioners, medical specialists and surgeons, and physiotherapists).

2. Income replacement—which provides 80% of earnings up to a maximum weekly limit. This was originally called Earnings-Related Compensation (ERC) and is now called weekly compensation.

3. Other entitlements—these are paid quite separately from whether the claimant is receiving ERC/weekly compensation. They include modifications to houses (such as wheelchair ramps, remodelling kitchens or bathrooms, etc), vehicle modifications (most often replacing a manual transmission with an automatic one, but also providing vehicles which paraplegics and tetraplegics can drive), attendant care, home help (i.e. someone to help with housework and home maintenance such as mowing the lawns), and child care. Vocational re-training is also available, but the criteria are now more stringent, e.g. while it can cover university tuition, it is now focused more on improving employment prospects so that the case can be closed.

4. Lump-sum payments were previously paid for permanent impairment, and for pain and

suffering. They were abolished by the 1991 Act that came into force in July 1992, and replaced by a weekly Independence Allowance. Projections indicated that over the life of an average claim this allowance would probably provide more funding than the amount previously paid for impairment, but would not cover the amount previously allocated for pain and suffering. The initial payment for the Independence Allowance was made on the basis of disability (essentially the WHO 1980 definitions which were adopted by this Act), and the maximum payment was $40 per week. An amendment to the Act meant that the assessment has now reverted to Impairment, and the maximum amount is raised to $60 per week. The Independence Allowance is reviewed regularly, paid quarterly, and may continue for the claimant's life-time, or until they reach retirement age and are moved to social security retirement pension.

In addition to providing comprehensive no-fault coverage the ACC scheme has also funded injury prevention and research. The costs of administering the scheme have been about 9 cents per dollar, including injury prevention and research.

Although the 'no-fault' ACC system originally side-stepped the question of whether or not the problem was work related, the key issue for debate was then the question of whether or not a health problem was an 'injury'. Initially, this depended on the claimant describing a discrete, finite precipitating event occurring within 3 days of onset of symptoms, and the ACC medical officer accepting a causal link. This led to a decade of bitter legal dispute, and by 1984 the definition was relaxed to the extent that any event occurring within 3 months of the onset of symptoms was acceptable as causal. In practice, >99% of claims were then accepted, so that virtually anyone with back pain could seek and get benefits from ACC. Under the 1981–1982 Act, the lump-sum payments for permanent impairment could be up to $17,000, and for pain and suffering up to $10,000, but the appeal courts always tended to give the maximum awards. Moreover, these limits applied to each incident, and awards could be given for multiple incidents. The result was that the system got out of control, with escalating costs.

Since its inception, the ACC system has always been something of a 'political football', although in view of escalating costs reforms were also inevitably financially driven. The fourth Labour government that served two terms between 1984 and 1990 made plans to integrate the ACC system with the social welfare system. This was intended to ensure there were no inequities between the benefits paid to those with illnesses and those who had experienced personal injuries. However, the incoming National government reversed this policy in 1990 and subsequently turned the ACC scheme into a *de facto* insurance system with the introduction of the Accident Rehabilitation and Compensation Insurance Act (1991). On 1 July 1992 the ACC was replaced by the Accident Rehabilitation Compensation and Insurance Corporation (ARCIC). Funding was Pay-As-You-Go with a separate Employers' Account, Motor Vehicle Account and No-earners' Account (which was government funded). ARCIC, like ACC, covered wage replacement, medical costs and social and rehabilitation costs. Non-earners got the minimum national wage. Lump-sum payments were abolished and replaced by a weekly allowance. There was to be regular reassessment and provision for a Work Capacity Test which would provide an exit from benefits, but this was not fully implemented. These reforms provoked vigorous political opposition, with the formation of a Coalition on ACC (COACC) lobby group.

In March 1994, a case management system was introduced to facilitate rehabilitation. Case managers were charged with ensuring an integrated delivery of services, and empowered to make the majority of purchasing decisions.

ACC accepted a total of 1.5 million new claims in the 1997/98 financial year. Direct payments to claimants were $1.29 billion for weekly compensation (by far the most costly), home help, child care, attendant care, and transport assistance. ACC also paid for a total of 6.98 million medical treatments:

- 2.8 million GP visits
- 2.9 million physiotherapy treatments
- 188,000 visits to medical specialists
- 344,000 visits to radiologists.

It also paid for 771,000 visits to other health professionals such as chiropractors, osteopaths, etc. ACC has paid for treatments provided by chiropractors for many years but payment for treatment by osteopaths only more recently.

In 1997–1998, ACC accepted 21,184 new claims for injuries to the spine which cost a total of $55.2 million:

- 3984 were for the neck/cervical spine region, and cost a total of $8.9 million
- 17,200 were for the lower back or mid-back region, and cost a total of $46.3 million.

In 1997–1998, ACC also paid for a further 27,037 ongoing claims for injuries to the spine at a cost of $411.2 million:

- 4337 were for the neck/cervical spine region, and cost a total of $93.3 million
- 22,700 were for the lower back or mid-back region, and cost a total of $317.8 million.

The major cost of back injuries for ACC comes from those with long-term or chronic problems. Only about 10% of costs go to new claims (which approximates to 'acute injuries') and about 90% to ongoing, chronic claims. This is why ACC has taken such an interest in the prevention of chronicity.

The 1998 Accident Insurance Act came into force on 1 July 1999. Much of the political pressure for this change came from employers and the political goal was to transform the ACC scheme to allow for more market-driven competition. The new Act removed the ACC monopoly for work-place insurance, and established a state-owned enterprise called 'Work Insurance' to compete with private insurers. Those employers who do not arrange cover with a private insurer will by default obtain cover from this organisation. The self-employed will also remain covered by ACC. It is too early to determine if the cost of levies or premiums for employers will be cheaper, as the government hopes. Some early indications suggest that the cost of personal injury insurance could instead rise considerably.

A particular feature of the new Act is that any injury which occurs outside of the work-place, but results in the claimant not being able to work, will still be covered by the ACC.

It is anticipated that the work-relatedness of injuries will be contested, as never before in New Zealand. Perhaps a new case law regarding injury causation will emerge over the next few years. The result of this situation might mean that fewer cases are 'captured' by private insurers than anticipated, and more cases will actually remain under the ACC scheme. Some commentators have pointed out that this situation may be used by the government to provide an excuse effectively to privatise the remainder of the ACC scheme. However, the political nature of accident insurance in New Zealand will inevitably mean that future developments depend on the political balance.

McNaughton et al (2000) studied 100 consecutive ACC claimants who were off work for 4 weeks with LBP. Forty-three claims remained open at 6 months and 30 at 12 months, which they considered compared unfavourably with recent European figures. The strongest predictor of failure to return to work was the receipt of ERC. However, 80% of the whole series received this but no details were provided of what was different about them. McNaughton et al (2000) commented that, perhaps because of the availability of compensation under the ACC scheme, most family doctors and their patients assume that back pain is (work) injury related and fill out claims forms on that basis. This approach has generally been supported by the New Zealand courts whenever claims have been contested. McNaughton et al (2000) suggested that 'New Zealand's unique accident compensation environment may discourage return to work for people with back pain', although in view of the absence of any direct controls this was entirely speculative.

ACC (originally the Accident Compensation Corporation and subsequently the Accident Rehabilitation and Compensation Insurance Corporation), like WorkCover in Australia, has played a leading role in public education and the development of clinical guidelines for back pain (Burton & Waddell 1998). In the late 1980s and early 90s, ACC undertook a public education programme, with 1 million pamphlets and a TV advertising campaign. This took an ergonomic approach and the message was 'don't use your back as a crane'. It included the anatomy and biomechanics of the spine and discs, ergonomic advice and encouragement to 'take care of your back'. This programme had no impact on ACC statistics for back injuries (N Kendall, personal communication, 1999).

The New Zealand Acute Low Back Pain Guide (ACC 1997) had a much stronger emphasis than any previous international clinical guideline on the need to prevent chronicity, and introduced the concept of psychosocial 'yellow flags'. A separate Guide to Assessing Psychosocial Yellow Flags in Acute Low Back Pain (Kendall et al 1997) provided guidance on assessment and management of those at risk. This formed the basis of a second extensive education programme over the next 18 months which reached a much higher proportion of those involved than any previous such effort. Approximately 6000 health professionals treat back pain in New Zealand, and 1000 of them attended a training programme. These meetings were held locally with the active involvement of professional opinion leaders. They were run by a clinical psychologist who was seen as having no vested interest. They dealt with acute back pain management, the assessment of psychosocial yellow flags and psychosocial approaches to preventing chronicity.

A booklet for patients seeking health care, similar to *The Back Book* in the UK (Roland *et al* 1996), was also produced for health professionals to distribute, and 1 million were printed for a population of 3.5 million. Only one physiotherapist felt unable or unwilling to use the leaflet for her patients. A survey by an independent market research organisation found patients were split in their acceptance of the booklet's messages. Many patients and members of the public misunderstood 'acute' and chronic as describing severity rather than duration of symptoms. Some people initially had a negative response but subsequently accepted the messages. A guide for employers, *Active and Working* (Kendall 2000) was produced later.

Evaluation of this campaign is still ongoing. Preliminary results suggested that the programme had a major impact on the key target of preventing chronicity. In workers who lost any time off work with a low back claim, the proportion who remained off work at 3 months (i.e. became chronic) averaged 45% for the 3 years up to February 1997 but fell steadily to 25% by mid 1999 (N Kendall, personal communication, 1999, with data extracted by ACC Information Services). However, no scientific reports have been published since this time on the impact of the educational programme. The ACC website (www.acc.co.nz) provides very limited statistics on back injury claims from 1996–1997 to 1998–1999 (those for 1999–2000 are not comparable because they do not include employees now covered by private insurers). These statistics show an *increase* of 10% in the number of back injury claims but a fall in the number of ongoing claims (i.e. chronic cases) but the data were insufficient to draw any conclusions.

There is again a footnote to this account (N Kendall, personal communication, May 2002). In the past few years there has been political change in New Zealand and a change in the senior management of ACC. The new management has looked for new initiatives that it considers might give short-term pay-offs. This has resulted in less interest and support for the previous educational approach: instead, it has now imported North American sickness management techniques and is looking at North American back school approaches.

Japan

Japan is a small, populous and wealthy country with a population of 125 million and one of the highest densities of people per square kilometre in the world. The birth rate has fallen sharply in recent years and this, coupled with the longest life expectancy in the world, has resulted in the most rapidly ageing population. Despite these changes, family structure has been slow to change. Income per capita is one of the highest in the world.

Situated on the border of east and west, for millennia Japan has shown the ability to learn from foreign cultures and ideas and to adapt them to its own circumstances. Traditional Chinese medicine was introduced to Japan in the 6th century AD. Japan was first exposed briefly to western medicine almost a 1000 years later, but then had a policy of isolationism up until 1867 and only after that was Japanese medicine progressively exposed to western influence.

Iglehart (1988) described the Japanese health-care system which, like that in most European and North American countries, is based on three main principles: ready access, high quality and reasonable cost. It reflects in some respects the entrepreneurial, market-driven nature of the Japanese economy, but conversely the ideas that hospitals should be organised on a non-profit basis, that all citizens should have access to health care irrespective of their ability to pay, and that physicians should place the patient's welfare above their own material gain. Iglehart (1988) stated that (at least at that time) there was cultural resistance to invasive medical procedures in Japan. Wherever possible, the Japanese preferred bed rest and medication to surgery.

Although by many indicators Japanese health has improved dramatically since World War II and is now the best in the world, the Japanese show the same increasing self-perception of sickness as people in Europe and the US. A national survey in 1985 found that 14.5% of people reported that they were experiencing 'any abnormality in physical or mental condition' at the time of the survey (Iglehart 1988). The Japanese pay close attention to their health, have ready access to health care, visit a physician frequently and physicians are revered figures in Japanese society. On average, a Japanese person visits his or her physician 15 times a year (compared with <4 times a year in the UK). Physicians see large numbers of patients for short consultations. Most doctors work privately, although the network of health insurance plans has led to a form of socialisation of medical care which now accounts for >90% of total medical expenditures. No data could be found on Japanese consultation rates for back pain for this review.

Brena et al (1990) and Sanders et al (1992) compared American and Japanese patients with LBP and reported similar biomedical findings, but Japanese patients were significantly less impaired in psychological, social and vocational functioning than the American patients. These authors suggested there might be significant cross-cultural differences in how Japanese and Americans reacted to LBP, particularly in the psychosocial and behavioural areas, although this required further confirmation in larger samples.

In the late 1800s Japan, like most European countries, imitated the German experience and gradually developed various forms of social protection for workers and citizens. The present structure of social insurance is largely based on the Health Insurance Act of 1922, and all Japanese and their families are covered for the direct and indirect costs of illness. With American occupation after World War II, there was imposition of a constitutional democracy and some further westernisation of health-care and social security institutions, although these changes were reversed to some extent from the 1950s onward as Japan regained political independence. However, a US style Workers' Compensation system was introduced and still remains.

Hadler (1994, 1995, 1997, and personal communication) reviewed the current situation in Japan and discussed how the different health-are and compensation systems have affected back pain and disability. As in any other country, a Japanese worker with back pain may either go off sick or report an injury. If they go sick, they receive health insurance of about 60% of basic wages (excluding bonuses) after being off work for 3 days, and this continues for up to 5 years even if the worker loses their job. They then revert to a pension from the national social security scheme, which is less generous and carries more social stigma. In practice, non-specific back pain rarely qualifies for a pension and usually only leads to a lump sum payment of <$1000 for partial permanent disability. This is the path of least resistance, which most Japanese workers with back pain follow. Alternatively, the worker or their physician may report the back pain to the employer as an injury, but this involves proving causality and over-coming administrative hurdles. Both worker and employer must testify that it was a work-related 'injury' which is a very special category reserved for external force events. Short of such an event, the worker must recruit co-workers to assert that the back pain started suddenly at work while doing something that was physically demanding. This is unlikely to make the worker popular in the work place and is subject to investigation by the Labour Office who may even interview co-workers. Those who are accepted as having compensable injuries receive 60% of wages from their employer for the first 3 days. They then receive about 80% replacement from the workers' compensation system with some additional allowance for usual bonuses for as long as they are under medical care, and they cannot be fired. Whichever path is chosen, acute medical care is readily available for the worker with back pain and carries little stigma, but is at the discretion of the (authoritative) physician, is conservative, and usually consists of frequent, brief, doctor–patient contacts. There is little inducement for physicians to prolong treatment, and they do not encourage it. Expectation of healing and rapid return to work is facilitated by the culture and the lack of a comparably appealing alternative.

In this very different culture and system in Japan, Hadler (1994, 1997) stated that the impact of back pain remained remarkably constant for many years. Health insurance had covered about 24 million days of care for LBP each year since 1970. The incidence of claims for work-related back injuries remained stable at under 10,000 per year from 1973 through 1990, or about 5% of all workers' compensation claims.

However, isolated and fragmentary reports by Japanese authors give a different perspective. Kuwashima et al (1997) analysed a sample of 5820 cases of LBP reported to the Japanese Labour Standards Inspection Offices in 1986 and 7346 cases in 1988, from the national 'Report on Workers' Casualties'. They agreed that the incidence of back injury claims was very low: only 1.5 per 1000 workers per annum for men and 0.4 per 1000 for women but suggested that back injuries accounted for about half of all workers' casualty claims.

Nevertheless, there was sufficient concern about back pain in Japan for the Labour Standards Bureau to issue *Guidelines on Worksite Prevention of Low Back Pain* in September 1994, subsequently published in English by Yamamoto (1997a). Yamamoto (1997b) described the background to these guidelines and gave data on trends (Table 4.91). These confirmed Hadler's account that the incidence of occupational back pain had not risen and according to these more recent data had actually fallen. However, like Kuwashima et al (1997), Yamamoto (1997b) also stated that back pain accounted for 60% of the total number of officially recognised cases of occupational disease, compared with Hadler's figure of 5%. Despite correspondence with Hadler and unsuccessful attempts to contact various of the

TABLE 4.91   Annual incidence of officially recognised cases of occupational LBP causing at least 4 days off work

	Number of cases of occupational low back pain
1987	8635
1988	7952
1989	8281
1990	7981
1991	7222
1992	6747
1993	6299
1994	5935
1995	5573
1996	5162

From Yamamoto (1997b).

Japanese authors it has not been possible to resolve this discrepancy, or to obtain any other Japanese statistics from official sources.

According to Hadler, the Japanese benefits system is generous in the short-term to those with compensable back injuries, but it is under very strict controls and is generally restrictive and in the long-term is very harsh by European standards. Under this system, there has not been any rise in health insurance or workers' compensation for back pain in Japan. However, these various figures seem to suggest that it is the claims rate for compensation that is very low and stable, rather than that back pain is not a problem in Japan. This obviously to a large extent reflects the structure of the compensation system, but it should not be over-interpreted simplistically as solely an effect of this system. Cultural attitudes and traditions, physician attitudes and medical management, and the compensation system all act in concert. The benefits system may reflect other, more fundamental cultural attitudes that non-specific LBP is not a generally acceptable basis for permanent total disability.

It is difficult to get an accurate picture about what is happening in the social security system in one's own country, never mind in any other country, but this is especially so in Japan. Hadler (personal communication) also warns that it is exceedingly difficult to find out or understand what is happening in Japan, even when he was in residence and able to interview Japanese experts, social security officials and mid-level bureaucrats, with the assistance of Japanese colleagues who had done some of their training in the US and seemed willing to try to bridge the language and cultural divide. Moreover, the economic situation and the workers' compensation system is changing in Japan, just as elsewhere, and some of the above information may now be out of date. There is no evidence available on whether or not there has been any change in back pain trends in Japan during the past few years of economic crisis. Given all of these caveats, interpretation or extrapolation of these findings from a very different western perspective must be very cautious.

5 Special issues

Three issues have recurred throughout this review: early retirement; unemployment; and the incentives and controls of the social security system. This final section includes some relevant material which seems to be more general in nature rather than fitting into the review of any one country. This chapter describes material retrieved during the course of the main review and is not a systematic or comprehensive review of these issues.

Early retirement

Health-care and social security spending rise rapidly after age 60. UK data for 1991 showed a five-fold increase in spending between the ages of 50–55 and 85–90 years (Hills 1997).

Population forecasts for Europe suggest that the proportion of the population aged 65+ is likely to increase by 3–7% by 2020, but fears of a 'demographic time-bomb' are often over-stated (Hills 1997). This increase could raise health and pension expenditure by about 15–20%. Any demographic effect on retirement is likely to have less effect than actual working and retirement patterns, political decisions about taxation in general, and policy and administrative changes in the social security system. There have already been major changes in all of these areas over the past 35 years, and any impact of an ageing population over the next 20 years is likely to be much less. However, this does not allow for the problem of increasing numbers of the very old (aged 85+), many of whom need institutional care at some point, which could mean large increases in these particular costs. One of the common political responses to these demographic trends has been to argue for an increase in the state pension age, although some countries such as Sweden and Italy are introducing a more flexible pension age with financial inducements to deferring retirement.

Table 5.1 shows the official state retirement pension arrangements in various European countries.

The age at which people actually stop working and leave the labour force is often quite different from the official state retirement age, and since the early 1980s increasing numbers of people have retired early before they become eligible for the state retirement pension. Table 5.2 shows official statistics for labour force participation in different age groups in various European countries. Overall, only 30% of men in Europe now work beyond age 60 and <40% of women beyond age 55, but there is marked variation in different European countries. Sweden has by far the highest European participation rates among older workers, with 59% of men and 50% of women aged 60–64 years still working. In the UK and Denmark, over 40% of men and 20–25% of women aged 60–64 are still working. In most other European countries, only 10–25% of men and 5–15% of women continue working

TABLE 5.1 Retirement arrangements in different European countries

Entitlement	Basic pension level ECU *		Entitlement	Basic pension level (ECU)[1]	Average actual pension (%)[2]
	Men	Women			
UK	65	60 rising to 65 between 2010 and 2020	Based on National Insurance contributions for most employees	3952	39
Ireland	65	65	Based on National Insurance contributions for most employees	5252	
Sweden	65	65	National pension: all residents Supplementary pension: all employees and self-employed with pension carrying income	4057	
Norway	67	67	National pension: all residents Earnings- related old-age pension		57
Finland	65	65	National pension: all residents Employment pension: all employees and self-employed	4356	74
Denmark	67	67	National pension: all resident nationals Supplementary pension: employees, sick and unemployed	6173	
The Netherlands	65	65	All residents	8316	
Belgium	60–65[3]	60–65[3]	All employees	8452	
France	60	60	Employees and assimilated	5875	63
Germany	60–65[3]	60–65[3]	Industrial and non-industrial staff	Average net wages	74

* Single male with 40-years contribution

[1] Replacement ratios net of social and tax deductions for a qualified, private sector worker with dependent partner, and full career under compulsory and general benefits plus company schemes in selected countries (ISSA 1995a).

[2] Arrangements for early pensions before standard age of 65 if sufficient years of contributions and either incapacity or unemployment.

From MISSOC (1996, 1998).

TABLE 5.2   Work participation rates by age

	Men (age group)				Women (age group)			
	45–49	50–54	55–59	60–64	45–49	50–54	55–59	60–64
UK	86.0	80.3	67.9	43.0	76.2	67.6	52.0	24.8
Sweden	86.2	85.8	76.8	58.5	85.6	83.3	73.7	49.5
Finland	74.5	72.7	46.4	22.1	75.5	74.1	47.6	18.0
Denmark	88.8	83.6	74.1	41.3	79.6	68.5	51.8	19.2
The Netherlands	88.7	81.2	58.8	19.6	57.5	46.3	28.8	9.1
Belgium	86.5	77.4	47.0	17.2	53.0	37.7	19.2	5.0
France	87.8	83.6	55.7	11.0	70.6	63.3	40.5	11.2
Germany	87.9	83.8	63.8	26.1	68.2	60.2	41.9	10.3
Total EU15	87.3	80.8	61.8	30.0	62.1	53.1	36.6	14.1

From Eurostat Labour Force Survey (1996). More recent Eurostat Labour Force Surveys and the International Labour Organisation do not provide such detailed age breakdown. Eurostat LFS (1996) did not have comparable work participation rates by age for Ireland.

after age 60 years. The US has always had a higher work participation rate among older people and higher average retirement age, although one recent Canadian survey found that the average *desired* retirement age is now 58 years (Cloutier 2000).

Before considering early retirement, it is worth looking at the effect of ageing on workers (Cloutier 2000). Ageing inevitably leads to varying rates and degrees of physical, cognitive and psychological decline, but to counter-balance this, there is also acquisition of experience and skills which may enable the older worker to adapt his or her working practices to compensate for these diminishing capacities. However, this adaptation requires a certain flexibility and freedom for older workers to change how they do their work, in certain situations or at certain times they may need some tolerance or assistance from fellow workers, and at times it may reduce some aspects of their productivity. Unfortunately, modern changes in work organisation and management and the emphasis on 'efficiency' often increase work intensity and stress and reduce the very flexibility and freedom older workers require to do their jobs. In the demand to deliver efficiency, employers and fellow workers may be less tolerant of older workers.

The complex balance of diminishing capacities, increasing experience, changing work practices and changing attitudes may affect occupational health and accidents. Cloutier (2000) found that the incidence of work-related accidents fell with age, but older workers were likely to be off work longer (in this particular example of fire fighters, 'older' was taken to be >35 years which emphasises that age is relative). Accidents to younger workers were more likely to involve specific physical demands at work and their inexperience might be a contributory factor. Accidents to older workers were more likely to demonstrate their increasing physical and cognitive vulnerability. The physical demands of work, work intensity, work stress and the psychosocial aspects of work might all have a differential impact on older workers, which might affect the pattern of their occupational health, sickness and disability. Cloutier (2000) concluded that the impact of ageing on occupational health varies with the physical and psychological demands of each job. It is necessary to look at health status and subjective health complaints such as pain and stress as well as work 'accidents'.

Work organisation must allow sufficient flexibility for older workers to adapt their working practices, and in view of changing demographics, 'age management planning' is essential to utilise the skills and experience of older workers.

In more general terms, Scales & Scase (2000) found that people in their 50s are now much more comparable in their attitudes, activities and behaviour to people in their 30s and 40s, they no longer regard themselves as 'older' and it is only in their 60s that they change.

Hayden *et al* (1999) made a qualitative study of the attitudes and aspirations of older people (age 50 and above) in the UK. Attitudes to work and early retirement varied with gender, income and employment status. Nevertheless, most people in their 50s felt they got a lot out of work and did not necessarily feel ready to stop work either before or at the state pension age. They thought there should be opportunities to continue working in some form after retirement—albeit in different jobs, often part-time, and either paid or voluntary. Notwithstanding positive attitudes to work, many felt there was discrimination against older people in the work force and a lack of respect for age and experience. There was lack of the active support and understanding required for workers (and particularly older workers) to adapt to changing working patterns. Among those who had retired, work in retirement was seen as different from pre-retirement, with benefits such as more flexibility, less commitment and responsibility, and a better balance between work and other activities.

Scales & Scase (2000) provided a very broad and comprehensive review of social, occupational and economic trends among adults in their 50s. They found:

- Those over 50 now account for one-fifth of the UK population but own 80% of the wealth and are the most likely to vote in general elections
- From a broadly homogenous group, the over 50s have become fragmented into a number of diverse groups depending on type of employment, occupational pensions, marital status and financial commitments such as children and mortgages
- The number of men aged 50–59 in full-time employment has fallen from 93% in the 1975 to approximately 74% in the early–mid 1990s, and since then has stabilised around 77% in 2000 (Labour Force Survey 2000). For women this figure has remained constant at around 60%
- The proportion of men working is stable at about 85% from 45 to 50 years of age and then progressively falls to <60% by age 60. For women, the proportion gradually falls from 80% at age 45, to 75% at age 50, to 53% at age 58, to 32% at age 60 years (Labour Force Survey 2000)
- Twice as many men in their 50s compared to those in their 30s report their health is poor. For women, the pattern is less pronounced
- GP visits are not significantly greater for most of those in their 50s, although they are higher for those living alone and particulary for those who are economically inactive
- Men in their 50s are more likely to experience longer periods of economic inactivity and ill health but there are occupational differences
- Unemployment leads to low motivation, depression and a general disengagement from active social participation

- Moving out of employment reduces stress and improves health levels for those in managerial and professional occupations but increases stress and is associated with deteriorating health for those in manual unskilled occupations. Professional women who remain in employment are likely to show an increase in stress

- 'Age' is being re-defined. Life-styles and leisure patterns of those in their 50s are now similar to those in their 30s and 40s. It is only in the 60s that age generally begins to impact on life-style activities

- Attitudes towards the family, gender roles, the economy and the welfare state are similar to those in their 30s and 40s but those in their 50s show more concern about unemployment (particularly women) and the environment

- Those in work are most likely to be satisfied with their social life (79%) followed by those inactive and in receipt of a pension (68%). Only 46% of those with no pension say they are happy. Conversely, 22% of those in work are not satisfied with the amount of leisure time they have compared with 12% of those who are economically inactive. Satisfaction with life overall runs at 86% (working), 80% (inactive, in receipt of a pension) and 48% (inactive, no pension)

- For men and women in managerial and professional occupations, an expectation of early retirement has become entrenched and will be difficult to change. Only about a third of inactive men and about 20% of inactive women in their 50s would like to have a regular job, and only 20% and 15% respectively would like to return to full-time work; 25–30% of those in 'white collar' jobs and about 40% of those in manual jobs would give up their job if they could afford to do so, although 65% overall would not like to give up working completely

- Increasing numbers of younger employees expect to have work careers of 25–30 years' instead of 40 years' duration. Life after work is seen to offer a period of about 30 years when personal talents and skills can be developed free from the demands of work. The idea of mere subsistence in retirement is, for most, unthinkable

- For many people in their 50s from professional occupations, early withdrawal from the labour market is a choice based upon access to an occupational or private pension income. However, for manual workers it is more likely to be early retirement on grounds of ill health

- 50% of non-working professionals report that they are financially comfortable compared to <20% of former blue collar workers, 60% of whom are finding things quite or very difficult compared to 30% of inactive professionals.

From this they predicted:

- Those who are released from financial commitments—mortgages paid, children have left home, etc—are likely to exit the labour market in their 50s, creating a labour market shortage of those with managerial, professional and other expert skills. The 50s age group is therefore likely to polarise into affluent early retirees and those compelled to work because of financial necessity

- Many will find they have saved nowhere near enough to have a comfortable retirement

- Pressures for those divorced and separated to maximise their earning capacities and future pensions by deferring retirement and for those already retired to seek part-time employment

- Increased tendency for those in ill health to seek publicly provided social security and welfare support.

The lessons for social policy were:

- Notwithstanding government policy, a social and work culture has emerged with the expectation and desire for early retirement
- The wide degree of social polarisation that arises from life-time earnings trajectories and transitions in marital status
- Harsh economic realities show a mismatch between people's expectations of early retirement and expectations in retirement versus the lack of state or personal financial provision for this.

Ginarlis (2000) disagreed to some extent with this analysis and prediction of likely future social trends. He suggested that over the last 20 years powerful structural and organisational factors had driven early retirement:

- Older employees tend to be more senior and expensive and therefore there are greater savings by removing them
- 'Mechanisms' of early retirement are easier and meet less resistance than some other forms of redundancy
- Under most pension schemes, the financial burden of early retirement has been transferred from the company to the (more or less separate) pension fund. In times of booming stock markets and high interest rates, pension funds were over-funded and therefore were able and willing to absorb early retirement costs
- Public sectors similarly shifted the costs of early retirement from departmental budgets to central government funds
- Pension rules are 'all or nothing' and prohibit or limit any combination of early retirement and continued part-time work with the same company
- The corporate boom in the 1990s meant that many employers could afford to offer attractive additional incentives for early retirement.

The economic landscape at the start of a new millennium has changed dramatically and Ginarlis (2000) argued this is likely to reverse many of these structural and organisational factors and so act against early retirement in future. There are emerging shifts in the next generation's age pattern of financial commitments for children, mortgages and pensions which are also likely to delay when retirement becomes possible.

If increasing numbers of people retire early before being entitled to state pensions, they obviously need some alternative form of financial support to cover the intervening period. This has been partly supplied by employment pension plans and special arrangements associated with industrial re-organisation, and probably to a lesser extent by personal pension plans and private savings. For those who do not have access to such financial support, the only alternative is some form of social security benefit. Whatever, increasing numbers of people are clearly not dependent on the state pension and one way or another are in a position to take early retirement without it. So raising the state pension age or changing the state retirement pension inducements may not have much effect, but may simply transfer more of the cost of retirement provision to these other sources (MISSOC 1995).

Aarts et al (1996) summarised various possible routes from work to retirement (Figure 5.1).

In most European countries the numbers receiving short-term sickness benefits rises with increasing age, from somewhere between age 45 and 55 in men and 40–50 in women (Table 5.3). In most European countries the number more or less doubles between the 30s and 50s, in men and women, which is what might be expected from the epidemiology of illness. However, in contrast to every other country and the expected epidemiology of illness, there is virtually no increase in sickness over this age range in Belgium. The number receiving long-term invalidity benefits shows a similar pattern (Table 5.4). The fall in the sickness benefit rate in some countries after age 55–60 probably reflects a healthy worker effect with varying numbers changing from sickness benefits to invalidity or retirement pensions. In most countries women show slightly higher short-term sickness benefit rates but much lower long-term invalidity benefit rates, which may reflect entitlement. Back pain shows the same pattern of sick certification with age (Table 5.5).

There is no clear inter-relationship between work activity rates, unemployment rates and both short- and long-term work incapacity with increasing age in different countries (Table 5.6). Sweden, Denmark and the UK have the latest retirement in practice, but despite this have relatively low rates of unemployment, sickness absence and long-term incapacity among older workers. In Germany there are several ways of early exit from the labour force (see Chapter 4 for review of individual countries). Men can get an early old-age pension once they have paid pension contributions for 35 years, and women who have paid contributions for 10 out of 20 years of work. There are also relatively high rates of unemployment

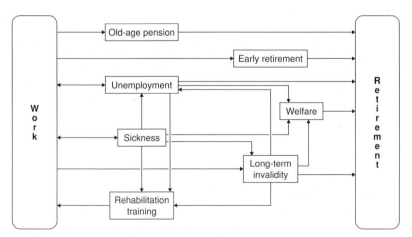

Figure 5.1 Alternative routes from work to retirement

Adapted from Aarts et al (1996)

TABLE 5.3   Short-term sickness and employment injury benefits by age and gender in 1995 (%)

Age	UK	Sweden	Denmark	The Netherlands	Belgium	Germany
Men						
16–19	3.6	1.3	1.0	2.9	2.8	3.1
20–24	2.6	2.0	2.8	4.2	2.7	3.7
25–29	3.3	2.5	4.6	3.9	2.6	3.4
30–34	2.6	3.0	4.5	4.1	3.1	3.9
35–39	3.1	3.5	5.0	5.0	3.0	4.4
40–44	2.8	3.7	6.1	4.7	3.5	4.8
45–49	3.1	4.1	7.0	5.8	3.6	5.7
50–54	4.2	5.1	8.2	5.2	4.0	7.2
55–59	5.1	6.7	9.6	8.2	3.0	8.1
60–64	5.1	8.0	7.2	5.2	1.3	11.1
Women						
16–19	1.0	1.5	0.7	4.2	2.5	3.1
20–24	3.8	2.9	3.3	6.3	3.2	3.6
25–29	2.6	3.8	5.0	6.7	3.1	3.3
30–34	3.8	4.6	6.8	6.5	3.4	3.6
35–39	4.3	4.9	8.8	6.9	5.5	4.1
40–44	5.1	5.2	10.5	6.1	6.3	4.8
45–49	4.4	5.7	12.3	7.2	5.3	5.6
50–54	5.9	6.6	13.6	6.7	5.1	7.0
55–59	6.8	(7.9)	15.6	11.2	2.8	7.5
60–64	—	9.5	—	—	2.5	9.5

among older workers. In the Netherlands the very high level of long-term or permanent incapacity appears to be the most common mechanism of early retirement. Thus older workers who stop working in Germany may be classified (and paid) as unemployed or as ordinary retirements, whereas in the Netherlands they are classified (and paid) as early retirements due to sickness or disability pensions. Belgium, with one of the earliest retirement patterns, has among the lowest levels of unemployment, and both short- and long-term sickness absence among older workers, which may be because the low retirement age means that these alternative mechanisms of funding are not required. However, Denmark, with the oldest official retirement age, does not have particularly high levels of unemployment or sickness absence and only average long-term incapacity among older workers. Germany, despite its more flexible exits from the labour market, still has the highest level of unemployment in older workers.

There is no biomedical explanation for these differences between different countries or for rising trends of early retirement, which appear to have more to do with social factors. In principle, differences in the structure of the social security systems and the presence of alternative 'exits' from the labour market would be expected to influence the different levels of early retirement due to incapacity in different countries. The increase has to a large extent coincided with changes in the general economic situation, labour market forces and reduced employment opportunities which have certainly made it more difficult for

TABLE 5.4 Long-term incapacity rates by age and gender in 1990 (%)

Age	UK	Sweden	Denmark	The Netherlands	Belgium	Germany
Men						
16–19	0.0	0.8	0.5	0.1	0.0	0.0
20–24	0.3	0.7	0.9	0.6	0.3	0.0
25–29	0.8	0.9	1.4	1.4	0.7	0.2
30–34	1.3	1.4	2.1	3.0	1.6	0.5
35–39	1.9	2.1	2.7	5.3	2.6	1.0
40–44	2.9	2.7	3.6	9.3	4.0	1.9
45–49	4.3	3.7	4.5	13.0	6.3	3.7
50–54	7.8	6.8	7.4	22.1	10.4	7.5
55–59	13.1	13.4	12.0	32.9	15.7	17.7
60–64	26.0	30.4	27.0	67.6	23.4	41.6
Women						
16–19	0.0	0.6	0.2	0.1	0.0	0.0
20–24	0.5	0.6	0.7	0.9	0.2	0.0
25–29	1.3	0.8	1.2	2.9	0.7	0.1
30–34	1.9	1.3	2.0	4.5	1.7	0.6
35–39	2.4	2.1	2.6	5.5	3.2	1.2
40–44	2.7	3.2	4.1	8.4	5.3	2.0
45–49	4.0	4.9	5.2	12.7	8.5	3.3
50–54	8.2	8.8	9.3	21.2	13.3	6.3
55–59	14.8	15.5	15.4	32.7	18.7	18.3

From Einerhand et al (1995).

TABLE 5.5 Age distribution of sick certification for back pain

Age	% with sick certification in last 4 weeks	% with sick certification for complete last 4 weeks
16–24	1.1	0
25–44	1.4	1.0
45–54	3.0	2.7
55–64	3.0	3.0

Based on data from Mason (1994).

older workers to retain or obtain jobs. The labour market may push people out of work involuntarily, e.g. redundancy, increasing unemployment, or structural changes in the demand for labour such as fewer jobs for unskilled workers. Some workers who retire early get various pension packages or redundancy payments as part of industrial re-organisation. Other factors may increase the attractiveness of early retirement, e.g. more liberal criteria for granting disability pensions or social security benefits, or higher financial payments. In most European countries during the 1980s and 90s, the original strict medical grounds for early retirement were relaxed to include increasing numbers of people with more non-specific health problems and incapacities. There was increasing allowance for age, unemployment and the difficulty of obtaining work. At the same time, once people were on long-term benefit there was less effective monitoring, fewer came off benefit, and it became accepted

TABLE 5.6 Relationship between retirement, official retirement age, unemployment, sickness and invalidity by gender in different EU countries

	Employment rate (in rank order) (%)		Official retirement age	Unemployment rate 55–59 (%)	Short-term sickness absence age 55–59 (%)	Long-term work incapacity age 55–59 (%)[1]
	Age 55–59	Age 60–64				
Men						
Sweden	76.8	58.5	65 (1993)	8.7	6.7	13.4
Denmark	74.1	41.3	67	6.1	9.6	12.0
UK	67.9	43.0	65	9.9	5.1	13.1
Germany	63.8	26.1	60–65	13.4	8.1	17.7
The Netherlands	58.8	19.6	65	3.6	8.2	32.9
Belgium	47.0	17.2	60–65	4.9	3.0	15.7
Women						
Sweden	73.7	—	65	6.6	(7.9)	15.5
Denmark	51.8	—	67	6.8	15.6	15.4
UK	52.0	—	60	4.2	6.8	14.8
Germany	41.9	—	60–65	16.4	7.5	18.3
The Netherlands	28.8	—	65	5.6	11.2	32.7
Belgium	19.2	—	60–65	—	2.8	18.7

[1] 1990 data.

Based mainly on 1995–1996 data from Tables 1.1, 1.3, 1.4 and Einerhand et al (1995), Prins et al (1998).

that they would remain on benefits more or less permanently until retirement age. In effect, early retirement on health grounds gradually became an acceptable means of earning a living while awaiting the ordinary retirement pension at age 65. To the individual, this was perhaps a realistic attitude towards the prospects of rehabilitation and re-employment in the current economic and labour market situation. To employers, it was a convenient method of shifting any further responsibility for these workers. To politicians, it helped to reduce the politically sensitive unemployment figures. The social security system, the taxpayer and society were left to foot the bill.

There is considerable other evidence on early retirement in the medical literature, some particularly relevant to back pain, which was reviewed by Waddell & Norlund (2000).

Since the 1970s, economists have carefully examined retirement patterns and trends, and sought to identify and measure the factors which influence the timing of retirement, although much of this research is fairly technical and inaccessible to non-specialist readers. Leonesio (1996) provides a non-technical review of this economic evidence.

Astrand & Isacsson (1988) studied 391 male employees in a Swedish pulp and paper company in 1961 and then followed them for 22 years. Sick leave in their sample was low. There were 30 cases of early retirement with a diagnosis of back disorder on the retirement certificate. Perhaps surprisingly, report of back pain at baseline did not predict early retirement due to back pain although back abnormalities on physical examination was a weak predictor.

Hasenbring et al (1994) in Germany studied a selected group of 111 consecutive patients with sciatica and proven lumbar disc prolapse. The best predictors of application for disability pension at 6-months follow-up were age, duration of symptoms, depression and stress at work, but none of the other biomedical data about their back condition.

Junge et al (1995) made a prospective study of pre-operative predictors of outcome in 381 patients from Germany and Switzerland who had lumbar disc surgery. On multivariate analysis, the best predictors of a poor outcome at 12 months included severity of pain and disability, multiple pain sites, duration of sickness absence and considering or applying for a disability pension. However, the published data and interpretations about disability pension appear inconsistent and it has not been possible to obtain any further clarification from the authors.

Rothenbacher et al (1997) also carried out a longitudinal study of prognostic factors for early retirement among employees in the construction industry in Germany. Reported back pain or sciatica led to a relative risk of 1.6 (95% CI 1.3–2.1) of early retirement. An abnormal clinical finding in the spine led to a relative risk of 1.8 (1.4–2.2) and a recorded medical diagnosis of a back condition to a relative risk of 1.5 (1.2–1.8). Siebert et al (2001) followed 10,809 male workers in the construction industry in Germany from 1986 to 1994. During this period, 2472 workers changed employment and 359 were granted disability pension on health grounds. A wide range of chronic diseases was associated with increased rates of early retirement and mortality but not occupational mobility. However, disorders of the back and spine (ICD-9 codes 720–724) were common reasons for both occupational mobility ($n = 41$, RR 1.17, 95% CI 1.04–1.32) and early retirement ($n = 39$, RR 1.50, 95% CI 1.20–1.88). Differential occupational mobility preceded differential early retirement by more than a decade. These findings demonstrated a healthy worker effect. Hartvigsen et al (2001) also demonstrated that low back pain for >30 days in the past year produced a healthy worker effect among workers with heavy physical work who were more likely to move to sedentary work.

Hagen et al (2000) reported an 11-year prospective observational study of the entire insured population of Norway. Between 1983 and 1993 the annual incidence of early disability retirement attributed to non-inflammatory low back pain was 0.15% which accounted for about 15% of all disability pensions. Of these, 51% were in the lower back, 20% in the neck and the remainder in multiple or unspecified areas of the back. Socio-economic status was strongly associated with early retirement due to non-inflammatory low back pain (for unskilled workers: men OR 3.1, 95% CI 2.6–3.7; women OR 2.1, 95% CI 1.7–2.5) but only moderately associated with early retirement due to inflammatory low back pain. Each year of formal education was independently associated with a decreased risk of early retirement due to both non-inflammatory and inflammatory low back pain. No other variables were studied, so the relative importance of these predictors could not be assessed.

Eden et al (1994) in Sweden studied 453 early retirement pensioners and compared them with matched controls. Low socio-economic status, lower educational level, heavy manual work and immigrant status were associated with increased early retirement. Eden *et al* (1995) found that early retirement was followed by a deterioration in self-reported health status in men of all ages and in women aged 25–54 years, although health status improved in women aged 55–64. However, these studies did not provide separate data on back pain. Berg *et al* (1988) found no significant difference in the prevalence of back or neck symptoms in male manual or office workers before and after retirement. Ostberg & Samuelsson (1994) found that women aged 62–64 had improved subjective health and fewer musculoskeletal symptoms after retirement, and the prevalence of back complaints fell from 47 to 31%.

Harkapaa (1992) in Finland followed 476 patients with chronic low back pain for 4.5 years and found that back pain accounted for 51% of the early retirements. Older age and psychological measures were the best predictors of early retirement, irrespective of the initial level of low back disability or treatment. Mansson & Israelsson (1987) undertook health screening of 123 men aged 48–50 and reviewed them again 4–8 years later after they had received early disability pensions, most commonly for musculoskeletal disorders (41%), mental illness (17%) and cardiovascular disease (16%). The most striking difference from the control group was the number of pensioners with raised gamma-glutamyl-transferase suggesting high alcohol intake. The highest enzyme levels were associated with increased reports of back pain, both before and even more so after retirement.

Baldwin *et al* (1996) analysed first return to work and subsequent work loss in 8690 WCB patients in Canada who were injured in 1974–1986 and examined by a physician in 1989–1990 for permanent partial disability assessment. All else being equal, back injuries were associated with longer first work absences than other injuries in men but not in women, and with a higher chance of failing ever to return to work, more repeat absences and higher chance of eventually giving up work in both men and women. All else being equal, increasing age was associated with longer duration of first absence, higher chance of failing ever to return to work and higher chance of multiple absences and eventually giving up work in both men and women.

The first comprehensive database on retirement was the US Social Security Administration's *Retirement History Study* of approximately 11,000 Americans who were aged 58–63 in 1969 and who were followed for 10 years until 1979, by which time most of them had retired. Leonesio (1996) provided a comprehensive review of retirement in the US, based on the *Retirement History Study* and other data. 1995 data showed a fairly even pattern of retirement between age 55 and 70, although for men this accelerated as they entered their early 60s, with slight peaks of retirement about age 62 and 65. Labour force participation fell from 81% at age 55 to 20% at age 70 for men, and from 62 to 11% for women. Since World War II there had been a trend to retire earlier, although by 1995 the median retirement age in the US was still 62. The major change had been in the number who continued working well after age 65: labour force participation by all men aged 65 or older fell from 49% in 1948, to 22% in 1974, to about 10% in 1995. Perhaps surprisingly from a European perspective, however, in 1995 about 7% of US men and 3% of US women were still working at age 75. Moreover, many male household heads who had spent most of their adult life working with a single employer only partially retired in their later working years, and a quarter of those who did retire subsequently took other employment. Overall, about a third of US adults worked part-time at some stage of their later working life, for an average of about 20 hours per week over an average of 5 years.

An increasing amount of data are now becoming available from the US Social Security Administration's *Health and Retirement Study* (Juster & Suzman 1995, Willis & Suzman 2000). This longitudinal study of approximately 5000 couples and 2400 unmarried individuals aged 51–61 was set up in 1992 and samples have been re-interviewed every 2 years. Several additional groups have since been added and the *Health and Retirement Study* is now a representative sample of >22,000 Americans over age 50. The *Health and Retirement Study* is intended to provide data for researchers, programme planners and policy makers regarding patterns of retirement, health, savings and social provision. It is designed to gather data to:

- Explain the antecedents and consequences of retirement
- Examine the relationship between health, income and assets over time
- Examine life-cycle patterns of savings and expenditure
- Monitor patterns of work disability
- Examine how the distribution and mix of economic, family and programme resources affect key outcomes, including retirement, savings, health decline and institutionalisation.

The variables include:

- Demographic characteristics
- Health status and health care
- Occupation, employment and employment history
- Economic circumstances such as income, assets and pension data
- Housing and living arrangements
- Family relationships and support.

Several hundred documents based on the *Health and Retirement Study* have now been published (Willis & Suzman 2000) and a detailed list can be obtained at www.umich.edu/~hrswww/pubs/biblio.html.

There are obvious economic constraints on when retirement becomes an option: however, decisions about work, retirement and leisure are not solely economic, but all part of how people decide to use their time. The basic work–leisure choice and the secondary decision about how much to work depend on the balance between the financial and other rewards of work, alternative sources of income available, financial needs, and the other attractions but also financial needs for retirement and leisure activities. Economists produce statistical models and empirical analyses to support this kind of decision-making framework (Gustman et al 1994, Leonesio 1996). Job opportunities, social pressures and health also influence the decision, and it must be viewed in a dynamic model as part of a whole life-cycle. However, retirement, and particularly early retirement, is nowadays often a voluntary decision, and there may be wide variation in how individuals respond to these various influences.

Leosenio (1996) reviewed a number of empirical studies which suggested that the availability of social security pension was a major factor in the timing of retirement, although the actual level of payments had a relatively modest effect. For example, a 10% increase in retirement benefit might lower the average retirement age by about 1 month. The best estimate was that the Social Security Administration structure accounted for the current popularity of retirement at age 62 and 65 in the US and, overall, had probably reduced the average age of retirement for men by several months. An earlier analysis in the UK (Zabalza et al 1980) reached similar conclusions: people do respond to economic incentives, but age, gender and poor health have much stronger influence.

However, most of these social security analyses failed to allow for private pensions, which are a key source of retirement income for a significant portion of the population to whom the structure of their pension plan may be much more important than social security benefits. Kotlikoff & Wise (1989) studied one US Fortune 500 company and suggested that the provisions of the firm's pension plan were the major factor in the timing of early retirement, much greater than any social security considerations, although social security conditions might also contribute to the peak in retirements at age 65. The influence of financial incentives varied with health status: poor health might lead to higher financial benefits; persons in poor health were more likely to respond to financial incentives; persons in poor health were more sensitive to bad job characteristics. Moreover, these economic studies seemed to accept health as a completely independent variable and assumed cause and effect. They failed to allow for the interactions between psychosocial aspects of work, financial incentives and health complaints. Nevertheless, overall, age and health again appeared to overshadow financial incentives in the decision to retire.

Gustman et al (1994) reviewed economic research on company pensions in the US which suggested that many issues were important (Table 5.7), although they concluded there was insufficient evidence to determine the relative weight to attach to these.

The percentage of women working in the US rose from 28% in 1940 to 57% in 1991, and women now make up 45% of the US labour force. However, until recently most of

TABLE 5.7 Behavioural motivations for employer-provided pensions

Worker motivations	Tax preferred retirement savings, often inflation proofed
	Convenience and economies of scale
	Insurance against incapacity and other contingencies
	Union preference
Employer motivations	Human resource tool:
	− regulate retirement
	− reduce worker turnover other than retirement
	− productivity incentive
Outcomes of supply–demand interactions	Pension plan structure and conditions
	Patterns of retirement
	Worker selection, motivation, turnover
	Wage bargaining

the research on retirement has been about men, and there are relatively few studies on the retirement decisions of older women. Weaver (1994) reviewed 13 studies, but urged that the results should be interpreted with caution because of the limited data, much of which were already quite dated, and methodological weaknesses. Generally, these studies showed that married women's decisions about retirement seemed to be related more to the financial rewards of work, but not to the levels of financial benefits after retirement. This might be partly explained by a lack of linkage between earnings and benefits for many married women, which might act as a deterrent to retirement. Husbands and wives might often reach joint retirement decisions, and a married woman was less likely to continue working once her husband retired, just as a married man was less likely to continue working once his wife retired. The family, the presence of dependent children or parents, and the husband's health appeared to play little part in a woman's decisions to retire. This was perhaps surprising, but might be due to conflicting influences: increased need for the woman in the home versus increased financial need for her to work and increased attractiveness of getting out of the home. There were virtually no data available on the relationship of women's health to retirement decisions, and very little data on unmarried women, although their retirement decisions might be more similar to those of men. The current US *Health and Retirement Study* of couples should in due course provide much better data on all these issues, as should the US *National Longitudinal Survey of Mature Women*, which has now been running for about 30 years, with many of the subjects now of about retirement age.

A Department of Social Services study in the UK (Erens & Ghate 1993) studied 1545 new recipients of long-term sickness benefits. 'Among recipients aged 50+, their health condition appeared to be only one of several considerations in determining their attitudes towards returning to work. Attitudes to work appear to change quite dramatically around aged 50. It would appear that personal considerations and labour market conditions play a prominent role in shaping the attitudes of recipients aged 50+'. Once again, the changes seemed to be more social than biomedical (CSAG 1994a). Older people may have more difficulty coping with back pain, with heavy physical work, and especially with the combination. However, any biological changes in the back with age seem to be only part of the story. Early retirement due to back pain is not limited to workers with heavy jobs. Over the last two decades in which there has been a marked increase in sickness benefits and early retirement attributed to back pain, there is no evidence of any change in back pain and the number of people in heavy manual jobs has fallen.

The UK Retirement Survey (Disney et al 1997) was a longitudinal study of 3500 people aged 55–69 when they were first interviewed in 1988–1989, and two-thirds were interviewed again in 1994. This confirmed the trend to earlier retirement, particularly in men. By 1994, the average UK retirement age was 62.3 for men and 59.5 for women. The state pension age (65 for men and 60 for women) was still the most common retirement age, but about half of men and nearly one-third of women retired earlier. There was a progressive fall in the employment rate of men aged 60–64, reflected in successive age cohorts: the number of men still working at age 60 fell from 85% of those born in 1913–1917, to 66% of those born in 1918–1922, to 58% of those born in 1923–1928. Men in professional and white-collar occupations with an occupational pension scheme retired on average 2.5 years earlier than men in manual work who were dependent on the state pension. Eighty-one per cent of men and 42% of women had at some time been in an occupational pension scheme but this was not necessarily 'for life'. One-third of men and nearly one-tenth of women had been in more than one scheme. However, some schemes had been cashed in or the rights 'lost' and 14% of men and 30% of women who had at some time been in a scheme would never actually receive a pension. The net effect was that only about 70% of working men and about 30% of working women would actually receive any occupational pension. Although the number of men in occupational pension schemes was now only rising slightly, there was a considerable increase in the value of the pensions paid (Table 5.8).

TABLE 5.8 Median weekly occupational pension 1994

Age	Men (£)	Women (£)
60–64	102	33
65–69	60	26
70–74	45	29

From Disney et al (1997).

Table 5.9 lists the main reasons people gave for early retirement, which may be divided into four main categories. The first group were those where early retirement appeared to be instigated by the firm; the second were those who gave ill-health as the main reason for early retirement; the third group were those who appeared to have made a more or less voluntary decision to retire early, and most of them gave positive reasons for leaving employment; and the reasons for the fourth group retiring early were miscellaneous and

TABLE 5.9 Main reason for early retirement (as % of those retiring early)

	Men	Women
By reason		
Own ill health	26.0	27.7
Ill health of others	4.1	7.3
Fixed retirement age	10.3	0.7
Involuntary redundancy	15.0	13.7
Voluntary redundancy—reasonable financial terms	23.6	7.1
Spend more time with family	2.5	10.7
Enjoy life while young and fit	5.8	5.4
Fed up with work/wanted a change	4.4	6.9
Retire at same time as partner	0.3	6.4
By category		
Firm-instigated	14.1	12.7
Ill health	28.3	32.3
Voluntary decision	36.2	35.7
Other	21.4	19.3

unclear. Men and women in professional and white-collar occupations with an occupational pension scheme were slightly more likely to retire voluntarily, while those in unskilled manual work dependent on a state pension were slightly more likely to retire on health grounds. Women and self-employed men were more likely to continue working after the official state retirement age.

The main change in the relatively short period between 1988–1989 and 1994 was the number attributing early retirement to ill health, rising from 27 to 34.4% for men and from 30.3 to 39.4% for women aged 60–64 at the time of each survey. Approaching the problem differently and asking all people of working age who were not employed why they were not working, three-quarters of men aged 55+ attributed it to ill health and half of women aged 55+ attributed it to looking after their home and family. The UK Retirement Survey also included a more detailed analysis of disability in 1988–1989 and 1994 using the disability scales of the 1985–1986 ONS Disability Surveys. This focused mainly on care needs rather than working capacity, and showed that the majority of recipients of Invalidity Benefit had much lower severity scores than those receiving Disability Living Allowance.

The UK Retirement Survey also looked at expectations about retirement. In 1988–1989, 60% of men and 40% of women expected to retire at the state retirement age (65 for men and 60 for women) while most of the rest expected to retire earlier; 15% still did not know when they would retire even though they were already aged over 55. On follow-up, 40% of men and 20% of women actually retired earlier than they had expected, but only a small percentage later than expected.

Poole (1997) assessed the process and outcome of retirement due to ill health in six large organisations in the UK. Rates of retirement due to ill health varied from 2–25 per 1000 contributing members per annum. In different organisations the rate of early retirement rose progressively after age 40 or 45 years, but in two organisations which provided gender-specific data, women showed a more even spread with another slight peak in their late 20s and early 30s. Musculoskeletal and minor psychiatric illnesses were the most common medical reasons given for early retirement. In four organisations the modal age and length of service at retirement coincided with enhancement in benefits. Hobbs (1997) studied sickness absence and medical retirement in the police service in England and Wales with very similar findings. He found a high level of sickness absence of about 5.5% of days lost in both police officers and civilian support staff and a very high level of retirement on medical grounds, most commonly due to musculoskeletal conditions and stress-related disorders. In 1996–1997 between 16 and 77% of all police retirements in different police forces were on medical grounds, reflecting wide variation in management and culture in different forces. After government concern, medical retirement in the police fell from a national average of 59% in 1991 but was still 43% in 1996–1997. This was partly because there was no formalised alternative to assist departure from the police and Hobbs (1997) identified a particular problem of retirement on medical grounds which pre-empted disciplinary proceedings. Retirement on medical grounds was also closely related to pension entitlement. Bourne (1997) made a parallel study of the London Metropolitan Police Service, with similar findings, and discussed approaches to the management of long-term sickness absence.

Poole (1999) provided an overview of current ill-health retirement in the UK. There has been a major increase in early retirement on grounds of ill health in the last 20 years, but with wide variation from <10 to nearly 70% in different occupational settings. Of local government employees, 39% now retire early on health grounds compared with 10–20% in the private sector. The reasons for ill-health retirement vary with occupation, although there is a disproportionate increase in minor psychiatric and musculoskeletal conditions. 'Psychiatric' grounds account for 50% of early retirement in teachers, 4% in construction workers and 25% in the police, while musculoskeletal conditions show the opposite pattern.

Poole (1999) pointed out that the granting of ill-health retirement is often not determined solely by illness but may consist of 'medicalising occupational dissatisfaction'. There is a concurrence of early retirement with enhanced benefits. Different organisations make more or less use of early retirement on health grounds as a method of terminating employment, or alternative methods of redundancy whether compulsory, voluntary or forced, disciplinary proceedings or early retirement on non-health grounds. Doctors may be subject to organisational pressures and conflicts of interest in reaching these decisions. There are conflicts of interest between the employer and employee and between clinical management and occupational health. Medical judgements on ill-health retirement are unreliable and inconsistent, and are often based on whether the employee is likely to return to work rather than whether he or she meets the criteria for ill-health retirement.

O'Donnell (1999) reviewed ill-health retirement in the National Health Service in England. Twenty per cent of all retirements were early on health grounds, although the rate varied in different NHS Trusts from 4 to 17 per 1000 employees per annum. Forty per cent of applications for early retirement were for musculoskeletal disorders of which 62% were granted, 24% for mental health disorders of which 53% were granted, compared with 5% for neoplasms of which 80% were granted. Many of those with a primary musculoskeletal disorder had a secondary mental health diagnosis. Medical assessment for the NHS pension scheme has now been privatised, but there is some suggestion that the number of ill-health retirements is already falling slowly, possibly by about 50% in the last 5 years.

Poole (1999) suggested that the first criteria for retirement on medical grounds should be whether the employee's medical condition is permanent. They must have had appropriate and adequate treatment. Are they fit for similar or comparable work? Would they be fit for modified or alternative work, bearing in mind the provisions of the Disability Discrimination Act? Only then and quite separately, are there grounds for dismissal and do they meet the criteria of the particular pension scheme for ill-health retirement and benefits? O'Donnell (1999) pointed out some of the practical problems in decision making:

● Poor evidence
● What is the meaning of permanent?
● What do we mean by reasonable treatment options?
● Long waiting lists for treatment (and specialist assessment)
● Achieving fair and reliable decisions.

O'Donnell (1999) also suggested some ways in which ill-health retirement in the NHS could be improved:

- Tighten the mechanism of applying for ill-health retirement through the occupational health department
- Include the provisions of the Disability Discrimination Act in the scheme rules
- Separate the management of long-term sickness absence from ill-health retirement
- Educate managers and doctors on ill-health retirement scheme rules.

However, Poole (1999) also considered the implications of tightening up on ill-health retirement—these employees would then revert to being a managerial problem. Management would need to be prepared to dismiss on capability grounds and make arrangements for non-health-related severance or premature retirement packages. They should avoid 'medicalising dissatisfaction'; they should ask treating doctors about diagnosis, treatment and prognosis but not about 'fitness to work'; and they should avoid multiple medical opinions. O'Donnell (1999) pointed out this might require better training for managers in dealing with workplace issues, improving psychosocial aspects of work and improving staff relations.

Summary

Many of these studies suggest that the worker's medical condition is only one and often not the most important element in early retirement on health grounds. Early retirement attributed to 'back pain' is often associated with co-morbidities, psychological problems and social factors, including psychosocial aspects of work. On the present data it is not possible to determine the relative importance of these various elements linking employment status, low back disability and early retirement. It is probably always multifactorial and the relative importance of different elements varies in each individual. Back pain and disability may contribute to incapacity for work and job loss. Conversely, the physical demands and psychosocial aspects of work may influence back complaints and how workers cope. There are major gender differences in early retirement patterns. The physical, mental and social ill-effects of loss of employment may interact with and aggravate low back pain and disability. There may be social and financial advantages to sick certification, sickness benefits and retirement on medical grounds. Or the common bodily symptom of back pain may be used to cover other reasons for sickness absence or early retirement. On the evidence available, the balance of probabilities is that the physical state of the back is often the least important.

There is, however, a fundamental question about whether or to what extent early retirement is forced upon people by labour market forces or a matter of personal choice. Over the past few decades, there have been major changes in attitudes to work and retirement and a large proportion of people now want and expect to retire before the official state retirement age. The amount of early retirement is likely to depend on the balance between individual attitudes and expectations, labour market forces and the pension and social security systems. This involves social and political issues about how long people should be expected to work, the social and financial mechanisms society should provide for retirement, and whether subjective health complaints like low back pain should be acceptable grounds for early retirement. These questions are still unresolved, but the solution depends on addressing these social and political issues rather than biomedical questions or health care for back pain, or indeed medical assessment for sick certification and incapacity or disability benefits.

Unemployment

In current western society, work plays a major role in most people's lives. The primary purpose of work may be to provide for financial needs and security, but it also defines the individual and their role in society (Waddell 1998). Work provides:

- Income (should this come first or last?)
- Activity
- Occupies and structures time
- Creativity/mastery
- Social interaction
- Sense of identity
- Sense of purpose.

All workers get these to varying degrees, though their relative importance varies with the individual and the job.

If work is such an important part of the modern social fabric, it is not surprising that loss of work and unemployment are catastrophic. Unemployment causes loss of all the financial, social and psychological benefits of work. It undermines the individual's whole social position and status and is one of the greatest personal failures in a material society. Welfare status may also involve loss of social value, loss of (self-)respect and isolation. So it is not surprising that unemployment causes pessimism, depression and fatalism. Unemployment, poverty and social deprivation lead to poor physical and mental health, with increased suicide and mortality rates, as reviewed systematically by Janlert (1997). A large, prospective, 10-year study in Denmark showed that the mortality rate among the unemployed was 2–3 times higher in all age groups, mainly through violent deaths (accidents and suicide) and alcohol-related deaths, although also from cardiovascular disease (Iversen & Sabroe 1988). Lack of work causes loss of physical fitness and weight gain, psychological distress and depression, and loss of work-related attitudes and habits, all of which are associated with low back disability. Janlert (1997) pointed out this is not entirely a question of unemployment causing ill health: ill health also increases the chance of unemployment. However, Martikainen (1990) in Finland found that even allowing for health status at the start of unemployment and considering only the 'healthy unemployed', the relative risk for death was still doubled. So there was an element of health selection among those who became unemployed, but unemployment then also caused deterioration in health. This was in a time of relatively low unemployment, but unemployment in Finland then rose rapidly from 3.2% in 1990 to 11.6% in 1992. Martikainen & Valkonen (1996) found that the mortality ratios for men and women unemployed for the first time in 1990 were 2.11 (95% CI 1.76–2.53) and 1.61 (1.09–2.36) respectively, but for those unemployed for the first time in 1992 the corresponding ratios fell to 1.35 (1.16–1.56) and 1.30 (0.97–1.75). They suggested that the association between unemployment and poor health had weakened as the general unemployment rate increased, when there was less selection involved in becoming unemployed and unemployment became more socially 'normal'.

As part of the long-term, prospective Whitehall II study of civil servants in the UK, Ferrie et al (2001) studied how health outcomes varied with employment status after job loss. Baseline data were collected in 1985–1988 and this particular subgroup were followed up until 18 months after their department was privatised in 1992. Rumours reached the work force 2–3 years before privatisation and during this 'anticipation' phase there was a deterioration in self-reported health compared with baseline and other control departments. Eighteen months after job loss, those in secure re-employment had no significant change in health status compared with baseline. Those who remained unemployed and also those in insecure re-employment had significantly increased minor psychiatric morbidity and more consultations with their family doctor. Those who permanently exited the work force reported a higher rate of 'long-standing illness' (which may have formed the basis for getting early retirement) but their self-reported health status, symptoms and GP consultations were otherwise very similar to those in stable re-employment.

Table 5.10 gives standardised (by age and sex) unemployment rates from 1985 to 2001 for all of the countries in this review. Overall, unemployment rates in Europe remained below 3% from 1960 until the early 1980s. They then rapidly increased to about 10%, although the rise occurred at different times in different European countries. It occurred first in the Netherlands, Belgium, France and the UK, and to a lesser extent in Denmark and Germany in about the early 1980s. In Sweden and Norway it occurred later in the early 1990s and was to a lesser degree. In Finland, the rate increased slightly to about 5% in the early 1980s, remained fairly constant until the early 1990s, rocketed to almost 17% by 1993, since when it has gradually fallen to about the European average. Since 1985, average European unemployment rates have fluctuated between 8 and 11%. US unemployment rates have always been lower than in Europe, fluctuating between 5.5 and 7% from the mid 1980s to mid 1990s and since then falling to 4–4.5%. Australian rates have generally been comparable to or slightly lower than in Europe, fluctuating between 6 and 11%. New Zealand rates were much lower at about 4% in the mid 1980s, rose to over 10% by the early 1990s and since then have fallen to about 6–7%. Japanese rates remained <3% from the 1960s to the mid 1990s but since then have crept up to 4.9%.

It should however be noted that these are all official figures for recipients of unemployment benefit, which is not the same as the number who are actually available for and seeking work but who are unable to obtain employment. A UK study (Beatty et al 1997) suggested that the true unemployment rate may be about double these figures for the number receiving unemployment benefits.

TABLE 5.10   Standardised OECD unemployment rates

	1985	1986	1987	1988	1989	1990	1991	1992	1993	1994	1995	1996	1997	1998	1999	2000	2001
Sweden	2.9	2.7	2.2	1.8	1.5	1.7	3.1	5.6	9.1	9.4	8.8	9.6	9.9	8.3	7.2	6.1	4.9
Norway	2.7	2.0	2.1	3.2	5.0	5.3	5.6	6.0	6.1	5.5	5.0	4.9	4.1	3.3	3.2	3.5	—
Finland	6.0	6.7	4.9	4.2	3.1	3.2	6.6	11.6	16.4	16.7	15.2	14.5	12.6	12.6	10.2	9.7	8.8
Denmark	7.1	5.4	5.4	6.1	7.3	7.7	8.4	9.2	10.2	8.2	7.2	6.8	5.6	5.2	5.2	4.8	4.6
The Netherlands	8.3	8.3	8.1	7.6	6.9	6.2	5.8	5.6	6.6	7.1	6.9	6.3	5.2	4.1	3.3	2.9	2.4
Belgium	10.4	10.3	10.1	9.0	7.5	6.7	6.6	7.2	8.8	10.0	9.9	9.7	9.4	9.5	9.1	6.9	6.8
France	10.2	10.3	10.5	10.0	9.4	9.0	9.5	10.4	11.7	12.3	11.7	12.4	12.3	11.8	11.3	9.5	8.5
Germany	7.2	6.5	6.3	6.2	5.6	4.8	4.2	4.5	7.9	8.5	8.2	8.9	9.9	9.4	8.8	7.9	7.8
UK	11.5	11.6	10.6	8.7	7.3	7.1	8.9	10.0	10.5	9.6	8.7	8.2	7.0	6.3	6.1	5.3	5.0
Total EU15	10.5¹	10.5¹	10.3¹	9.7¹	8.7¹	8.1¹	8.2	9.2	10.7	11.1	10.7	10.8	10.6	9.9	9.2	8.2	8.2
US	7.2	7.0	6.2	5.5	5.3	5.6	6.8	7.5	6.9	6.1	5.6	5.4	4.9	4.5	4.2	4.0	4.5
Australia	8.3	8.1	8.1	7.2	6.2	6.9	9.6	10.8	10.9	9.7	8.5	8.5	8.5	8.0	7.2	6.1	6.9
New Zealand	4.2	4.0	4.1	5.6	7.1	7.8	10.3	10.3	9.5	8.2	6.3	6.0	6.6	7.5	6.8	—	—
Japan	2.6	2.8	2.8	2.5	2.3	2.1	2.1	2.2	2.5	2.9	3.1	3.4	3.4	4.1	4.7	4.7	4.9

Standardised unemployment as defined in the ILO as a percentage of civilian labour force.

¹Only non-standardised data available for these countries for these years.

Based on data from OECD *Quarterly Labour Force Statistics* (2000) and *Labour Market Trends* (2001).

Unemployment benefit rates are highest in the 20–24-year-old age group and then progressively fall with increasing age in most European countries (Table 5.11) (Eurostat Labour Force Survey 1996). There is a slight rise in unemployment benefit rates at age 55–59, most marked in Germany and Finland, and to a lesser extent in Sweden and the UK. The slightly higher proportion of unemployment benefits over age 60 in Sweden and the UK probably simply reflects the higher proportion still working in this age group (Table 5.2). However, in older workers it is particularly important to stress that these data are only for unemployment benefits paid. It seems that most people in their 50s or early 60s who are faced with loss of their job take other options and do not appear in official unemployment (benefit) figures. Such people may not be technically 'unemployed' but they are still of working age, many are fit for some form of work, many would prefer to continue working if they had the choice, but they are without a job, nonetheless.

Table 5.12 shows little difference in the prevalence of back pain whether employed or unemployed. The unemployed seek slightly more health care for back pain, but the most dramatic increase is in sick certification. The UK social security statistics show that nearly half the benefits paid for back pain go to people who were not employed when they started these benefits. These statistics should however be interpreted with caution as some claimants might have lost their jobs because of back pain before starting Incapacity Benefit and it is not possible entirely to separate cause and effect.

TABLE 5.11 Unemployment benefit rates by age groups

	Men (age group)				Women (age group)			
	45–49	50–54	55–59	60–64	45–49	50–54	55–59	60–64
Sweden	6.2	6.2	8.7	9.9	5.1	4.5	6.6	8.8
Finland	12.1	11.4	20.1	—	11.8	9.1	15.6	—
Denmark	5.3	4.7	6.1	5.6	5.5	6.4	6.8	—
The Netherlands	3.9	4.3	3.6	—	8.4	6.5	5.6	—
Belgium	5.6	5.0	4.9	—	9.0	6.7	—	—
France	7.5	8.0	9.3	2.8	9.1	8.8	9.1	4.1
Germany	6.8	7.5	13.4	8.2	8.8	10.3	16.4	5.4
UK	5.8	7.2	9.9	9.0	3.9	4.4	4.2	1.2
Total EU15	6.4	7.2	9.9	6.6	8.1	8.0	10.3	4.2

From Eurostat Labour Force Survey (1996). More recent Eurostat Labour Force Surveys and the International Labour Organisation do not provide such detailed age break-down.

TABLE 5.12 Relationship of back pain to lack of employment

	Employed (%)	Not employed (%)
Prevalence of back pain:		
— point prevalence	11	9
— 1-year prevalence	37	42
— life-time prevalence	65	62
Medical care for back pain in the past year	13	20
Sick certification for the last 4 weeks because of low back pain	1	20

Sanderson et al (1995) studied a selected group of patients at one orthopaedic surgeon's problem back clinic. They found that disability (as measured by the Oswestry disability questionnaire) was related to both employment status and litigation, but unemployment was the more important: 79% of the unemployed had an Oswestry score >40 compared with 40% of those who were still employed, but it was not possible to distinguish cause and effect.

Selander et al (1996) in Sweden analysed Social Insurance data on 915 people who were sick-listed for 90 days or more in Stockholm during 1992. Twenty per cent were already unemployed when they first reported sick. The odds of going on to temporary disability pension was about 3 times greater for the unemployed, with a particularly high risk for younger people aged 16–39 years (crude odds ratio 6.88 calculated from published data). The greatest difference in the unemployed was the frequency of psychiatric diagnoses— 50% in unemployed men and 37% among unemployed women. This study gave very limited information on a small sub-sample of people with back pain which did not permit any more detailed analysis, but did not show any significant difference in the number of unemployed who were sick certificated for back pain.

The above two clinical studies dealt with small groups of individual patients, but there are also a number of population-based studies.

Enterline (1966) showed that the general sickness absence rate over time was inversely proportional to the unemployment rate. At that time, he found that on an average day about 7% of US workers were not at work—either unemployed or sick. As unemployment rates rose, so sickness rates fell, and vice versa. Brooker et al (1997) made a similar analysis of macro-economic forces ('the business cycle') and back claim rates in Ontario from 1975 to 1993. Both back pain claims and other acute musculoskeletal claims increased during boom times and fell during periods of recession, inversely with unemployment rates. The relationship was slightly more clear using a combination of the current unemployment rate and the unemployment rate for the previous 3 months. It was similar in different industry sectors. Hager (1997) also showed that US workers' compensation claims and costs in 35 states between 1980 and 1995 were fundamentally dependent on the US economic environment and real GDP. Specifically, claims' frequency and costs tended to rise during periods of economic expansion and to fall during periods of economic stagnation or decline, and the magnitude of this effect was generally underestimated. Hager (1997) hypothesised that in times of expansion firms took on more workers (increasing the number at risk) who were also new, less experienced and from a shrinking poll of available labour, all of which would make them more liable to injury. However, there was no empirical evidence to confirm that and Hager (1997) appears to have assumed uncritically that it was entirely a matter of 'injury' causing sickness absence without considering whether labour market conditions might influence reported symptoms and claims.

Rupp & Stapleton (1995) analysed the growth of Social Security Administration (SSA) disability programmes and reported that earlier analyses in the mid 1970s had shown a relationship to the business cycle, although they did not give any details. Their own analysis of SSA data from 1988 to 1993 showed that the strongest relationship was with the business cycle as measured by unemployment rates, but unlike the three studies by Enterline (1966), Brooker et al (1997) and Hager (1997), Rupp & Stapleton (1995) found the correlation was positive. The effect was stronger on Social Security Disability Insurance than on Supplemental Security Insurance and stronger for applications than for awards. The effect began during the year in which unemployment changed but then progressively increased over the next 2 years in a 'lagged' effect. The effects of unemployment remained remarkably stable from the mid 1970s to the early 1990s. They suggested there might also be more subtle effects of the business cycle in addition to the availability of jobs, e.g. the 'discouraged worker effect'. One major problem was that workers who entered the disability roles during economic down-turns might then stay there even when the economy improved. Rupp & Stapleton (1995) reviewed other studies and estimated that a 1% rise in the unemployment rate led to a rise of anything from negligible to 4% in the numbers receiving SSA disability benefits, although a few estimates were as high as 7%. These effects were greatest for mental and musculoskeletal impairments. The actual level or wage-replacement rate of disability benefits appeared to have a relatively weak effect, although the relative value of alternative or complementary benefits was more significant.

During the past decade the unemployment rate in Sweden has risen to levels that had not been seen since the 1920s, and sickness absence rates have also changed. RFV statistical analysis in 1993 found that each 1% increase of unemployment was associated with 4% decrease of days of sickness absenteeism, or −0.9 days. However, a more recent RFV analysis covering the period 1987–1993, found this relationship was only significant for levels of unemployment between 1 and 5%, i.e. the levels that used to be normal in Sweden before the 1990s [data quoted by Waddell & Norlund (2000)].

There are several other North American studies of unemployment and back pain. Volinn et al (1988) carried out a small area analysis in Washington State, which showed that disabling back pain was related to the local unemployment rate, the percentage receiving food stamps, and income. Clemmer & Mohr (1991) found that sickness absence due to low back strains, but not due to low back impact injuries or non-low back injuries, increased during times of worker layoffs. Cheadle et al (1994) also found that unemployment was a significant factor in multivariate analysis of the duration of work loss in 28,472 workers' compensation claims in the same State. Hurwitz & Morgenstern (1997) analysed the 1989 US National Health Interview Survey and found that the unemployed had an odds ratio of 1.33 (1.16–1.53) for a disabling back condition, but in that cross-sectional analysis it was not possible to distinguish cause and effect. Eshoj et al (2001) carried out multivariate analysis of long-term sickness absence (>10 weeks) in 481 Danish workers compared with 1326 controls and found that unemployment within the past 3 years (men OR 1.7, women OR 1.5) and 'much back pain' in the past 3 years (men OR 2.1, women OR 1.8) were significant predictors, together with level of education, heavy physical work and various psychosocial aspects of work. Long-term absence was socially skewed and particularly associated with the combination of most of these factors in men over the age of 50 years.

Thomason (1993) found that an interaction between increased benefit levels and the unemployment rate was related to the transition from temporary to permanent disability status in the workers' compensation system. Cheadle et al (1994) reviewed five studies, including their own which showed higher duration of sickness absence in areas with high unemployment rates, although all of these studies were about sickness absence for all causes and the effect was modest (0.88, 95% CI 0.82–0.95).

The Department for Work and Pensions (personal communication 2002) have made a small area analysis of age adjusted Incapacity Benefit (IB or Severe Disablement Allowance) and local unemployment rates in the UK. The unemployment rate for men aged under 50 years was taken as the best measure of local job availability: the total male unemployment rate is distorted by the high prevalence of early retirement and of disability benefit receipt in men over 50; while the female unemployment rate under 50 is distorted by the number of non-working women and lone parents. The regression coefficients of $r^2 = 0.63$ for men and $r^2 = 0.55$ for women suggested that more than half the variance in claims for incapacity benefits reflected the local unemployment rate. Strictly, all cross-sectional studies only demonstrate variance in common or association and do not establish cause and effect— this could equally be due to shared causes or trends. Nevertheless, it could be concluded that 'sickness and disability benefit receipt is an economic phenomenon'. The outliers, with high or low disability benefit rates relative to labour market conditions, shared some interesting social characteristics although these were difficult to interpret.

Waddell & Norlund (2000) quoted RFV data from Sweden which showed that local unemployment had a high negative correlation for the outcome of male long-term sickness absence: a weak labour market was associated with longer sick-listing. One explanation might be that attempts at rehabilitation were considered less meaningful in times of high unemployment. For women, higher rates of unemployment were associated with increased risk of early retirement. The explanation of these different results for men and for women might be their employment in different sectors of the economy, i.e. more men were employed in the private sector and more women in the public sector. The different effects from unemployment might be interpreted as one of societal economic development (i.e. the state of the market) for men, but as one of structural problems for women (i.e. women tended to stay unemployed for longer periods since market changes only slowly affect the public sector).

Stopping work because of a condition like back pain is ultimately a decision made by the worker, with or without the advice or agreement of a health professional or employer (even if such formal, professional legitimisation may be required at some, possibly later, stage). Enterline (1964, 1966) suggested that when a worker fell ill, he or she was more likely to stay off work if there was:

- Little risk of losing their job (because of low unemployment and labour shortage)
- Little or no economic loss (because of continued pay or good wage replacement rates)
- Little or no disapproval from fellow workers and supervisors, which was closely linked to little or no disruption of their work.

Trends in disability benefits must also be set in a broader social context. Brooker *et al* (1997) discussed alternative hypotheses about how the economic climate might influence the composition of the work force, the work environment, work stress and the risk of injury. According to the economic model, the decision to stay off work depends on the relative attractiveness and price of the alternatives. Higher unemployment rates produce greater competition for available work and higher selection criteria by employers. More jobs are also now shorter term with greater turnover of labour, which increases the frequency with which workers must seek and gain jobs. Any degree of mental or physical incapacity, whether due to age or illness, or a poor sickness record, may make it harder to get or hold work than in better economic times when work is more readily available. A mild degree of incapacity may then result in a person adopting the sick role who would otherwise have been able to continue to work without their symptoms being a 'health problem'.

Berthoud (1998) also suggested that trends in disability benefits form part of much wider and systematic shifts in employment patterns and in particular depend on two simultaneous and interacting social changes:

- As the supply of labour has expanded faster than demand, employers have become more selective in their choice of staff. Marginal workers, such as disabled people, have been disadvantaged and excluded
- Social attitudes about work and who should work have changed. It has become accepted that if people have health problems and if these make it difficult for them to work, they need not work and social security benefits are an entitlement with less stigma than previously. Disabled people now demand the same recognition and status as pensioners.

Grimshaw (1999) reviewed the changing world of work. The UK among other countries was cited by OECD (1997a) as a role model for improving labour market performance since the 1980s through wide-ranging structural reform including benefit cuts, reduced job protection and industrial relations legislation. However, whatever the economic benefits (about which there is some dispute among academics), this has had a high social cost for the most disadvantaged members of society. The main problem for the unemployed is the poor quality and insecurity of the jobs they are able to get. Gregg & Wadsworth (1997) analysed Labour Force Survey data from 1994 to 1995 on the jobs taken by people leaving unemployment: 50% were part-time; 27% were temporary; and the median wage was only £86 per week.

Autor & Duggan (2001) carried out one of the most recent and comprehensive analyses of the rise in disability recipients and its relationship to labour market forces in the US, and showed two main effects. First, more liberal control mechanisms and higher benefit levels directly reduced the level of labour force participation among potential beneficiaries. The second was an interaction effect. Potential recipients may not apply for disability benefits so long as they are employed, but if they become unemployed for labour market reasons they then apply—'conditional applicants'. So the combination of a more liberal disability programme and deteriorating labour market conditions has greater impact than either alone.

Autor & Duggan (2001) analysed these trends across states between 1979 and 2000. Following liberalisation in 1984, Social Security Disability Insurance application and receipt rates became two to three times more responsive to changes in labour demand. Contemporaneously, if labour demand fell, male and female high-school drop-outs became more likely to remain outwith the labour force via disability benefits rather than being categorised as unemployed. They estimated that disability benefits among the low-skilled unemployed had effectively reduced the US unemployment rate by two-thirds of 1%.

These economic analyses focus on the financial aspects of labour market and disability benefit trends. However, over the past decade or two there has also been a change in attitudes to disability which has become much more socially acceptable. This has been supported by policy attempts to improve the social facilities and status of disabled people. For disabled people, this has clearly been helpful. It means, however, that entry to disability status has also become more socially acceptable. It may be hypothesised that sickness and disability are now more socially acceptable than unemployment. Over the same period, pain *per se* has also become acceptable as a basis for chronic disability and benefits (Fordyce 1995). Enterline (1966), from a US perspective, commented that since the 1950s and 60s 'the right not to go to work when feeling ill appears to be part of a social movement that has swept across Europe'. Sickness benefits are generally financially better than unemployment benefits and may have less social stigma, and there are suggestions that many doctors collude to help their patients by giving sick certificates for social rather than medical reasons (Ritchie et al 1993).

Summary

Four longitudinal analyses in earlier times of relatively low unemployment (<5–6%) showed an inverse relationship between unemployment and sickness absence or claim rates. Conversely, three more recent longitudinal analyses and numerous cross-sectional analyses show that in more recent times with generally high unemployment, increased unemployment rates are associated with increased numbers of social security recipients. This suggests that unemployment may have different effects in different situations. In earlier times of low unemployment, when unemployment rose and job security fell, there may have been more pressure on workers to stay at work when they felt unwell and this perhaps reduced absenteeism associated with a subjective health complaint like back pain. However, in times of high unemployment the individual may be more vulnerable to market forces outwith their control. Those with poorer health might be more disadvantaged at retaining work or re-entering the labour force. Once someone is under threat of layoff or loses their job, there are social and financial incentives to sickness and disability benefits, which might tend to increase sick certification and claims for incapacity and disability benefits. This may all have a more specific effect on social security benefits.

This is not only a matter of unemployment. Waddell & Waddell (2000) reviewed the literature regarding social influences on back pain and found strongly suggestive evidence that low back pain and disability, sick certification, and disability and incapacity benefits are all linked to social disadvantage. This raises broader issues of education, training and skills; availability of employment; the physical demands of work; economics; social disadvantage; social exclusion and marginalisation; life-style and behaviour that may affect health and working capacity (Marmot 1999). However, this is hardly surprising if the primary goals of social security are to provide support to those in need and to alleviate poverty.

Incentives and controls

We all respond to economic incentives and disincentives, and social security benefits unquestionably affect behaviour.

Waddell & Norlund (2000) considered the theoretical basis of social security incentives and controls. Both the labour market and the social security system provide incentives to individuals and employers, which can be analysed within a framework of financial risk and control. In principle, benefits which provide 100% wage replacement maximise the welfare of the individual, while perfect controls safeguard the interests and minimise the cost to employers and society, and with perfectly efficient administration are completely fair. In practice, no social security system can provide 100% compensation for all risks so the individual is always exposed to some loss; it is generally impossible to achieve perfect control so there is always some risk of abuse or even fraud; and no system is ever 100% efficient or fair. The structure and practice of the disability and incapacity benefit system can then be considered in terms of financial self-risk for the individual versus the effectiveness of the control mechanisms for society. Theoretically, the average worker or claimant may be considered as 'the economic man', whose behaviour is to at least some extent influenced by financial considerations, which should not to be misinterpreted as selfishness or greed. Nor should these general economic considerations be confused with moral judgements about the motivation of individual workers. The key question is simply what financial (dis)incentives are offered by the benefit system.

From a somewhat loaded US perspective, Osterweis et al (1987) considered the central question to be whether wage replacement in any form may act as a disincentive which undermines motivation to work:

- The availability of benefits may act as an incentive for workers with marginal disabilities to drop out of the work force and seek incapacity benefits instead
- The receipt of benefits may act as a disincentive for the recipient to return to work
- The receipt or potential receipt of benefits may act as a disincentive to rehabilitation.

This could lead to conflict between two competing social goals:

- Providing economic security to disabled people
- Keeping as many people as possible in the work force, and returning as many people as possible to work through rehabilitation.

The review of individual countries showed that most social security systems vary between a combination of generous benefits and weak controls, and lower benefit levels and tighter controls. Using statistical definitions, the former is a type II-error, i.e. a social security structure which facilitates abuse, and the latter is a type I-error, i.e. a social security structure which deprives the sick and needy (Waddell & Norlund 2000). It may be a matter of moral or political perspective whether over-utilisation is regarded as abuse or fraud or, alternatively, as inefficient administration of the system due to weak structure or poor decisions. Ideally, incapacity benefit systems should provide a reasonable balance between security and incentives for the individual employee to provide for his or her own economic support. If the benefit system is too restrictive, with high financial self-risk on the claimant and excessively tight controls, there is a risk that some sick people will be forced unreasonably to go to work. Conversely, if the benefit system is too lax, with little or no self-risk for the claimant combined with inadequate controls, this will probably encourage some claimants to stop work unreasonably with minor health complaints. Setting the balance between these two extremes is a matter of society's and political choice, and not only economics. However, unless the goals and strategies are consciously considered and planned, the risk is that there will be problems of under- or of over-utilisation, with all the implications either can have on sick and disabled individuals or on society as a whole.

The relative value of different benefits and alternative sources of income may also provide the wrong incentives. Indeed, from a purely economic perspective, the surprising thing is that so many low-paid workers do choose to work at all for such marginal financial gains. The first problem is that low earnings may be little better or even lower than certain benefits. Various attempts have been made to overcome such 'benefit traps', although these have often made only marginal difference, were clumsy and inefficient, and did not work in practice. To have any real impact, such schemes need to be simple to operate and produce sufficient financial differential to provide a real incentive. Many claimants on long-term benefits, however, have no realistic prospect of returning to work and the second problem is then the relative value of alternative social security benefits. In particular, disability and incapacity benefits are generally higher than alternatives such as unemployment benefits and income support in all the countries reviewed. Apart from meeting the prime requirement of 'sickness' or 'incapacity for work' (which is usually relatively easy), incapacity benefits often have less stringent conditions: they are not means tested; in one form or another they are effectively not time-limited; they carry less social stigma; there is little or no conditionality; and there is less pressure to return to the labour force. The third problem is that benefits for long-term incapacity are often higher than those for short-term sickness, which provides increasing financial reward for prolonged incapacity, which is theoretically the wrong incentive if the aim is to encourage early return to work. The present pattern is based on the premise that long-term sickness and disability is associated with increased costs, but conversely it may be argued that financial needs are probably greatest with short-term sickness when outlays remain set at pre-sickness levels. They may then be more likely to fall with long-term incapacity when the person no longer has to meet the various costs associated with working, their life-style may be more constrained because of their disability, and they have time to adjust.

Against this theoretical background, there is considerable evidence throughout this review that financial incentives are important: 'money matters'. The review of workers' compensation studies showed that a 10% increase in compensation levels was associated with a 1–11% increase in the number of claims and a 2–11% increase in the duration of claims, which is a very clear although actually quite modest effect. The present review of social security trends in individual countries provided extensive evidence that disability and incapacity benefit systems have a powerful impact on the amount of sickness absence and claims for benefits in each country and over time. Many authors try to relate sickness absence in different countries to the financial levels of benefits, but these analyses are usually over-simplified and Table 3.15 shows there is no simple relationship. Rather, the balance of the evidence suggests that the structure of the social security system and the availability and ease or difficulty of getting sickness and invalidity benefits (i.e. the control mechanisms: eligibility criteria, the definition and assessment of incapacity, and the claims, adjudication and appeals procedures) have more impact than the actual financial level of the benefits (i.e. the financial self-risk for the individual) on the number of claims and the number and duration of benefits paid. The most powerful means of modulating the number and costs of disability and incapacity benefits is by modifying the regulations and control mechanisms of the social security system. However, using these mechanisms to control the number of claims and awards of benefit may produce an irreconcilable tension between making benefits readily available to those who are entitled and who often have least social skills for dealing with the system, and at the same time discouraging a rising number of claims that are not equally deserving.

Most economic analyses focus on overt incentives and controls, but the 'culture' of the social security system is probably more important. It may be hypothesised that varying cultural and social attitudes to work, sickness and benefits are what matters, even if these are difficult to define or measure and there is little direct evidence. Changes in sickness benefit levels and wage replacement rates and in social security control mechanisms may not be the direct *cause* of variation in sickness absence and claims rates, but may *reflect* national values and customs that have a more direct effect on sickness absence.

Summary

These three aspects of unemployment and social disadvantage, early retirement, and the (dis)incentives and control mechanisms of the social security system are inter-related. From a social security perspective, neck and back pain are not a discrete health problem, but are only a symptom of much more fundamental social problems. Progressively lower employment rates and earlier retirement of older workers may be due to labour market forces and lack of employment opportunities, or to changed attitudes to work, retirement and benefits, and a matter of both economic forces and personal decision. The inter-action and relative importance of these forces may vary in different social classes and situations. In the more socially and economically advantaged groups there may often be a greater element of personal decision. These individuals are likely to have more financial resources to support this choice, even if there may still be other psychosocial consequences. In the socially, educationally, work skills and financially disadvantaged, it may be more a matter of labour market forces over which they have no control. There may then be few alternative job opportunities and these individuals are likely to have no other financial options but to make the best use of the available social security options. These people become trapped into a situation from which there is no ready escape, and face major problems of social exclusion and disadvantage. Health care for neck or back pain will not solve this problem, but may actually reinforce and perpetuate invalidity.

6   Conclusion

The aim of this book was to review the literature, available data and trends on back pain, incapacity for work and social security benefits in the UK, Sweden, Norway, Finland, Denmark, the Netherlands, Belgium, France, Germany, the US, Australia, New Zealand and Japan. This is not the place and it is not the authors' remit to offer an extended discussion or personal recommendations. Nevertheless, it seems reasonable to identify certain key issues from this review which require consideration in any future welfare debate.

Back pain typifies current social security and workers' compensation problems in most countries. Also, some of the issues raised in this review may be equally relevant to several common social security problems, such as other chronic pains, musculoskeletal complaints, stress-related disorders and chronic fatigue.

From a health-care perspective, back pain is not a disease but a common bodily symptom, and chronic low back disability depends more on psychosocial factors than on physical pathology or impairment. From an epidemiological perspective, back pain is not a discrete health problem, but is often associated with other pains, co-morbidities, psychological and stress-related symptoms, and work-related or other social problems. From a social perspective, trends of incapacity for work attributed to back pain and social security benefits paid for back pain form a social phenomenon which is related to the economic and labour market situation. These perspectives are not mutually exclusive, but may represent different views of a complex set of interacting forces. What is beyond dispute is that from a social security perspective, back pain is not simply a health problem, but often raises more fundamental psychosocial issues.

The medical and epidemiological evidence suggests that there is little, if any, change in the physical basis, health status or overall level of back pain and disability in any of the countries reviewed during recent decades. There is now extensive evidence that psychological and psychosocial factors play a dominant role in the development of chronic pain and disability. Social security and compensation trends appear to have more to do with social issues than with any change in physical disease.

There has been a radical change in medical understanding and management of back pain during the past decade. The traditional biomedical model regarded back pain as due to spinal injury or degenerative changes, often assumed to be work-related, which caused permanent damage. The main strategy of management was by rest, and it was often advised that activity should be limited until the pain settled completely. It was assumed that pain is equivalent to disability, and subjective reports of continued pain after a simple back strain were accepted as the basis for permanent disability, often in the absence of any demonstrable physical abnormality. A century of research and investigation has failed to demonstrate any permanent structural damage in non-specific LBP. It is now hypothesised that continued pain may be more a question of disturbed function in which the back is simply not moving and working as it should but is stiff, unfit or out of condition.

Back pain can be occupational in the sense that it is common in adults of working age, frequently affects capacity for work, and presents for occupational health care, but there is increasing scientific question about the extent to which it is actually *caused* by work. The scientific evidence shows that physical demands of work (bending and twisting, lifting, manual materials handling, and exposure to whole body vibration) can be associated with increased back symptoms and reported 'injuries' but they do not generally produce lasting damage. Overall, they are less important than other individual, non-occupational and unidentified factors. There is now extensive evidence that psychosocial factors are more important than any physical changes in the back for the development and maintenance of chronic pain and disability. As pain and disability become chronic, these psychological, social and occupational factors may become 'obstacles to recovery'. It is increasingly accepted that low back disability is best understood and managed according to a biopsychosocial model.

There is now good evidence that rest is not an effective treatment but may actually delay recovery and lead to physical de-conditioning and a disuse syndrome. Physical dysfunction and illness behaviour are mutually re-inforcing. There is good evidence that continuing ordinary activity as normally as possible leads to faster recovery from the acute attack, *fewer* recurrent problems and less chronic disability. This implies that:

- Chronic pain and disability are not an inevitable consequence of a simple low back strain
- Good clinical and occupational health management often means supporting patients to stay at work or return to work as quickly as possible and does not necessarily require sick certification
- The individual should share some responsibility for his or her own management and outcome.

This review demonstrates the difficulty that almost all social security systems have dealing with a subjective health complaint like back pain, in which it is difficult to define any objective medical condition and psychosocial issues are important. It illustrates the need to distinguish pain, disability and incapacity for work, which are clearly related but only weakly, and it raises questions about the balance between health care and social support. Health care for back pain is rightly directed primarily to the relief or control of symptoms, although there is increasing recognition that it should also be directed to the secondary prevention of chronic pain and disability, and must avoid causing iatrogenic disability. Optimistically, UK data provide some evidence that improved management for back pain is beginning to have an impact on social security trends. Nevertheless, perhaps incapacity for work and social support are separate issues that need to be addressed independently of health care and reconsidered on different grounds.

There is almost unanimous agreement throughout this review that support for those who are disabled or incapacitated for work due to sickness or disability is one of the hallmarks of a civilised society, and that the state social security system should provide a large portion of this support, particularly for those members of society who are not in a financial position to make provision for themselves. There is wide public and political consensus on the need for, and willingness to pay for, adequate social support for those who are 'really' incapacitated for work due to sickness and disability.

The broad aims of social security are generally described as:

- To help provide social protection to all members of society against the traditional risks of sickness and disability (and old age and unemployment)
- To alleviate poverty, which often involves some degree of deliberate redistribution of wealth
- To help promote a flexible and healthy economy, which benefits all members of society and produces the wealth to provide that social security.

The development and structure of social security systems are intertwined with and cannot be separated from the ethical foundations and moral principles of social support. However, planning and legislation are often based on implicit rather than explicit assumptions. Social security planning and expenditure are inevitably subject to political and budgetary constraints.

In every country reviewed, the social security structures and regulations that cover disability and incapacity are complex. This is partly historical because they have developed piecemeal to cover different categories of disability and incapacity, and partly because legislation has evolved and increased in complexity to cover every possible entitlement and to withstand legal scrutiny. However, it is probably also because some of these benefits started from different principles, many have now developed beyond their original conceptual basis, and there is often a lack of clear, unifying principles. This complexity produces considerable variation and some iniquities in the entitlement and levels of benefit for people with different categories of disability or incapacity. It also imposes difficulties for claimants trying to understand the social security system and claim benefits, with estimates that only 40–75% of disabled people in the UK actually claim and receive the Disability Living Allowance to which they would be entitled. Although these problems are well recognised and there have been many attempts to simplify and improve the efficiency of social security systems, none of the countries reviewed here has managed to achieve the universal goal of a simple, fair and user-friendly social security system.

There appears to be a natural social security 'cycle'. Benefits are set by legislation to meet perceived needs, but the benefit structure and regulations and the levels of benefits depend on a political process which reflects democratic pressures and compromises. The availability of benefits provides an incentive to claim and benefits are delivered by a system whose primary ethos is to control the benefits paid and to direct them to those claimants who are entitled under the regulations. This is counter-balanced by constant pressure from claimants, an appeals system, and tribunal or judicial decisions which tend gradually to broaden entitlement and benefit decisions beyond the original legislative intent. The net effect of these various pressures has been a steady tendency to increasing numbers and costs of social security benefits in most western countries, although the extent of this varies in different countries and is not as great as sometimes claimed. This rise has been countered by periodic revision of the legislation to tighten the scope of benefits, or revision of the structure, regulations and practice of the benefits system to increase controls and make it more difficult to get benefits. This all occurs against a background of rising social expectations and demands, and greater social acceptability of social security benefits as a 'right'.

Most of the social security and compensation systems reviewed here share common problems, even if these vary with local circumstances, in degree and over time. Comparison with other countries' experiences may help to illustrate general principles and possible approaches, although none of the countries reviewed here has managed to solve the common problems. Simply attempting to import a solution from another system may not work in the same way when applied to the very different system and circumstances in another country but may lead to undesirable and even counter-productive effects. Any attempt to import other approaches must make due allowance for local circumstances.

Most social security and compensation systems for sickness and disability were designed primarily for serious physical and mental disease, severe disability and handicap. Claimants with these severe problems now account for about 20–25% of all sickness and incapacity benefits, their prevalence is not increasing significantly, their disability is relatively easy to define and assess, and they are not a major problem in any social security and compensation system. There is general public support for benefits for these severely disabled people, there is no political dispute about the need for these benefits, and any debate is about whether current support is appropriate and adequate.

At the same time, increasing numbers of people on disability and incapacity benefits, in the absence of any corresponding change or increase in physical disease, suggests that some people are now receiving benefits who are not equally incapacitated for work. Almost all social security and compensation systems have had a considerable increase in the number of people receiving these benefits over the past few decades, even if the degree, timing and reasons vary in different countries, and it may be due to varying combinations of increasing numbers of people claiming or receiving benefits, people staying on benefit longer, and fewer people coming off benefits. Most of this increase is accounted for by less serious medical conditions compared to those for which the system was originally designed, and more subjective health complaints which are largely dependent on self-report and may be influenced by psychological and social factors.

This discrepancy raises issues of targeting sickness and incapacity benefits to those who 'really' need financial support from society and the tax-payer. It also inevitably involves moral and political judgements about who 'deserves' this support and about society's willingness to pay.

Underlying the trends in disability and incapacity benefits over the past few decades has been a progressive shift from a strict medical definition of disability due to serious medical conditions to a more liberal definition of incapacity attributed to more non-specific and subjective health problems. Addressing this requires re-definition of illness, disability and incapacity for work and how they should be assessed.

The primary purpose of disability and incapacity benefits is to provide income and support for adults of working age who are incapable of work due to long-term physical or mental illness or disability. In recent years, there has been increasing agreement in most of the countries reviewed that incapacity should return to being based on medical rather than social grounds, but this requires careful definition and also efficient and reliable assessment. Currently, many social security and workers' compensation systems attempt to control rising trends by adjusting entitlement, but the more fundamental need is to improve methods of defining and assessing disability and particularly incapacity for work. Most systems are more effective at gate-keeping to control entry to benefits rather than helping people to get off benefits and back into work. Health care, also, is better at providing short-term symptomatic relief rather than getting patients with chronic low back pain (LBP) back to work. Once someone is incapacitated and on benefits for a prolonged period (>6–12 months) health care, rehabilitation and social security initiatives, or at least most of those that have been tried in practice so far, are quite ineffective at getting them back to work. In some circumstances, the health-care and social security systems may actually act as obstacles to recovery. The challenge is to devise assessment processes which emphasise the remaining functional capacity of the disabled worker rather than focus negatively on incapacity, and to develop health care and social security systems which effectively assist him or her to return to work.

The practical problem is how to assess 'real' incapacity for work, and this review suggests that the major issue is the extent to which subjective health complaints should form the basis for social support. Only the sufferer can experience and report his or her personal pain and suffering, and this may reasonably be a sufficient basis for health care. However, health care and social support are, or perhaps should be, different issues. Subjective health complaints may need to be distinguished from medical conditions, and do not necessarily fulfil the criteria of 'medical incapacity'. Once an individual seeks social and financial support from society, society has every right to question the need for that support. Human nature being what it is, society may reasonably seek some kind of check or confirmation, and indeed in the interest of the tax-payer is obliged to do so. The challenge then is to develop fair, efficient and acceptable methods of assessment.

Sickness and incapacity benefits cannot be considered in isolation, but must be considered in the context of the underlying health and social issues, and the options open to these claimants including their prospects of work and alternative sources of income available. Over the past few decades, most western countries have gone through, and are still going through, major social change including demographics, patterns of employment and post-industrial restructuring. Many older workers have been shed and many of them are at a disadvantage in gaining re-employment, whether or not this has anything to do with any 'degenerative changes' in their backs. The single, greatest social security problem in all of the countries in this review is the increasing number of people taking early retirement on health grounds, and non-specific LBP is one of the most common reasons given. This is a particular problem in those over about age 50, for whom disability pensions and incapacity benefits provide one mechanism of exit from the labour force and bridge the financial gap before retirement pension. This is not unique to back pain but forms part of a much larger social issue.

This review also provides evidence that LBP and disability, sick certification, and disability and incapacity benefits are linked to social disadvantage. This is partly but not only a matter of unemployment. It also involves issues of education, training and skills, labour market forces, the physical and psychological demands of work, social disadvantage, social exclusion and marginalisation, life-style and behaviour that may affect health and working capacity. Ultimately it is largely a matter of relative poverty. The problems of social disadvantage and poverty inescapably raise issues of taxation and re-distribution of wealth which society and politicians must address. Again, this is not unique to LBP but forms part of a much larger social issue.

This review also shows that a large proportion of people on incapacity benefit are not employed, many were not working immediately before they started incapacity benefits, and most of those on long-term incapacity benefits (particularly those aged over about 50 or who have been on benefits for >1–2 years) have very little prospect of returning to work even if their health improved and they came of incapacity benefits.

Everyone responds to economic incentives and disincentives, and social security benefits and compensation unquestionably affect behaviour. This review suggests, however, that:

- The financial level of benefits has a relatively small effect on the number of claims and the duration that people stay on benefits
- The availability and ease or difficulty of getting sickness and invalidity benefits, i.e. the control mechanisms, have a much greater impact on the number of claims and the number and duration of benefits paid. The greatest rises and falls in the number and costs of sickness and incapacity benefits have resulted from such changes in benefit systems.

However, such discussions are largely about overt incentives and controls. Underlying 'cultural' changes in attitudes and behaviour in society, the social security system and claimants are probably more important.

Adjusting the incentives and controls of the social security system will only be effective if people come off benefits and return to work, and this is only possible if employment is available. Otherwise, they will simply move to some other form of social support and probably sink further into social disadvantage and poverty. The related issue is how to support and facilitate (re-)employment, and to develop effective rehabilitation and mechanisms for return to work. This requires adequate occupational health and rehabilitation services and resources. The underlying issue is for society to develop a fair and equitable distribution of work for all its citizens, whatever their (dis)abilities and skills. Labour markets must become more accommodating of disabled people, and both labour markets and society in general must provide opportunities which enable disabled people to fulfil their potential in as full and normal a life as possible.

Back pain is a very real, physical problem which causes a great deal of human suffering and disability. Social and social security issues may *influence* back pain and disability, but this does not imply the symptoms are not real, nor that they are imaginary or faked. Sickness and incapacity benefits are designed to meet a very real need. But disability and benefit trends are not only a matter of physical pathology: this review shows they also depend on psychosocial issues. A biopsychosocial model of pain and disability may offer a framework for a renewed debate about the medical basis for incapacity for work and social security benefits. Sickness and incapacity benefits cannot be considered in isolation, but must be considered in the context of the underlying health and social issues. Society must address the underlying social issues before it will be possible to develop just policies and structures for the social security system. Ultimately, fundamental cultural changes in attitudes and behaviour about sickness, health care, disability, (in)capacity for work and social support may be more important than structural changes in the social security benefit system for incapacity, but they are likely to be much more difficult to contrive.

References

AAOS (1962). *Manual for Orthopaedic Surgeons in Evaluating Permanent Physical Impairment*. Chicago: American Academy of Orthopaedic Surgeons

Aarts LJM, Vurkhauser RV, de Jong PR (1996). *Curing the Dutch Disease*. International Studies of Social Security, Vol I. Aldershot: Avebury

ACC (Accident Rehabilitation and Compensation Insurance Corporation) and the National Advisory Committee on Health and Disability (1997). *New Zealand Acute Low Back Pain Guide*. Wellington, ACC

Acheson D (1998). *Inequalities in Health Report*. London: The Stationery Office

Allan DB, Waddell G (1989). An historical perspective on low back pain and disability. *Orthop Scand* **234**(60) (Suppl): 1–23

AMA (1958). *AMA Guides to the Evaluation of Permanent Impairment*, 1st edn. Chicago: American Medical Association

AMA (1993). *AMA Guides to the Evaluation of Permanent Impairment*, 4th edn. Chicago: American Medical Association

Arthur S, Corden A, Green A *et al* (1999). *New Deal for Disabled People: Early Implementation*. DSS Research Report No 106. London: The Stationery Office

Arthur S, Zarb G (1997). *Evaluation of the 1995 Changes to Disability Working Allowance*. DSS In-house Report 25. London: Social Research Branch, DSS

Astrand NE, Isacsson SO (1988). Back pain, back abnormalities and competing medical, psychological, and social factors as predictors of sick leave, early retiral, unemployment, labour turnover and mortality: a 22 year follow up of male employees in a Swedish pulp and paper company. *Br J Ind Med* **45**: 387–95

Atlas S, Chang Y, Kammann E *et al* (2000). Long-term disability and return to work among patients who have a herniated lumbar disc: the effect of disability compensation. *J Bone Joint Surg* **82A**: 4–15

Australian Commonwealth Department of Family and Community Services (1998). *Customers: Statistical Overview*. Canberra: Commonwealth of Australia

Australian Commonwealth Department of Family and Community Services. *Annual Reports*. Canberra: Commonwealth of Australia (www.facs.gov.au/dss)

Australian Department of Social Security. *Annual Reports*. Canberra: Commonwealth of Australia

Autor DH, Duggan MG (2001). *The Rise in Disability Recipiency and the Decline in Unemployment*. NBER Working Paper Series. Cambridge, MA: US National Bureau of Economic Research

Aylward M (2000). Chronic fatigue and its syndromes: historical perspectives. (www.eumass.com/CFS2.htm)

Aylward M, Dewis P, Henderson M (eds) (1998). *The Disability Handbook. A Handbook on the Care Needs and Mobility Requirements likely to arise from Various Disabilities and Chronic Illnesses*, 2nd edn. London: The Stationery Office

Baldwin ML, Johnson WG, Butler RJ (1996). The error of using returns-to-work to measure the outcomes of health care. *Am J Ind Med* **29**: 632–41

Ball RM, Bethell TN (1997). Bridging the centuries: the case for traditional social security. In: Kingson ER, Schulz JH (eds) *Social Security in the 21st Century*. New York: Oxford University Press, 259–94

Ballantyne DS (1999). *Dispute Prevention and Resolution in Workers' Compensation: A National Inventory*. Cambridge, MA: The Workers' Compensation Institute, 3–309

BAMS (1999). *Incapacity Benefit Handbook for Medical Services Doctors*. London: Benefits Agency Medical Services

Barth PS (2000). Workers' compensation systems and benefits for permanent partial disabilities. In: Mayer TG, Gatchel RJ, Polatin PB (eds) *Occupational Musculoskeletal Disorders*. Philadelphia: Lippincott Williams & Wilkins, 747–54

Batavia AI (1998). Unsustainable growth; preserving disability programs for Americans with disabilities. In: Rupp K, Stapleton D (eds) *Growth in Disability Benefits; Explanations and Policy Implications*. Kalamazoo, Michigan: WE Upjohn Institute for Employment Research, 325–36

Beatty C, Fothergill S, Gore T, Herrington A (1997). *The Real Level of Unemployment*. Sheffield: Centre for Regional Economic and Social Research

Becker N, Hojsted J, Sjogren P, Eriksen J (1998). Sociodemographic predictors of treatment outcome in chronic non-malignant pain patients. Do patients receiving or applying for Disability Pension benefit from multidisciplinary pain treatment? *Pain* **77**: 279–87

Beljaars P, Prins R (1996). *Combating a Dutch Disease; Recent Reforms in Sickness and Disability Arrangements in The Netherlands*. Leiden: AS/tri

Beljaars P, Prins R (2000). Disability programme reforms and labour market participation in The Netherlands (1990–2000): principles, measures and outcomes in a decade of combating high disability rates. The Year 2000 International Research Conference on Social Security. Helsinki: 25–27 September

Bellamy R (1997). Compensation neurosis. *Clin Orthop* **336**: 94–106

Berg M, Sanden A, Torell G, Jarvholm B (1998). Persistence of musculoskeletal symptoms: A longitudinal study. *Ergonomics* **31**(9): 1281–5

Bergendorff S, Hansson E, Hansson T et al (1998). Work incapacity & reintegration—a summary of the first report from the Swedish project. Stockholm: Rikforsakringsverket (RFV) (National Social Insurance Board)

Bergenudd H (1989). Occurrence and incidence of some common locomotor complaints in 55-year-old men and women. In: Talent, Occupation and Locomotor Discomfort. PhD Thesis, Malmo, Chapter 6

Bergenudd H, Nilsson B (1994). The prevalence of locomotor complaints in middle age and their relationship to health and socioeconomic factors. *Clin Orthop* **308**: 264–270

Berkowitz ED (1997). The historical development of social security in the United States. In: Kingson ER, Schulz JH (eds) *Social Security in the 21st Century*. New York: Oxford University Press, 22–38

Berkowitz M (ed) (1990). *Forging Linkages: Modifying Disability Benefit Programs to Encourage Employment*. New York: Rehabilitation International, 1–15

Berkowitz M, Dean D, Mitchell P (1987). *Social Security Disability Programs: An International Perspective*. New York: World Organisation for Disability Prevention and Rehabilitation & World Rehabilitation Fund

Berthoud R (1998). *Disability Benefits. A Review of the Issues and Options for Reform*. York: Joseph Rowntree Foundation

Beveridge W (1942, reprinted 1984). *Social Insurance and Allied Services*. London: HMSO Cmd 6404

Beveridge W (1944). *Full Employment in a Free Society*. London: Allen & Unwin

Bigos S, Bowyer O, Braen G et al (1994). *Acute Low Back Problems in Adults*. Clinical practice guideline no. 14. AHCPR publication no. 95-0642. Rockville, MD: Agency for Health Care Policy and Research, Public Health Service, US Department of Health and Human Services

Binder LM, Rohling ML (1996). Money matters: a meta-analytic review of the effects of financial incentives on recovery after closed head injury. *Am J Psychiatr* **153**: 7–10

Bixby AK, DiSimone RL, Grundmann H et al (1993). Social Security programs in the United States, 1993. *Soc Secur Bull* **56**(4): 3–82

Bloch FS (1994a). Disability benefit claim processing and appeals in six industrialized countries. ISSA Occasional Papers on Social Security. Geneva: ISSA

Bloch FS (1994b). Assessing disability: a six nation study of disability pension claim processing and appeals. *Int Social Security Rev* **47**(1): 15–35

Bloch FS, Prins R (eds) (2001). *Who Returns to Work and Why?* International Social Security Series (ISSA). New Brunswick: Transaction Publishers

Boden LI (1996). Work disability in an economic context. In: Moon SD, Sauter SL (Eds) *Beyond Biomechanics: Psychosocial Aspects of Musculoskeletal Disorders in Office Work*. London: Taylor & Francis, 287–93

Bolderson H (1991). *Social Security, Disability and Rehabilitation: Conflicts in the Development of Social Policy 1914–1946*. London: Jessica Kingsley Publishers

Bolderson H, Mabbett D, Hudson J et al (1997). *Delivering Social Security: A Cross-national Study*. Social Security Research Report No 59. London: The Stationery Office

Bourne J (1997). *The Management of Sickness Absence in the·Metropolitan Police Service*. London: The Stationery Office

Bradshaw J (1992). Social security. In: Marsh D, Rhodes RAW (eds) *Implementing Thatcherite Policies: Audit of an Era*. Buckingham: Open University Press, 81–99

Brena SF, Chapman SL (1984). Pain and litigation. In: Wall PD, Melzack R (eds) *Textbook of Pain*. Edinburgh: Churchill Livingstone, 832–8

Brena SF, Sanders SH, Motoyama H (1990). American and Japanese chronic low back pain patients: cross-cultural similarities and differences. *Clin J Pain* **6**: 118–24

Brooker A-S, Frank JW, Tarasuk VS (1997). Back pain claims rates and the business cycle. *Soc Sci Med* **45**: 429–39

Buchbinder R, Jolley D, Wyatt M (2001a). Effects of a media campaign on back pain beliefs and its potential influence on management of low back pain in general practice. *Spine* **26**: 2535–42

Buchbinder R, Jolley D, Wyatt M (2001b). Population based intervention to change back pain beliefs and disability: three part evaluation. *BMJ* **322**: 1516–20

Burns JW, Sherman ML, Devine J et al (1995). Association between workers' compensation and outcome following multidsciplinary treatment for chronic pain: roles of mediators and moderators. *Clin J Pain* **11**: 94–102

Burton AK, Waddell G (1998). Clinical guidelines in the management of low back pain. *Bailliere's Clin Rheumatol* **12**: 17–35

Butler RJ (2000). Workers compensation concepts and economics. In: Mayer TG, Gatchel RJ, Polatin PB (eds) *Occupational Musculoskeletal Disorders*. Philadelphia: Lippincott Williams & Wilkins, 9–23

Butler R, Durbin D, Helvacian N (1996). Increasing claims for soft tissue injuries in worker's compensation: Cost shifting and moral hazard. *J Risk Uncertainty* **13**: 73–87

Carron H, DeGood DE, Tait R (1985). A comparison of low back pain patients in the United States and New Zealand: psychosocial and economic factors affecting severity of disability. *Pain* **21**(1): 77–89

Carter JT, Birrell LN (eds) (2000). *Occupational Health Guidelines for the Management of Low Back Pain at Work—Principal Recommendations*. London: Faculty of Occupational Medicine

Central Statistical Office (2000). *Family Expenditure Survey UK 1989*. London: HMSO

Cheadle A, Franklin G, Wolfhagen C et al (1994). Factors influencing the duration of work-related disability: a population-based study in Washington State Workers' Compensation. *Am J Public Health* **84**: 190–6

Chew CA, May CR (1997). The benefits of back pain. *Fam Pract* **14**: 461–5

Chitty C, Elam G (eds) (1999). *Evaluating Welfare to Work*. Papers from the joint DSS and National Centre for Social Research Seminar, June 16th 1999. DSS In-house Report 67

Clemmer DI, Mohr DL (1991). Low back injuries in a heavy industry II: labor market forces. *Spine* **16**: 831–4

Cloutier E (2000). Ageing workforce: how to turn a potential problem into an occupational health and safety asset. Presented to the Association of Workers Compensation Boards of Canada Congress, June 28. Charlottetown, Prince Edward Island

Cocchiarella L, Andersson GBJ (eds) (2000). *AMA Guides to the Evaluation of Permanent impairment*, 5th edn. Chicago: American Medical Association

Cohen M, Nicholas M, Blanch A (2000). Medical assessment and management of work-related low back or neck/arm pain. *J Occup Health Safety Aust NZ* **16**: 307–17

Collie J (1913). *Malingering and Feigned Sickness*. New York: Paul B Boeber

Commission of the European Communities (1995). *The Future of Social Protection: A Framework for a European Debate*. COM(95) 466 final Documents EN 05. Brussels: CEC

Conn HR (1922). The acute painful back among industrial employees alleging compensable injury. *JAMA* **79**: 1210–2

Craig P (1996). *Disability Follow-up to the Family Resources Survey: Aims, Methods and Coverage*. DSS In-house Report 19. London: Department of Social Security

Craig P, Greensdale M (1998). *First Findings from the Disability Follow-up to the Family Resources Survey*. Research Summary No 5. London: Department of Social Security

Croft P (2000). Is life becoming more of a pain? (editorial). *BMJ* **320**: 1552–3

CSAG (1994a). *Back Pain*. Report of a Clinical Standards Advisory Group Committee. London: HMSO

CSAG (1994b). *Epidemiology Review: The Epidemiology and Cost of Back Pain*. Annex to the Clinical Standards Advisory Group's Report on Back Pain. London: HMSO

Curry J (1986). *Report of the Commission on Social Welfare*. Dublin: Stationery Office

Danson PM (1993). The determination of workers' compensation benefit levels. In: Durbin D, Borba PS (eds) *Workers' Compensation Insurance: Claims Costs, Prices and Regulation*. Boston: Kluwer Academic, 1–24

Dean DH, Dolan RC (1991). Assessing the role of vocational rehabilitation in disability policy. *J Policy Anal Manage* **10**: 568–87

Department of Employment (1990). *Employment and Training for People with Disabilities: Consultative Document*. London: Department of Employment, 1–108

Department of Health (1999). *The Prevalence of Back Pain in Great Britain in 1998*. Based on the Office of National Statistics Omnibus Survey module. London: Department of Health, Statistics Division 3 (www.doh.gov.uk/public/backpain.htm)

DHHS (1992). *The Social Security Disability Insurance Program: An Analysis*. ('709 Report') Report of the Department of Health and Human Services (DHHS) pursuant to a request from the Board of Trustees of the Federal OASI and DI trust funds

Disability Rights Handbook, 21st edn. London: Disability Alliance

Disler PB, Pallant JF (2001). Vocational rehabilitation (editorial). *BMJ* **323**: 121–3

Disney R, Webb S (1990). Why social security expenditure in the 1980s has risen faster than expected: the role of unemployment. *Fiscal Studies* **11**: 1–20

Disney R, Webb S (1991). Why are there so many long-term sick in Britain? *Economic J* **101**: 252–62

Disney R, Grundy E, Johnson P (eds) (1997). *The Dynamics of Retirement*. DSS Research Report No 72. Leeds: Corporate Document Services

DoH/HSE (2001). UK Department of Health/Health & Safety Executive Back in Work Pilot Initiatives Final Conference, London, 17 October

Donceel P, Du Bois M (1998). Fitness for work after surgery for lumbar disc herniation: a retrospective study. *Eur Spine J* **7**: 29–35

Donceel P, Du Bois M, Lahaye D (1999). Return to work after surgery for lumbar disc herniation. A rehabilitation oriented approach in insurance medicine. *Spine* **24**: 872–6

Dorsett R, Finalyson L, Ford R et al (1998). *Leaving Incapacity Benefit*. DSS Research Report No 86. London: The Stationery Office

Drewry WF (1896). Feigned insanity: report of three cases. *JAMA* **27**: 798–801

DSS Project Team (1992). *In-house Report on Short Term Benefits (including RMS) Review*. London: DSS

DSS (1993). *The Growth of Social Security*. London: HMSO

DSS (1998). Bulletin from the Chief Medical Adviser Department of Social Security to All Certifying Medical Practitioners on Incapacity for Work and Medical Certification (November)

DSS (2000a). *Social Security Statistics 2000*. London: Department of Social Security, Table 19

DSS (2000b). *Family Resources Survey Great Britain 1998–99*. London: HMSO

Dworkin RH, Handlin DS, Richlin DM et al (1985). Unravelling the effects of compensation, litigation and employment on treatment response in chronic pain. *Pain* **23**: 49–59

DWP. *Incapacity Benefit and Severe Disablement Allowance.* Quarterly Summary Statistics. London: Department of Work and Pensions (www.dwp.gov.uk/asd)

DWP (2001). *Incapacity Benefit and Severe Disablement Allowance.* Quarterly Summary Statistics (February). London: Department of Work and Pensions

DWP (2001). *Incapacity Benefit Key Fact Sheet.* London: Department of Work and Pensions

Eardley T, Bradshaw J, Ditch J et al (1996). *Social Assistance in OECD Countries: Country Reports.* Department of Social Security Research Report No 47. London: HMSO

Eden L, Ejlertsson G, Lamberger B et al (1994). Immigration and socio-economy as predictors of early retirement pensions. *Scand J Soc Med* **22**: 187–93

Eden L, Ejlertsson G, Leden I (1995). Health and health care utilisation among early retirement pensioners with musculoskeletal disorders. *Scand J Prim Health Care* **13**: 211–16

Einerhand HGK, Kool G, Prins R, Veerman TJ (1995). *Sickness and Invalidity Arrangements: Facts and Figures from 6 European Countries.* Den Haag: Ministrie van Sociale Zaken en Wergelegenheid

Elgie R (1995). History of Workers' Compensation: Problems and Directions. Lecture delivered at the Workers' Compensation College, Halifax, Nova Scotia. October 16 (www.wcb.ns.ca/elgie.htm)

Emanuel H (1994). *Controlling Admission To and Stay in Social Security Benefit Programmes.* ISSA Research Meeting—Social Security: A Time for Redefinition? Geneva: ISSA

Enterline PE (1964). Sick absence in certain Western countries. *Indust Med Surg* **33**: 738–41

Enterline PE (1966). Social causes of sick absence. *Arch Environ Health* **12**: 467–73

Erens B, Ghate D (1993). *Invalidity Benefit: A Longitudinal Study of New Recipients.* Department of Social Security Research Report No 20. London: HMSO

Eshoj P, Jepsen JR, Nielson CV (2001). Long-term sickness absence—risk indicators among occupationally active residents of a Danish county. *Occup Med* **51**: 347–53

European Commission (2000). *Social Protection in Europe 1999* COM(2000)-163 (http://europa.eu.int/comm/employment_social/soc-prot/social/com163/com163_en.pdf)

European Commission Communication (1995). *The Future of Social Protection: A Framework for a European Debate* COM(95)-466

European Commission Communication (1997). *Modernising and Improving Social Protection in the European Union* COM(97)-102 (http://europa.eu.int/comm/employment_social/soc-prot/social/com97-102/com102_en.pdf)

European Commission Communication (1999). *A Concerted Strategy for Modernising Social Protection* COM(99)-347 (http://europa.eu.int/comm/employment_social/soc-prot/social/com99-347/com99-347_en.pdf)

European Council Recommendation (1992). *Convergence of Social Protection Objectives and Policies* 92/442/EEC

Eurostat (1995). *Disabled Persons Statistical Data*, 2nd edn. Luxembourg: Office for Official Publications of the European Communities

Eurostat (1996). *Labour Force Survey 1996.* Brussels: European Commission

Eurostat (2000). *Social Protection Expenditure and Receipts 1980–98.* Luxembourg: European Commission

Ferrie JE, Martikainen P, Shipley MJ et al (2001). Employment status and health after privatisation in white collar civil servants: prospective cohort study. *BMJ* **322**: 17

Fishbain DA (1994). Secondary gain concept: definition problems and its abuse in medical practice. *Am Pain Soc J* **3**: 264–73

Fishbain DA, Rosomoff HL, Cutler RB, Rosomoff RS (1995). Secondary gain concept: a review of the scientific evidence. *Clin J Pain* **11**: 6–21

Fisher G, Upp M (1998). Growth in federal disability programs and implications for policy. In: Rupp K Stapleton D (eds) *Growth in Disability Benefits; Explanations and Policy Implications.* Kalamazoo, MI: WE Upjohn Institute for Employment Research, 289–97

Foley KM (1986). *Report of the Commission on the Evaluation of Pain.* US Department of Health and Human Services, SSA Pub No 64-031

Folkesson H, Larsson B, Tegle S (1993). *Health Care and Social Services in Seven European Countries.* Stockholm: Socialstyrelsen (National Board of Health and Welfare)

Fordyce W (ed) (1995). *Back Pain in the Workplace.* Report of an IASP Task Force. Seattle: IASP Press

Frank A (Chairman) (2000). *Vocational Rehabilitation: The Way Forward.* Report of a Working Party commissioned by the British Society of Rehabilitation Medicine. London: British Society of Rehabilitation Medicine

Galizzi M, Boden LI (1996). *What Are the Most Important Factors Shaping Return to Work? Evidence from Wisconsin.* Cambridge, MA: Workers' Compensation Research Institute

Gallacher RM, Williams RA, Skelly J et al (1995). Workers' compensation and return to work in low back pain. *Pain* **61**: 299–307

Gardiner J (1997). *Bridges from Benefit to Work: A Review.* York: Joseph Rowntree Foundation

Gardner HH, Butler RJ (1996). A human capital perspective for cumulative trauma disorders. In: Moon SD, Sauter SL (eds) *Beyond Biomechanics: Psychosocial Aspects of Musculoskeletal Disorders in Office Work.* London: Taylor & Francis, 233–49

Gardner J (1989). *Return to Work Incentives: Lessons for Policy Makers from Economic Studies.* WC-89-2. Cambridge, MA: Workers' Compensation Research Institute

Geurts S, Kompier M, Grundemann R (2000). Curing the Dutch disease? Sickness absence and work disability in the Netherlands. *Int Social Security Rev* **53**: 79–103

Ginarlis J (2000). Commentary on Fit & Fifty. In: Scales J, Scase J (eds) *Fit and Fifty?* A report prepared for the Economic and Social Research Council. University of Essex, Institute for Social and Economic Research, 58–9

Glouberman S (2001). *Towards a New Perspective on Health Policy.* Canadian Policy Research Networks Study No H|03 (www.cpm.org/cpm.html)

Gluck JV, Olienick A (1998). Claim rates of compensable back injuries by age, gender, occupation and industry. Do they relate to return to work experience? *Spine* **23**: 1572–87

Grahame R (1998). *Disability Living Allowance Advisory Board Annual Report 1998.* London: Department of Social Security

Green H, Smith A, Lilly R et al (2000). *First Effects of ONE.* DSS Research Report No 126. London: The Stationery Office

Greenough CG, Fraser RD (1989). The effects of compensation on recovery from low back injury. *Spine* **14**: 947–55

Greenwood J (2000). Profile of workers' compensation administration. In: Mayer TG, Gatchel RJ, Polatin PB (eds) *Occupational Musculoskeletal Disorders.* Philadelphia: Lippincott Williams & Wilkins, 755–63

Gregg P, Wadsworth J (1997). A year in the labour market. *Employment Audit* Issue 4: 13–14

Grimshaw J (1999). *Employment and Health: Psychosocial Stress in the Workplace.* London: The British Library

Groen J (1994). The Netherlands—recent trends in cash benefits. In: Ploug N, Kvist J (eds) *Recent Trends in Cash Benefits in Europe.* Copenhagen: Danish Institute of Social Research, 103–16

Grundy E, Ahlburg D, Ali M et al (1999). *Disability in Great Britain: Results from the 1996/97 Disability Follow-up to the Family Resources Survey.* DSS Research Report No 94. Leeds: Corporate Document Services

Gustman AL, Mitchell OS, Steinmeier TL (1994). The role of pensions in the labor market: a survey of the literature. *Industrial Labor Relations Rev* **47**: 417–38

Gutberlet G (1994). Social security in Germany—recent trends in cash benefits. In: Ploug N, Kvist J (eds) *Recent Trends in Cash Benefits in Europe.* Copenhagen: Danish Institute of Social Research, 85–102

Hadler NM (1978). Legal ramifications of the medical definition of back disease. *Ann Intern Med* **89**: 992–9

Hadler NM (1984). *Medical Management of the Regional Musculoskeletal Diseases.* Orlando: Grune & Stratton

Hadler NM (1986). Industrial rheumatology. The Australian and New Zealand experiences with arm pain and backache in the workplace. *Med J Aust* **144**(4): 191–5

Hadler NM (1989). Disabling backache in France, Switzerland, and The Netherlands: contrasting sociopolitical constraints on clinical judgement. *J Occup Med* **31**: 823–31

Hadler NM (1994). Backache and work incapacity in Japan. *J Occup Med* **36**: 1110–14

Hadler NM (1995). The disabling backache: an international perspective. *Spine* **20**: 640–9

Hadler NM (1996). The disabled, the disallowed, the disaffected and the disavowed. *J Occup Environ Med* **38**: 247–51

Hadler NM (1997). Work incapacity from low back pain: the international quest for redress. *Clin Orthop* **336**: 79–93

Hadler NM (2001). Regional musculoskeletal injuries: a social construction. (www.rheuma21st.com/archives/cutting_edge_hadler_muscul_injuries.html)

Hadler NM, Carey TS, Garrett J (1995). The influence of indemnification by workers' compensation insurance on recovery from acute backache. North Carolina Back Pain Project. *Spine* **20**: 2710–5

Hagen KB, Holte HH, Tambs K, Bjerkedal T (2000). Socioeconomic factors and disability retirement from back pain. A 1983–1993 population-based prospective study in Norway. *Spine* **25**: 2480–7

Hagen KB, Thune O (1998). Work incapacity from low back pain in the general population. *Spine* **23**: 2091–5

Hager WD (1997). The state of workers' compensation: should we compensate for the economy? *J Workers' Compensation* **6**: 88–91

Halsey AH (2000). A hundred years of social change. *Social Trends* **30**: 15–20

Hansson TH, Hansson EK (2001). The effects of common medical interventions on pain, back function and work resumption in patients with chronic low back pain. A prospective 2-year cohort study in six countries. *Spine* **25**: 3055–64

Harkapaa K (1992). Psychosocial factors as predictors for early retirement in patients with chronic low back pain. *J Psychosom Res* **36**: 553–9

Hartvigsen J, Bakketeig LS, Leboeuf-Ide C et al (2001). The association between physical workload and low back pain clouded by the 'healthy worker' effect. *Spine* **26**: 1788–93

Hasenbring M, Marienfeld G, Kuhlendahl D, Soyka D (1994). Risk factors of chronicity in lumbar disc patients. A prospective investigation of biologic, psychologic and social predictors of therapy outcome. *Spine* **19**: 2759–65

Hashemi L, Webster BS, Clancy EA (1998). Trends in disability duration and cost of workers' compensation low back pain claims (1988–1996). *J Occup Environ Med* **40**: 1110–19

Hayden C, Boaz A, Taylor F (1999). *Attitudes and Aspirations of Older People: A Qualitative Study.* DSS Research Report No 102. London: The Stationery Office

Heads of Workers' Compensation Authorities (1998, 2000). *Comparison of Workers' Compensation Arrangements in Australian Jurisdictions.* Melbourne: Heads of Workers' Compensation Authorities

Hennessey JC (1997). Factors affecting the work efforts of disabled-worker beneficiaries. *Soc Secur Bull* **60**(3): 3–20

Hennessey JC (1996). Job patterns of disabled beneficiaries. *Soc Secur Bull* **59**(4): 3–11

Hennessey JC, Muller S (1995). The effect of vocational rehabilitation and work incentives on helping the disabled-worker beneficiary back to work. *Soc Secur Bull* **58**(1): 15–18

Hill JMM, Trist EL (1962). *Industrial Accidents, Sickness and Other Absences.* London: Tavistock Publications

Hill M (1990). *Social Security Policy in Britain.* Aldershot: Edward Elgar

Hillman M, Wright A, Rajaratman G et al (1996). Prevalence of low back pain in the community: implications for service provision in Bradford, UK. *J Epidemiol Commun Health* **50**: 347–52

Hills J (1997). *The Future of Welfare: A Guide to the Debate, Revised Edition.* Joseph Rowntree Foundation

Hobbs P (1997). *Lost Time: The Management of Sickness Absence and Medical Retirement in the Police Service.* HNIC Thematic Inspection Report

Hodgson JT, Jones JR, Elliott RC, Osman J (1993). *Self-reported Work-related Illness*. Research Paper 33. London: Health & Safety Executive

Hojsted J, Alban A, Hagild K, Eriksen J (1999). Utilisation of health care system by chronic pain patients who applied for disability pensions. *Pain* **82**: 275–82

Holmes P, Lynch M, Mohlo I (1991). An econometric analysis of the growth in numbers claiming invalidity benefit: an overview. *J Soc Policy* **20**: 87–105

Hoskins DD (1996). Social Security in the 90s: the imperatives of change. Report of the Secretary General to the 25th General Assembly of ISSA (Nov 1995). *Soc Secur Bull* **59**(1): 72–8

Hunt A, Barth P, McGinn R (1997). *'The Upjohn Report.' Victoria Workers' Compensation System: Review and Analysis*. Michigan: WE Upjohn Institute for Employment Research

Hurwitz EL, Morgenstern H (1997). Correlates of back problems and back-related disability in the United States. *J Clin Epidemiol* **50**: 669–81

Inglehart JK (1988). Japan's medical care system. *N Engl J Med* 319: 807–12

ISSA (1995a). *25th General Assembly Report II. Replacement Ratios: Comparability and Trends*. Geneva: International Social Security Association

ISSA (1995b). *25th General Assembly Report XII. Quality, Effectiveness and Efficiency of Rehabilitation Measures*. Geneva: International Social Security Association

ISSA (1996). *Social Protection in Europe 1996*. Geneva: International Social Security Association

Iversen L, Sabroe S (1988). Psychological well-being among unemployed and employed people after a company closedown: a longitudinal study. *J Soc Issues* **44**: 141–52

Jamison RN, Matt DA, Parris WC (1988a). Treatment outcome in low back pain patients: do compensation benefits make a difference? *Orthop Rev* **17**: 1210–15

Jamison RN, Matt DA, Parris WC (1988b). Effects of time-limited vs unlimited compensation on pain behavior and treatment outcome in low back pain patients. *J Psychosom Res* **32**: 277–83

Janlert U (1997). Unemployment as a disease and diseases of the unemployed. *Scand J Work Environ Health* **23**(Suppl 3): 79–83

Jensen I (1998). *Kartlaggning av Rehabiliterinsatser*. Karolinska Institute: Stockholm

Jensen IB, Bodin L, Ljungqvist T et al (2000). Assessing the needs of patients in pain: a matter of opinion? *Spine* **25**: 2816–23

Jones AB, Llewellyn LJ (1917). *Malingering or the Simulation of Disease*. London: William Heinemann

Junge A, Dvorak J, Aherns ST (1995). Predictors of bad and good outcomes of lumbar disc surgery. *Spine* **20**: 460–8

Juster FT, Suzman R (1995). An overview of the health and retirement study. *J Hum Resources* **30**(Suppl): S7–S56

Kearney JR (1997). The work incapacity and reintegration study: results of the initial survey conducted in the United States. *Soc Secur Bull* **60**(3): 21–32

Kendall N (2000). *Active and Working: Managing Acute Low Back Pain in the Workplace. An Employer's Guide*. Wellington: Accident Rehabilitation & Compensation Insurance Corporation of New Zealand and the National Health Committee, 1–18

Kendall NAS, Linton SJ, Main CJ (1997). *Guide to Assessing Psychosocial Yellow Flags in Acute Low Back Pain: Risk Factors for Long-term Disability and Work Loss*. Wellington: Accident Rehabilitation & Compensation Insurance Corporation of New Zealand and the National Health Committee, 1–22

King A, Coles B (1992). *The Health of Canada's Youth: Views and Behaviours of 11-, 13- and 15-Year Olds from 11 Countries*. Ottawa: Health and Welfare Canada

King HD (1915). Injuries of the back from a medical legal standpoint. *Texas State J Med* **11**: 442–5

Kingson ER, Schulz JH (eds) (1997). *Social Security in the 21st Century*. New York: Oxford University Press

Kornfeld R, Rupp K (2000). The net effects of the Project NetWork return-to-work case management experiment on participant earnings, benefit receipt, and other outcomes. *Soc Secur Bull* **63**(1): 12–33

Kotlikoff LJ, Wise DA (1989). Employee retirement and a firm's pension plan. In: Wise DA (ed) *The Economics of Ageing*. Chicago: University of Chicago Press

Kreuger A (1990). Incentive effects of workers compensation insurance. *J Public Economics* **41**: 73–99

Kuptsch C, Zeitzer IR (2001). Public disability programs under new complex pressures. In: Hoskins DD, Dobbernack D, Kuptsh C (eds) *Social Security at the Dawn of the 21st Century*. International Social Security Series Volume 2. New Brunswick, London: Transaction Publishers, 205–30

Kuwashima A, Aizawa Y, Nakamura K *et al* (1997). National survey on accidental low back pain in workplace. *Ind Health* **35**: 187–93

Labour Force Survey (1996–97, 1997–98). London: The Stationery Office

Labour Force Survey (Summer 2000, Winter 2000/01). Quarterly Supplement. London: The Stationery Office

Labour Force Survey (1998). Technical report. Disability data from the Labour Force Survey: Comparing 1997–98 to the past. *Labour Market Trends* **106**: 321–5

Labour Market Trends (2001). London: The Stationery Office

Labour Ministers' Council (1998). *Comparative Performance Monitoring: Occupational Health and Safety and Workers' Compensation*. Canberra: Commonwealth of Australia

Lafuma A, Fagnani F, Vautravers P (1998). Management and cost of care for low back pain in primary care settings in France. *Rev Rhum Engl Ed* **65**: 119–25

Lampman RJ, Hutchens RM (1988). The future of workers' compensation. In: Burton JF (ed) New Perspectives in Workers' Sompensation. New York: ILR Press, 113–35

Lappegaard O, Bruusgaard D (1997). [Healthier population or stricter physicians? An analysis of reduced sick leave in a small community. In Norwegian only.] *Tidsskr Nor Laegeforen* **117**: 1447–50

Larsson TJ, Bjornstig U (1995). Persistent medical problems and permanent impairment five years after occupational injury. *Scand J Soc Med* **23**(2): 121–8

Lau EMC, Egger P, Coggon D *et al* (1995). Low back pain in Hong Kong: prevalence and characteristics compared with Britain. *J Epidemiol Commun Health* **49**: 492–4

Lazar H, Stoyko P (1998). The future of the welfare state. *Int Soc Secur Rev* **51**: 3–36

Leavitt F (1992). The physical exertion factor in compensable work injuries. A hidden flaw in previous research. *Spine* **17**: 307–10

Leavitt F (1990). The role of psychological disturbance in extending disability time among compensated back injured workers. *J Psychosom Res* **34**: 447–53

Leboeuf-Yde C, Lauritsen JM (1995). The prevalence of low back pain in the literature: a structured review of 26 Nordic studies from 1954 to 1993. *Spine* **20**: 2112–18

Leech C (1999). Medical evaluation of disability in DSCFA. Presented at Conference on Medical Evaluation of Disability, Dublin, 20 May

Lehto A-M, Sutela H (1998). *Tehokas, tehokkaampi, uupunut. Työolotutkimusten tuloksia 1977–1997*. Labour market 1998:12. Helsinki: Statistics Finland

Leigh H (2001). *Characteristics of the Industrial Injuries Disablement Benefit (IIDB) Load*. DSS ASD Analysis. DSS Corporate Medical Group Internal Report

Leino PL, Berg MA, Puschka P (1994). Is back pain increasing? Results from national surveys in Finland. *Scand J Rheumatol* **23**: 269–74

Leonesio MV (1996). The economics of retirement: a nontechnical guide. *Soc Secur Bull* **59**(4): 29–50

Lewis J, Walker R (1999). What works in the delivery of welfare to work? In: Chitty C, Elam G (eds) *Evaluating Welfare to Work*, 7–32. DSS In-house Report 67. Papers from the joint DSS and National Centre for Social Research Seminar, June 16th

Lilley P (1993). Benefits and costs: securing the future of social security. 1993 Mais Lecture by the Secretary of State for Social Security. 23.6.93. DSS Press Release 93/114

Loeser JD, Henderlite SE, Conrad DA (1995). Incentive effects of workers' compensation benefits: a literature synthesis. *Med Care Res Rev* **52**: 34–59

Loeser JD, Sullivan M (1997). Doctors, diagnosis and disability: a disastrous diversion. *Clin Orthop* **336**: 61–6

Lonsdale S (1993). *Invalidity Benefit: An International Comparison*. In-house Report No 1. DSS Social Research Branch (UK)

Lonsdale S, Aylward M (1993). Disability and incapacity benefits in Great Britain and their relevance for The Netherlands. Presented to a conference in the Tinbergen Institute, Rotterdam

Lonsdale S, Aylward MA (1996). United Kingdom perspective on disability policy. In: Aarts LJM, Vurkhauser RV, de Jong PR (eds) *Curing the Dutch Disease*. International Studies of Social Security, Vol I. Aldershot: Avebury

Main CJ, Spanswick CC (2000). *Pain Management: An Interdisciplinary Approach*. Edinburgh: Churchill Livingstone

Mair A (Chair) (1972). *Medical Rehabilitation: The Pattern for the Future*. Scottish Home and Health Department. London: HMSO, 1–102

Makela M (1993). *Common Musculoskeletal Syndromes. Prevalence, Risk Indicators and Disability in Finland*. Publications of the Social Insurance Institution

Mansson NO, Israelsson B (1987). Middle-aged men before and after disability pension. Health screening profile with special emphasis on alcohol consumption. *Scand J Soc Med* **15**(3): 185–9

Margoshes BG, Webster BS (1999). Why do occupational injuries have different health outcomes? In: Mayer TG, Gatchel RJ, Polatin PB (eds) *Occupational Musculoskeletal Disorders*. Philadelphia: Lippincott Williams & Wilkins, 47–61

Marmot M (1999). Importance of the psychosocial environment in epidemiologic studies. *Scand J Work Environ Health* **25**(Suppl 4): 49–53

Marsh D, Rhodes RAW (eds). *Implementing Thatcherite Policies: Audit of an Era*. Buckingham: Open University Press

Marshall TH (1950). *Citizenship and Social Class and Other Essays*. Cambridge: Cambridge University Press

Martikainen PT (1990). Unemployment and mortality among Finnish men 1981–5. *BMJ* **301**: 407–11

Martikainen PT, Valkonen T (1996). Excess mortality of unemployed men and women during a period of rapidly increasing unemployment. *Lancet* **348**: 909–12

Mashaw JL (1997). Disability: why does the search for good programs continue? In: Kingson ER, Schulz JH (eds) *Social Security in the 21st Century*. New York: Oxford University Press, 105–26

Mashaw JL, Reno VP (eds) (1996). *Balancing Security and Opportunity: The Challenge of Disability Income Policy*. Report of the Disability Policy Panel. Washington DC: National Academy of Social Insurance

Mason V (1994). *The Prevalence of Back Pain in Great Britain*. Office of Population Censuses and Surveys. Social Survey Division. London: HMSO

Matheson LN, Gaudino EA, Mael F, Hesse BW (2000). Improving the validity of the impairment evaluation process: a proposed theoretic framework. *J Occup Rehabil* **10**: 311–20

McGuirk B, King W, Govind J et al (2001). The safety, efficacy and cost-effectiveness of evidence-based guidelines for the management of acute low back pain in primary care. *Spine* **26**: 2615–22

McKeown T (1976). *The Role of Medicine: Dream, Mirage or Nemesis?* London: The Nuffield Provincial Hospitals Trust

McNaughton HK, Sims A, Taylor WJ (2000). Prognosis for people with back pain under a no-fault 24 hour cover compensation scheme. *Spine* **25**: 1254–8

Mendelsson G (1988). *Psychiatric Aspects of Personal Injury Claims*. Springfield, IL: Chas C Thomas

Mendelson G (1992). Compensation and chronic pain (editorial). *Pain* **48**: 121–3

Merskey R (1979). Pain terms: a list with definitions and notes on usage. *Pain* **6**: 249–52

Meyer B, Viscusi W, Durbin D (1995). Workers' compensation and injury duration: evidence from a natural experiment. *Am Econ Rev* **85**: 322–40

Miller JH (1976). *Preliminary Report on Disability Insurance*. To the Committee on Ways and Means of the US House of Representatives

MISSOC (Mutual Information System on Social protection in the member States of the European Union) (1994, 1995, 1996, 1998, 2000). *Social Protection in the Member States of the Union: Situation on July 1st (1995–2000) and Evolution*. Brussels: European Commission Directorate-General Employment, Industrial Relations and Social Affairs

Moffroid MT, Haugh LD, Hodous T (1992). *Sensitivity and Specificity of the NIOSH Low Back Atlas.* NIOSH Report RFP 200-89-2917 (P). Morgantown, WV: National Institute Occupational Safety & Health, 1–71

Moffroid MT, Haugh LD, Henry SM, Short B (1994). Distinguishable groups of musculoskeletal low back pain patients and asymptomatic control subjects based on physical measures of the NIOSH low back atlas. *Spine* **19**: 1350–8

Molloy AR, Blyth FM, Nicholas MK (1999). Disability and work-related injury: time for a change? (editorial). *Med J Aust* **170**: 150–1

Murphy PL, Volinn E (1999). Is occupational low back pain on the rise? *Spine* **24**: 691–7

Nachemson A (1991). *Ont i Ryggen: orsaker, diagnostik och behandling.* Stockholm: Swedish Council on Technology Assessment in Health Care (SBU)

Nachemson A, Jonsson E (eds) (2000). *Neck and Back Pain: The Scientific Evidence of Causes, Diagnosis and Treatment.* Philadelphia: Lippincott, Williams & Wilkins

Nagi SZ, Hadley LW (1972). Disability behavior: income change and motivation to work. *Ind Labor Relat Rev* **25**: 223–33

National Audit Office (1989). *Report on Invalidity Benefit.* London: HMSO

National Institute of Disability Management and Research (2000). *Code of Practice for Disability Management.* Port Alberni, BC (www.nidmar.ca/product22.htm)

NCCI (1992). *Workers' Compensation Back Claim Study.* Florida: National Council on Compensation Insurance, 1–25

Nelson WJ Jr (1994). Disability trends in the United States: a national and regional perspective. *Soc Secur Bull* **57**(3): 27–41

Nocon A, Baldwin S (1998). *Trends in Rehabilitation Policy.* London: King's Fund

O'Donnell J (1999). Ill health retirement—experience from the NHS pension scheme. Ill health retirement Meeting. Society of Occupational Medicine, London, 18 November

OECD (1997a). *Implementing the OECD Jobs Strategy: Lessons from Member Countries' Experience.* Paris: Organisation for Economic Co-operation and Development

OECD (1997b). *Labour Force Statistics.* Paris: Organisation for Economic Co-operation and Development

OECD (1997c). *Historical Statistics 1960–95,* 1997 edn. Paris: Organisation for Economic Co-operation and Development

OECD (2000a). *Historical Statistics 1970–1999.* Paris: Organisation for Economic Co-operation and Development

OECD (2000b). *Quarterly Labour Force Statistics,* No 4. Paris: Organisation for Economic Co-operation and Development

Office of Population Censuses and Surveys, Social Survey Division (1996). *General Household Survey 1996.* London: HMSO

O'Grady J (2000). Joint health and safety committees: finding a balaance. In: Sullivan T (ed) *Injury and the New World of Work.* Vancouver: University of British Columbia Press, 162–97

Olsson ASE, Hansen H, Eriksson I (1993). *Rapport till expertgruppen for studier i offentlig ekonomi. Social Security in Sweden and other European Countries—Three Essays.* Finans-Departementet Ds, 51

ONS Office of National Statistics (1993, 1996, 1998). Omnibus Survey back pain module. London: Department of Health, Statistics Division 3 (www.doh.gov.uk/public/backpain.htm)

Ostberg H, Samuelsson S-M (1994). Occupational retirement in women due to age—health aspects. *Scand J Soc Med* **22**(2): 90–6

Osterweis M, Kleinman A, Machanic D (eds) (1987). *Pain and Disability: Clinical, Behavioral and Public Policy Perspectives.* Institute of Medicine Committee on Pain, Disability and Chronic Illness Behavior. Washington DC: National Academy Press

Palme J (1994). Recent developments in income transfer systems in Sweden. In: Ploug N, Kvist J (eds) *Recent Rrends in Cash Benefits in Europe.* Copenhagen: Danish Institute of Social Research, 39–60

Palmer KT, Walsh K, Bendall H *et al* (2000). Back pain in Britain: comparison of two prevalence surveys at an interval of 10 years. *BMJ* **320**: 1577–8

Paoli P (1997). *Second European Survey on Working Conditions.* Loughlinstown, Co Dublin: European Foundation for the Improvement of Living and Working Conditions, 1–384 (www.eurofound.ie/themes/health/survey.html)

Parliamentary Written Answers 31 July 1998. HC Deb (1997–98) 317, col 759.

Pender P, Paita M, Benech JM (1993). Health Insurance Scheme figures on low back pain. Workshop on Epidemiology of Low Back Pain, Paris, October 1–2

Piachaud D (1986). Disability, retirement and unemployment in older men. *J Soc Policy* **15**: 145–62

Piercy Lord (Chair) (1956). *Report of the Committee of Inquiry on the Rehabilitation, Training and Resettlement of Disabled Persons.* Cmnd 9883. London: HMSO, 1–126

Ploug N, Kvist J (eds) (1994). *Recent Trends in Cash Benefits in Europe.* Copenhagen: Danish Institute of Social Research

Ploug N, Kvist J (1996). *Social Security in Europe: Development or Dismantlement?* The Hague: Kluwer Law International

Poole CJM (1997). Retirement on grounds of ill health: cross sectional survey in six organisations in United Kingdom. *BMJ* **314**: 929–32

Poole J (1999). Ill health retirement—the occupational physician's perspective. Ill Health Retirement Meeting. Society of Occupational Medicine, London, 18 November

Porter RW, Hibbert CS (1986). Back pain and neck pain in four general practices. *Clin Biomech* **1**: 7–10

Porter T (1997). *Early Customer Reactions to the Delivery of Incapacity Benefit.* In-house report 23. London: Department of Social Security, Social Research Branch

Prins R (1983). *Socio-medical Services and Labour Incapacity: An International Comparative Study.* Amsterdam: CCOZ

Prins R, Meijerink ECM (1997). *Return to Work Strategies: Foreign Experiences and Experiments.* An international exploration commissioned by the Dutch Ministry of Social Affairs and Employment. Leiden: AS/tri

Prins R, Veerman TJ (1998). *Disability due to Mental Disorders in the Netherlands.* Leiden: AS/tri

Prins R, Veerman TJ, Andriessen S (1992). *Work Incapacity in a Cross-national Perspective. A Pilot Study on Arrangements and Data in Six Countries.* Svr, Zoetermeer. The Hague: Ministerie van Sociale Zaken en Werkgelegenheid

Prins R, Veerman TJ, Koster MK (1998). Work Incapacity and Invalidity in 6 Countries: Facts and Figures 1980–95. Leiden: AS/tri

Rainville J, Sobel JB, Hartigan C, Wright A (1997). The effect of compensation involvement on the reporting of pain and disability by patients referred for rehabilitation of chronic low back pain. *Spine* **22**: 2016–24

Raspe HH (1993). Back pain. In: Silman AJ, Hochberg MC (eds) *Epidemiology of the Rheumatic Diseases.* Oxford: Oxford University Press, 330–74

RCGP (1996, 1999). *Clinical Guidelines for the Management of Acute Low Back Pain.* London: Royal College of General Practitioners

Ritchie J, Snape D (1993). *Invalidity Benefit: A Preliminary Qualitative Study of the Factors Affecting its Growth.* London: Social & Community Planning Research

Ritchie J, Ward K, Duldig W (1993). *A Qualitative Study of the Role of GPs in the Award of Invalidity Benefit.* Research Report No 18. Department of Social Security. London: HMSO, 1–72

Rohling ML, Binder LM, Langhinrichsen-Rohling J (1995). Money matters: A meta-analytic review of the association between financial compensation and the experience and treatment of chronic pain. *Health Psychol* **14**: 537–47

Roland M, Waddell G, Klaber-Moffett J et al (1996). *The Back Book.* Norwich: The Stationery Office

Rothenbacher D, Brenner H, Arndt V et al (1997). Disorders of the back and spine in construction workers. Prevalence and prognostic value for disability. *Spine* **22**: 1481–6

Rowlingson K, Berthoud R (1996). *Disability, Benefits and Employment.* Department of Social Security Research Report No 54. London: HMSO

Rupp K, Stapleton D (1995). Deteminants of the growth in the Social Security Administration's disability programs—an overview. *Soc Secur Bull* **58**(4): 43–70

Rupp K, Stapleton D (eds) (1998). *Growth in Disability Benefits; Explanations and Policy Implications.* Kalamazoo, MI: WE Upjohn Institute for Employment Research

Ruser J (1993). Workers' compensation and the distribution of occupational injuries. *J Hum Res* **28**: 593–617

Sainsbury R, Hirst M, Lawton D (1995). *Evaluation of Disability Living Allowance and Attendance Allowance.* Research Report No 41. London: Department of Social Security, Social Research Branch

Sander RA, Meyers JE (1986). The relationship of disability to compensation status in railroad workers. *Spine* **11**: 141–3

Sanders SH, Brena SF, Spier CJ et al (1992). Chronic low back pain patients around the world: cross-cultural similarities and differences. *Clin J Pain* **8**: 317–23

Sanderson PL, Todd BD, Holt GR, Getty CJ (1995). Compensation, work status, and disability in low back pain patients. *Spine* **20**: 554–6

Scales J, Scase J. *Fit and Fifty?* A report prepared for the Economic and Social Research Council. University of Essex: Institute for Social and Economic Research, 1–59

SCB (1997). *Statistiska centralbyran. Levnadsforhallanden Rapport nr 91 Valfard och ojamlikhet I 20-arsperspectiv 1975–1995.* Stockholm: SCB

Schechter ES (1997). Work while receiving disability insurance benefits: additional findings from the New Beneficiary Followup sSurvey. *Soc Secur Bull* **60**(1): 3–17

Scheel IB, Hagen KB, Oxman AD (2002a). Active sick leave for back pain patients: all the players on side, but still no action. *Spine* **27**: 654–9

Scheel IB, Hagen KB, Herrin J, Oxman AD (2002b). A call for action: a randomized controlled trial of two strategies to implement active sick leave for patients with low back pain. *Spine* **27**: 561–6

Scheel IB, Hagen KB, Herrin J et al (2002c). Blind faith? The effects of promoting active sick leave for back pain patients. *Spine* (in press)

Selander J, Mametoft S-U, Bergroth A, Ekholm J (1996). Unemployment among the long-term sick. *Eur J Phys Med Rehabil* **6**: 150–3

Shekelle P (1999). Point of view on "Murphy PL, Volinn E (1999) Is occupational low back pain on the rise? *Spine* **24**: 691–7". *Spine* **24**: 697

Siebert U, Rothenburg D, Daniel U, Brenner H (2001). Demonstration of the healthy worker survivor effect in a cohort of workers in the construction industry. *Occup Environ Med* **58**: 774–9

Siegelier E, Prins R (2000). Combating rising sickness and disability rates: lessons from abroad. Invitational Conference, The Hague, December 15

Silverstein B, Kalat J (1998). *Work-related Disorders of the Back and Upper Extremity in Washington State, 1989–1996.* Technical Report Number 1997:40-1. Olympia, WA: SHARP

Sim J (1999). Improving return-to-work strategies in the United States disability programs, with analysis of program practices in Germany and Sweden. *Soc Secur Bull* **62**(3): 41–50 [Note: misprinted as volume 59]

Simmonds M, Kumar S (1996). Does knowledge of a patient's workers' compensation status influence clinical judgments? *J Occup Rehabil* **6**(2): 93–107

Sjuk-och arbetsskadeberedningens expertgrupp (1997). *Sjukpenning, arbetsskada och fortidspension—forutsattningar och ehfarenheter.* Stockholm: SOU

Social Security Advisory Committee (1993). *Ninth Report.* London: HMSO

Soeters J, Prins R (1958). Health care facilities and work incapacity: a comparison of the situation in the Netherlands with that in six other West European countries. *Int Soc Secur Rev* **38**: 141–56

Sokoll G (2000). Managing medical and legal aspects of work injuries. Presented to the Association of Workers Compensation Boards of Canada Congress, Charlottetown, Prince Edward Island, June 28

South Australia Workcover Authority (1993). *Guidelines for the Management of Back-injured Employees.* Sydney: South Australia Workcover Authority

SSA. Annual Statistical Supplements. *Soc Secur Bull* (www.ssa.gov/statistics/supplement)

SSA (1996a). Report to congress on rising cost of Social Security Disability Insurance benefits. *Soc Secur Bull* **59**(1): 67–71

SSA (1996b). Social Security in the 90s: the imperatives of change. *Soc Secur Bull* **59**(1): 72–8

SSA (1996c). Executive summary of 'balancing security and opportunity: the challenge of disability income policy'. *Soc Secur Bull* **59**(1): 79–84

SSA (1999). *Social Security Programs Throughout the World 1999.* SSA Publication No 13-11805. Washington, DC: Social Security Administration.

SSA (2001). *Social Security Handbook.* Washington, DC: US Social Security Administration

Steuerle CE, Bakija JM (1997). Retooling Social Security for the 21st century. *Soc Secur Bull* **60**(2): 37–60

Strand L, Ljunggren AE, Haldorsen EMH, Espehaug B (2001). The impact of physical function and pain on work status at 1-year follow-up in patients with back pain. *Spine* **26**: 800–8

Sullivan T (ed) (2000). *Injury and the New World of Work.* Vancouver: University of British Columbia Press, 3–24

Svensson H, Brorsson J-A (1997). Sweden sickness and work injury insurance: a summary of developments. *Int Soc Secur Rev* **50**: 75–86

Swales K (1998a). *A Study of Disability Living Allowance and Attendance Allowance Awards.* In-house Report No 41. Social Security Research, Social Research Branch

Swales K (1998b). *Incapacity Benefit Tracking Exercise.* In-house Report No 44. Social Security Research, Social Research Branch

Swales K, Craig P (1997). *Evaluation of the Incapacity Benefit Medical Test.* DSS In-house Report No 26. London: Department of Social Security

Swales K, Davies R (1998). *Information on the Sick and Disabled.* DSS Analytical Services Division ASD5A

Sydsjo A (1998). Sickness Absence during Pregnancy. Linkopings University Medical Dissertation

Sydsjo A, Sydsjo G, Wijma B (1998). Increase in sick leave rates caused by back pain among pregnant Swedish women after amelioration of social benefits: a paradox. *Spine* **23**: 1986–90

Taylor H, Curran NM (1985). *The Nuprin Pain Report.* New York: Louis Harris and Associates, 1–233

Taylor VM, Deyo RA, Ciol M, Kreuter W (1996). Surgical treatment of patients with back problems covered by workers compensation versus those with other sources of payment. *Spine* **21**: 2255–9

Taylor VM, Deyo RA, Ciol M *et al.* Patient-oriented outcomes from low back surgery. A community based study. *Spine* **25**: 2445–52

Thomason T (1993). The transition from temporary to permanent disability: the evidence from New York State. In: Durbin D, Borba (eds) *Workers' Compensation Insurance: Claims Costs, Prices and Regulation.* Boston: Kluwer Academic, 69–97

Thornton P (1998). *International Research Project on Job Retention and Return to Work Strategies for Disabled Workers.* Geneva: International Labour Office

Thornton P, Sainsbury R, Barnes H (1997). *Helping Disabled People to Work: A Cross-national Study of Social Security and Employment Provisions.* Social Security Advisory Committee Research Paper 8. London: The Stationery Office

Titmuss R (1958). The social division of welfare. In: *Essays on the Welfare State.* London: Unwin

Tito F (2000). The consumer's perspective. In: *Law, Money and Medicine—Forum on Compensable Disability.* Sydney: Royal Australian College of Physicians

Tomlinson G (Chair) (1943). *Report of an Inter-departmental Committee on the Rehabilitation and Resettlement of Disabled Persons.* London: HMSO, 1–51

TUC (2000). *Consultation Document on Rehabilitation: Getting Better at Betting Back.* London: Trades Union Congress

Turk DC, Okifuji A (1996). Perception of traumatic onset, compensation status and physical findings: impact on pain severity, emotional distress and disability in chronic pain patients. *J Behav Med* **19**: 435–53

Tunbridge R (Chair) (1972). *Rehabilitation: Report of a Sub-committee of the Standing Medical Advisory Committee*. London: HMSO

Twomey B (2001). disability and the labour market: results from the summer 2000 LFS. National Statistics. *Labour Market Trends* **109**(5): 241–52

UK Government Green Paper (1998a). *New Ambitions for Our Country: A New Contract for Welfare*. Cm 3805. London: HMSO

UK Government Green Paper (1998b). *A New Contract for Welfare: Support for Disabled People*. Cm 4103. London: HMSO

UNUM (2001). *The Cost of Sickness Absence in UK*. London: UNUM

US General Accounting Office (1996). *SSA Disability: Program Redesign Necessary to Encourage Return to Work*. Washington, DC: Government Printing Office

Vandenbroucke F (Minister of Social Affairs, Belgium) (2000). The future of social security in Europe. Presented to the European Union of Medicine in Assurance and Social Security XIII European Congress, Gent, 7 April

Victoria Workcover Authority Annual Statistical Reports. (www.workcover.vic.gov.au)

Victoria Workcover Authority (1996). *Guidelines for the Management of Employees with Compensable Low Back Pain*. Melbourne: Victorian Workcover Authority

Volinn E, Lai D, McKinney S, Loeser JD (1988). When back pain becomes disabling: a regional analysis. *Pain* **33**: 33–9

Waddell G (1987). A new clinical model for the treatment of low back pain. *Spine* **12**: 632-44

Waddell G (1998). *The Back Pain Revolution*. Edinburgh: Churchill Livingstone

Waddell G (2002a). *Models of Disability, Using Low Back Pain as an Example*. London: Royal Society of Medicine Press.

Waddell G (2002b). Recent developments in low back pain. In: Giamberardino MA (ed) *Pain 2002— An Updated Review: Refresher Course Syllabus*. Seattle: IASP Press

Waddell G, Burton AK (2000). *Occupational Health Guidelines for the Management of Low Back Pain at Work—Evidence Review*. London: Faculty of Occupational Medicine

Waddell G, Main CJ (1984). Assessment of severity in low back disorders. *Spine* **9**: 204–8

Waddell G, Norlund A (2000). Review of social security systems. In: Nachemson A, Jonsson E (eds) *Neck and Back Pain: The Scientific Evidence of Causes, Diagnosis and Treatment*. Philadelphia: Lippincott, Williams & Wilkins, 427–71

Waddell G, Waddell H (2000). Social influences on neck and back pain and disability. In: Nachemson A, Jonsson E (eds) *Neck and Back Pain: The Scientific Evidence of Causes, Diagnosis and Treatment*. Philadelphia: Lippincott, Williams & Wilkins, 13–55

Waddell G, Sommerville D, Henderson I, Newton M (1992). Objective clinical evaluation of physical impairment in chronic low back pain. *Spine* **17**: 617–28

Walsh NE, Dumitru D (1988). The influence of compensation on recovery from low back pain. *J Occup Med* **3**: 109–21

Walsh K, Cruddas M, Coggon D (1992). Low back pain in eight areas in Britain. *J Epidemiol Comm Health* **46**: 227–30

Warton R, Walker R, Shropshire J, McKay S (1998). *Returning to Work: Characteristics of People with Disabilities*. Centre for Research in Social Policy, Loughborough University

Watson PJ (2001). *From Back Pain to Work*. A collaborative initiative between the NDDI and the Department of Behavioural Medicine, Salford Royal Hospitals Trust. Final report to DfEE

Weaver DA (1994). The work and retirement decisions of older women: a literature review. *Soc Secur Bull* **57**(1): 3–24

Weighill VE, Buglass D (1989). An updated review of compensation neurosis. *Pain Management* **2**: 100–5

Weill C, Ghadi V, Nicoulet I, Nguyen F (1998). *Back Pain in France: Epidemiology, Present Knowledge, Current Practice and Costs*. Paris: CD-Santé

Wemyss-Gorman P (1999). Getting back to work with back pain. Annual Meeting The Pain Society, Edinburgh, April

Wentworth ET (1916). Systematic diagnosis in backache. *J Bone Joint Surg* **8**: 137–70

Wesely S (2001). Historical perspectives. Conference on Malingering and Illness Deception, Woodstock, Oxford, 7–8 November

WHO (1980). *International Classification of Impairments, Disabilities and Handicaps.* Geneva: World Health Organization

WHO (2000). *International Classification of Functioning, Disability and Health (ICF).* Geneva: World Health Organization

Willis RJ, Suzman RM (2000). The Health and Retirement Study data set. *Soc Secur Bull* **63**(3): 54

Wood G, Morrison D, MacDonald S (1993). Factors influencing the cost of workers' compensation claims: the effects of settlement method, injury characteristics, and demographics. *J Occup Rehabil* **3**: 201–11

Working Backs Scotland. (www.workingbacksscotland.com)

Worrall JD (1983). Compensation costs, injury rates and the labor market. In: Worral JD (ed) *Safety and the Work Force.* Ithaca, NY: ILR Press, 1–17

Worrall JD, Durbin D, Appel D, Butler RJ (1993). The transition from temporary total to permanent partial disability: a longitudinal analysis. In: Durbin D, Borba PS (eds) *Workers' Compensation Insurance: Claims, Costs, Prices and Regulation.* Boston: Kluwer Academic, 51–67

Yamamoto S (1997a). Guidelines on Worksite Prevention of Low Back Pain. Labour Standards Bureau Notification No. 57. *Ind Health* **35**: 143–72

Yamamoto S (1997b). A new trend in the study of low back pain in workplaces. *Ind Health* **35**: 173–85

Yelin E (1997). The earnings, income, and assets of persons aged 51–61 with and without musculoskeletal conditions. *J Rheumatol* **24**: 2024–30

Zabalza A, Pissarides C, Barton M (1980). Social security and the choice between full-time, part-time work and retirement. *J Public Econ* **14**: 245–76

Index

Note: Page numbers in italics refer to information that is shown only in a table or figure on that page